the LONG-TERM CARE

CARE

HANDBOOK

3rd Edition

By Jeff Sadler

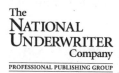

The
NATIONAL
UNDERWRITER
Company
PROFESSIONAL PUBLISHING GROUP

P.O. Box 14367 • Cincinnati, Ohio 45250-0367
1-800-543-0874 • www.nationalunderwriter.com

362.16

This publication is designed to provide accurate and authoritative information in regard to the subject matter covered. It is sold with the understanding that the publisher is not engaged in rendering legal, accounting or other professional service. If legal advice or other expert assistance is required, the services of a competent professional should be sought. – **From a Declaration of Principles jointly adopted by a Committee of the American Bar Association and a Committee of Publishers and Associations.**

ISBN: 0-87218-633-4

Library of Congress Control Number: 2003107218

3rd Edition

Copyright © 1996, 1998, 2003
The National Underwriter Company
P.O. Box 14367, Cincinnati, Ohio 45250-0367

Printed in U. S. A.

Acknowledgements

This seemed like it was going to be a smooth update, but timing is everything and the LTC market is volatile enough to give this 3rd Edition a substantial re-working. Yes, there's only one name on the front of the book, but scores of individuals who have helped me over the last several years in this specific field. I am indebted to the contributions of the following people: Eileen Mazur Abel, MSW, for the Doan story; Eileen Sadler for her patience and understanding during the writing of this book; Janet Strickland for an endless amount of resource material; the outstanding people on the Long-Term Care Working Group of the National Association of Health Underwriters and its chair, Ross Schriftman; Oklahoma Insurance Commissioner Carroll Fisher and his Senior Department Chief Bill Smith; and to my long-time editor, Deborah A. Miner, J.D., CLU, ChFC, for caring about these books as much as I do.

About the Author

Jeff Sadler began his career as an underwriter in the disability income brokerage division of the Paul Revere Life Insurance Company following his graduation from the University of Vermont in 1975. Disability income and long-term care insurance have been the primary focus of his career, leading to the founding of Sadler Disability Services, Inc. with his father in 1989.

Sadler Disability Services, Inc. specializes in national and international agent training, joint field work, and product development in both the disability income and long-term care markets. The company has been a nationally-known educator in the insurance field, conducting agent training classes, continuing education sessions, and client seminars on a regular basis.

Over the last several years, he has authored a number of insurance books, including *The Long Term Care Handbook* (2 editions – 1996 and 1998), *How To Sell Long Term Care Insurance* (2001), *Disability Income: The Sale, The Product, The Market* (2 editions – 1991 and 1995), and *The Managed Care and Group Health Handbook* (1997), all published by the National Underwriter. Other books include *Business Disability Income* (1993) and *Understanding LTC Insurance* (1992).

He has been very active in the industry, currently serving as a member of the National Association of Health Underwriters' Long-Term Care Working Group. He is a past president of the Central Florida Association of Health Underwriters, the Florida Association of Health Underwriters, and the Central Florida General Agents and Managers Association. He is a past winner of the Stanley Greenspun Health Insurance Person of the Year Award and the NAHU Distinguished Service Award.

Table of Contents

Chapter 1

The Doan Family

I t is a Norman Rockwell image of the typical American family: three generations all gathered around the table for Sunday dinner. You can see the joy on
the faces of the children, parents and grandparents. This has long been society's
picture of the ideal family.

In the 21st Century, the American family bears little resemblance to this
image. Adult children and their parents do not live in the same neighborhood;
often they do not live in the same state. The single-parent family has become as
prevalent as its two-parent counterpart. Parenthood itself is occurring much
later in life than in prior generations. In many instances, parents well into their
fifties and sixties are still rearing children.

In assisting today's adult children with financial planning – including preparation for an aging parent's illness or injury – a certain theme is often repeated:
disbelief that a parent could experience long-term medical problems. We cus-
tomarily think of our parents as powerful individuals who will always be there
for us and so we are caught off guard by the realities of aging and illness.

For planning purposes, we must overcome these preconceived ideas and help
our clients (and ourselves) focus on the preparation needed to ensure that plans
are in place to help pay for medical costs that are generally left uncovered by our
traditional third-party payors.

This planning often makes judicial use of long-term care insurance. The case of Karen Doan Parker and her 70-year-old mother, Betty Doan, clearly illustrates the importance of planning ahead.

The Doan Story

Vernon and Betty Doan, married for more than 48 years, have retired and lived for a number of years in Maitland, Florida, a suburb of Orlando. They have three children: Robert, Julie and Karen. Karen and Steve Parker have been married for 20 years. Karen, 41, is a third grade teacher and Steve is an electrical engineer. They live in Orlando, Florida with their three children: Kim, 13, James, 8, and Amy, 5. Karen's sister Julie, 43, lives nearby. Julie recently divorced Jim, her husband of 21 years, and has two children: Peter, 13, and Carly, 6. Karen and Julie's brother, Robert, 46, lives in San Diego, California with his wife Pam. Traditionally, Robert "visits the folks" once a year, usually in the spring. The Doan family tree appears in Figure 1.1.

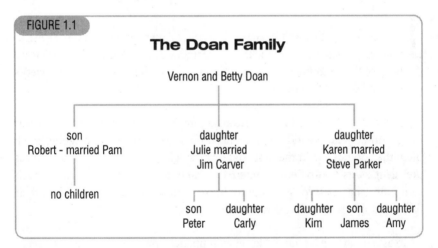

FIGURE 1.1

The Doan Family

Vernon and Betty Doan

son
Robert - married Pam

no children

daughter
Julie married
Jim Carver

son   daughter
Peter   Carly

daughter
Karen married
Steve Parker

daughter   son   daughter
Kim   James   Amy

When Karen was a girl, she was very close to her mother and sister. During the girls' teen years, however, Julie and Mrs. Doan were always at odds with each other. It seemed they were constantly arguing as Julie tested the limits of her mother's tolerance time and again. Julie grew to resent Karen, whom she viewed as her mother's "favorite." Karen, for her part, was only trying to learn from Julie's mistakes. The two sisters drifted apart.

After both were married, Karen and Julie once again developed a close relationship. They lived ten minutes apart and saw each other frequently. The two couples were often companions on Saturday nights out and their children played together. At least once a month they all gathered at their mother and father's house for Sunday dinner.

Suddenly, on one early evening following his customary after-dinner walk, Vernon Doan had a heart attack and died in the ambulance before reaching the hospital. Stunned and saddened by this loss of a loved one, the Doan family struggled to regroup.

Mrs. Doan and her husband had been married for 49 years when he died of a heart attack. While at first it was rough, the close proximity of her daughters enabled Mrs. Doan to make the transition to widowhood. Mrs. Doan joined a seniors' organization and remained active in her church. The pattern of Sunday get-togethers continued even after Vernon Doan's untimely death. Only now it was up to Karen and Julie to host the gathering. As their mother continued her emotional recovery, there were some traditions that were best looked after by others in the family.

Karen and Julie continued to visit on a weekly basis, often inviting their mother out to dinner or a social event. Mr. Doan's life insurance had left Mrs. Doan relatively comfortable financially. She had $62,000 in the bank and owned her own home. She often joked that "she was spending her grandchildren's inheritance." In the five years following Mr. Doan's death, Karen's husband, Steve, had taken care of his mother-in-law's financial arrangements, overseeing her investments and securities and helping with her taxes.

Over the past two years, the family's relationships have grown strained. Karen and Julie once more drifted apart. Following her divorce, Julie returned to work as a paralegal in one of the city's most prestigious law firms. Her ex-husband, Jim, was recently made a partner in his company. He typically works 12 hour days and rarely sees his kids. He continues to pay $1,000 a month in child support and the mortgage so that Julie and the kids can continue to live in their five bedroom, 3,000 square foot home. Julie and her children stopped coming regularly to Sunday dinners, which were now held exclusively at Karen's house.

One Wednesday morning while teaching reading to her third grade class, Karen received a summons from the principal assistant's office. Her mother had fallen while at the supermarket and was taken to Florida Hospital for treatment. Test results indicated that Mrs. Doan had broken her hip. The tests also revealed the presence of osteoporosis.

When Karen arrived at the hospital, she found her mother recovering from surgery and unable to communicate. She asked to see Mrs. Doan's doctor but was told he would not be back until the next morning. Steve called Julie and Robert to let them know of their mother's injury. Julie said she would try to get to the hospital after work. Robert asked Steve to "keep him posted."

Karen met with her mother's doctor the following morning. Dr. Ramon explained that her mother would require at least six months of skilled nursing rehabilitation care. She would also need to adhere to a special diet and exercise program and take calcium supplements to prevent further loss of bone. Should her hip fail to heal properly, the worst case scenario would result in the need for permanent home health care or placement in a nursing home.

Karen had promised her mother that under no circumstances would she ever have to go into a nursing home and if the need ever arose, she would see to her mother's care personally. Now, Karen was concerned about whether she would be able to provide the kind of care her mother needed and about the impact her mother's illness would have on Steve and the kids.

Unprepared to make the kind of decisions that would soon be necessary, Karen sought the advice of Mrs. Becker, the hospital's social worker and discharge planner. Because of the classification of Mrs. Doan's ailment, Medicare required that Mrs. Doan be discharged in 72 hours. Mrs. Becker assured Karen that she would help in any way to facilitate a smooth release for her mother from the hospital and discussed three possible discharge options available:

1.   Mrs. Doan returns home and receives 24-hour skilled nursing and skilled rehabilitative care;

2.   Mrs. Doan stays at one of her children's houses and receives private nursing care during the day for the next several months, with the family caring for her in the evenings; or

3.   Mrs. Doan is placed in a skilled nursing facility (nursing home) until fully recovered and able to return to her own home.

That evening Karen called Julie to discuss the alternatives, since Mrs. Doan's 72-hour hospital stay was drawing to a close. After hearing this, Julie tearfully confessed that with her job and the kids she could not take care of her mother. While it had been unspoken, the size of Julie's home could more easily accommodate their mother. Karen wanted to care for her mother, but felt she was squeezed for room in her three-bedroom house that would now have to house six people under its roof.

Karen then told Julie that "If she had a house as big as Julie's, she'd gladly take Mom in to stay with her." Naturally, this provoked both resentment and guilt in Julie, who responded angrily, saying, "You at least have a husband to help you out! I have to look after myself and the children. If I had someone to help me, I'd be able to have Mom come and stay, but it's too much by myself. If you can't get one of your children to give up his or her bed for a few months, then I suppose Mom will simply have to go into a nursing home." With that, Julie slammed down the phone.

Karen couldn't believe that Julie would even consider a nursing home as an alternative for her mother. Julie knew that her mother had made them both promise not even to consider that as an option. Karen decided to sleep on the decision, but knew that her mother would be coming to stay with her, even though it might mean significant difficulties for the Parker household.

Julie did not go to sleep right away that night. Instead, she drove to the hospital to explain to her mother why she could not stay with her and that Karen simply didn't have the room. She thought it best to explain this herself, rather than leave it up to the "good daughter, Karen." Julie informed her mother that since she could not live with her or Karen and, obviously could not live on her own, that a nursing home was the only practical solution.

Still in a great deal of physical pain, Mrs. Doan was stunned by Julie's visit. Distraught, she picked up the phone to call Robert and inform him of her daughters' betrayal. She knew her oldest child would not put up with the idea of his mother in a nursing home. All the stories of abuse and neglect! They call that care! She was convinced she would never leave a nursing home alive once she went in. She begged Robert, "Don't let them put me away!" He reassured her that it would never happen and hung up to call Karen.

Karen, blind-sided by Robert's call, could not calm her brother long enough to explain. Finally, she was able to assure Robert that she had no intention of putting their mother in a nursing home, that Mother would be coming to stay with her. Robert was still angry, but he was satisfied that he had changed the course of events for his mother.

Long-Term Care: More Than a Financial Decision

As you can see from the Doan story, a parent's illness or disability can result in a number of emotions in a family. If you believe this to be an isolated situation, you are mistaken. The dynamics of families dealing with these circumstances are at the heart of what long-term care is all about. Long-term care affects more than just the patient – it will surely have consequences for one or more other family members. An agent who works in this field should be prepared to balance the emotional and financial planning aspects of long-term care in developing a plan. Solving the long-term care need not only helps the individual needing care, but potentially many others within the family circle.

Another major lesson from the Doan story is the importance of advanced preparation. The family was caught completely off-guard by the hip fracture of the matriarch. Ownership of long-term care insurance could have helped the Doan family by reducing the possibility of the ultimate emotional flare-ups that occurred. Long-term care insurance provides flexibility and choice that might have made sorting through the care options that much easier. Given the time constraints (72 hours, in this case), advanced planning was the best way to ease the decision-making process.

Being caught unprepared puts the worst kind of pressure on families at the most difficult of times. Yet the job of the financial advisor is to help people confront this potential situation years in advance. Most people put off thinking about these possible future circumstances until they are actually confronted with them. Unfortunately, as we saw with the Doans, the decisions are then often clouded with emotion and are the hardest to make. Quite often, the wrong decisions are made.

It's not easy, but the agent must help people focus and plan ahead before these types of situations arise. By planning in advance for an injury or illness, the execution of pre-determined arrangements will be a much easier process. That's truly what financial planning is all about.

Thinking both emotionally and financially, let's evaluate Mrs. Doan's three care options.

Option #1: Mrs. Doan Returns Home and Receives 24-hour Skilled Nursing and Skilled Rehabilitative Care

This seems like the ideal solution. Being in her home gives Mrs. Doan both the security and independence she desires without unduly burdening any of her children. She feels loved by her family and not "abandoned" in a nursing home.

For Karen, this option allows her the peace of mind of knowing that she has lived up to her promise to her mother, without the necessity of displacing her husband and kids. Best of all, Karen can visit without feeling guilty. This solution also creates the least amount of strain between her and her siblings.

Julie is also pleased by this choice. She can continue to balance her life between work and home with minimal disruption.

Robert would also be encouraged by this option. Since his father died, Robert has felt that his mother tended to view him as a stand-in for his father. He resents his mother leaning on him and has difficulty saying no to his mother's requests. In this case, he would appear, in his mother's eyes, to have averted the potential nursing home disaster.

Emotional Verdict for Option #1: Overwhelmingly positive!

With everyone in agreement, Karen makes several phone calls to arrange for 24-hour private nursing care for Mrs. Doan. With Mrs. Becker's help, she contacts several home health care agencies. Karen soon discovers that the cost of full-time skilled nursing care and physical therapy is expensive – with estimates ranging as high as $300 a day.

Realizing that her mother's savings of $62,000 would virtually disappear in less than a year, Karen decides to pursue other financial sources. In fact, she's sure that Medicare will cover these necessary medical services.

But she soon finds that she is mistaken about what Medicare will and will not cover. One of the specific exclusions for home care reimbursement is *full-time* care. Since her mother needs someone around all the time in the event she has to get out of bed, or move around, full-time care is exactly what the family is needing. Karen sees that her mother's savings would not be up to six months of these costs.

Karen and Steve have read about Medicaid reimbursing for long-term care costs. When they contact a local Medicaid office, they discover that because Medicaid is a welfare program, Mrs. Doan, as a widow, would have to spend nearly all of her savings first before becoming eligible for any benefits. There would be no up-front money to pay for the full-time skilled nursing care that is critical to her mother's recovery.

The other possibilities fade out as quickly as they are recognized. Mrs. Doan's Medicare supplement insurance policy does not offer additional reimbursement for home health care. Furthermore, Mrs. Doan does not own any type of long-term care insurance. None of the children are in a financial position to assist their mother with the costs of full-time nursing care in her home.

Financial Verdict for Option #1: A disaster!

Option #2: Mrs. Doan Stays at One of Her Children's Homes for the Next Six Months and Receives Private Nursing Care During the Day With the Family Tending to Her Needs at Night

Because she would be cared for by one of her children at night, Mrs. Doan could contract for part-time home health services. Medicare would likely cover this since Mrs. Doan would be on the road to recovery. A normal recovery for Mrs. Doan would likely mean that the bulk of her long-term care expenses will be covered by Medicare. Her savings would be preserved and there would be no additional financial burden on the children.

Financial Verdict: Very positive!

However, where will Mrs. Doan go? Julie refuses to offer her home. Robert lives in California and there is no practical reason to transfer her there even if she could physically make the trip. By process of elimination, the youngest daughter Karen is left as the only possible host.

Karen knows both Julie and Robert are hoping that Karen will offer her home for their mother's recovery. The financial impact would be minimal to them (and their mother) and, more important, it keeps their mother out of a nursing home. Karen also understands that, given the choice, it is her home that her mother would rather stay. As much as Karen loves her mother, she realizes that bringing her mother into an already cramped living space would place a tremendous emotional burden on her own family.

In addition, after speaking further with the doctor, there is no guaranteed time frame for her mother's recovery. Six months is the estimate, but what if the rehabilitation process takes longer? How long can the family endure the changes thrust upon them? How long can Karen keep up a work schedule during the day and take care of her mother at night? Will she have time to see to all her children's needs? Can she get them to their activities, help with their homework, feed them their meals, and continue all the strong communication lines she's opened with them? Will Steve help out at all?

Emotional Verdict: Unsatisfactory for Karen!

Option #3: Mrs. Doan is Placed in a Nursing Home Until Fully Recovered and Able to Return Home

Option 1 is a financial mess. Option 2 is courting financial disaster with her own family. Reluctantly, Karen and Mrs. Becker check into skilled nursing facility placement for her mother. Karen's specific requirements are: private room, weekly beauty shop, and diet-conscious meals in a lovely dining room.

It takes Mrs. Becker more than two hours but she finds an available bed in a nursing home located 25 miles southwest of Karen's home and 40 miles away from Julie.

Emotional Verdict: Difficult, and could create a rift between Mrs. Doan and her children that may be difficult to mend.

Financially, Karen anticipated that Medicare would cover the majority of the costs of this care. But the reality turns out to be quite different.

Medicare pays for *skilled* nursing care in a nursing home, but only on a limited basis. Medicare would pay some of the cost if:

1. the nursing home was Medicare-certified;

2. the care needed is skilled (which it was);

3. the doctor certified the need for treatment;

4. there was at least a three-day hospital stay; and

5. Mrs. Doan's condition was improving.

As it happens, Mrs. Doan's situation and the nursing home Mrs. Becker found met every one of these requirements.

Medicare will pay for the first 20 days of skilled care in a nursing facility for a semi-private room up to an internal monetary limit. However, Karen requested and received a private room for her mother. Mrs. Doan will have to pay the difference between the cost of a semi-private room and the cost of a private room. Amazingly, the difference is only $25 per day.

After 20 days, Medicare continues to reimburse the costs of a semi-private room for an additional 80 days after Mrs. Doan makes a co-payment of $105 a day (2003 rules). After 100 days, there will be no further reimbursement from Medicare.

The cost for a private room in the nursing home facility is $150 a day. The semi-private room rate on which Medicare bases its reimbursements is $125/day. The payments break down as:

First 20 days:	Medicare: $125/day x 20	=	$2,500
	Mrs. Doan: $25/day x 20	=	$ 500
21st-100th day	Medicare: $20/day x 80	=	$1,600
	Mrs. Doan: $130/day x 80	=	$10,400 *
101-180 days	Medicare: -0-		
	Mrs. Doan: $150 x 80 days	=	$12,000

* partially reimbursed by Mrs. Doan's Medicare Supplement

Totals:	Medicare:	$4,100	(15.2% of costs)
	Med. Supp.:	$8,400	(31.1% of costs)
	Mrs. Doan:	$14,500	(53.7% of costs)

Karen was surprised that her mother would actually pay more of the expenses in the first 180 days than the other sources available. She was quite certain Medicare would pay the majority of bills, such as was the case with part-time home health care for her mother. Worse, what if her mother did not recover at six months as was hoped? Every additional day would be $150 more out of Mrs. Doan's savings. And Mrs. Becker said that the $150 per day only covered the room and board. There were additional costs for laundry, linens, beauty parlor, and a television that Karen did not yet have the chance to price out.

Financial Verdict: Much less than she had hoped for, given the negative emotional outlook.

After reviewing all three options, Karen is quickly coming to terms with the knowledge that the best financial option is the most difficult for her family emotionally. But, at this point, needing to make a decision as her mother was only a few hours from discharge, Karen feels she has little choice. She calls Mrs. Becker and tells her that she will pick up her mother. Would Mrs. Becker mind contacting the Medicare-approved home health agency not far from her home to discuss a treatment plan for her mother?

Long-Term Care: Both an Emotional and Financial Need

As an insurance and financial planner, you will be assisting your clients faced with situations like the one described above. You must not only be prepared to help people understand the financial burden of long-term care, but the potential emotional consequences as well. Karen's choice is one that is faced by non-voluntary caregivers across America every day. We are rapidly becoming a nation of "caregivers" because, without prior planning, we are left with no other choice financially or emotionally.

The Doan family circumstances suggests a number of issues that will be consistently addressed throughout this book, namely:

- The emotional aspect of caregiving.

- The financial analysis of a family's liquid net worth, cash flow, and discretionary income.

- How to determine when insurance is the right funding vehicle for a client.

- Family issues that inevitably surface during this emotional time.

- That long-term care involves many people, not just the individual needing the care.

- The role of government programs such as Medicare and Medicaid.

- The impact of the aging of America on all of our futures.

The Doans' story did not end with Mrs. Doan's move into Karen's three-bedroom house. Giving up his room was James, who thought it was a novelty to sleep on the couch for about 48 hours. The excitement of grandmother coming to stay was soon replaced by disappointment and resentment, as this was not the "Grandma" they knew and loved. The kids were also unhappy about the reduced attention their overworked mother was able to give them and the Parker family was troubled less than a week into the caregiving process.

Karen's husband Steve was upset that his household was disrupted when only five years earlier he and Karen had placed his mother in a nursing facility, where she died after a few months. Taking care of his mother-in-law has not been a pleasant experience for the family. If the children see less of their mother, Steve is once more removed from his spouse. After working all day, caring for her mother, and interacting with the children in the small amount of time left over, there's not enough left of Karen physically and emotionally to cater to Steve.

Julie visited twice a week to help out, but then reduced those visits to once a week and now once every two weeks. She and Karen don't speak much before, during or after Julie's visits. Julie's children have seen their grandmother only once since she was discharged from the hospital.

Mrs. Doan did not fully recover at six months. Nor seven. Or eight. It was more than ten months before the doctor pronounced Betty Doan fit to return to her own home. Then came the unexpected. Mrs. Doan was afraid to go home. She had not been in her home for so long she had developed a phobia about falling in her house. She had her bedroom on the second floor and she dreaded the trip up and down the stairs. She hung on at Karen's, less needy but still there, for another six weeks. Finally, she was persuaded to return home when Karen and Steve re-did a room on the first floor to be Mrs. Doan's bedroom, thus helping her avoid the second floor entirely.

Karen and Julie barely speak. Mrs. Doan and Julie barely speak. The marriage between Karen and Steve has deteriorated over the last year and though living under the same roof, things are not the same. James was glad to get his room back.

One person needing long-term care. Nine other lives affected, perhaps permanently.

Long-term care insurance has the power to provide choices, independence, and flexibility for millions of Americans. It is one of the keys to wealth (and emotional) protection as we look ahead to an America that is already represented by one in four adults being age 50 and over.

Today, thousands of people are seeing hard-earned assets eroding away as they struggle to meet the costs of needed long-term care services. Families are at odds with each other, succumbing to the pressures of caregiving. You can help! Long-term care is a market well worth pursuing because its growth over the next three decades will be substantial.

This book can be your guide to the future success of both you and your clients.

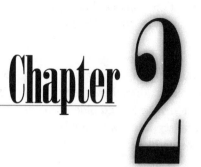

Chapter 2

Today's Changing Demographics

"Of all the self-fulfilling prophecies in our culture, the assumption that aging means decline and poor health is probably the deadliest."

– Marilyn Ferguson, The Aquarian Conspiracy

In this age of information, there is plenty of data available that can be overwhelming and confusing. The information associated with the "graying of America" is no different.

- The 2000 Census puts the age 65 and over population at 12.4% of the total U.S. population (34.9 million people).[1]

- The U.S. has more people over the age of 65 (nearly 35 million) than Canada has in its entire population (31.3 million).[2]

- More than 2.4 million grandparents are primary caregivers to a grandchild. The percentage of children living in a grandparent-headed home was 6.3 percent in 2000, up from 3.6 percent in 1980.[3]

- 50,454 Americans were age 100 in the year 2000, up 35 percent from 1990. The number of people age 90-94 increased 45 percent to 1.1 million. The number of Americans ages 80-84 surged 26 percent to 4.9 million.[4]

- Some census projections forecast that there could be as many as 1 million centenarians (age 100+) by 2050, when the oldest Baby Boomers would reach 100.[5]

- By 2020, one of out every six Americans will be age 65 or older, about 20 million more seniors than there are today. Further, by 2020, the number of Americans age 85 and older – the people most likely to use long-term care services – will double to 7 million, and double again to 14 million by 2040.[6]

- By the time the last Baby Boomers reach the retirement age of 65 in 2029, close to 22 percent, or 69.4 million people, will be over age 65.[7]

- Americans over age 50 control 70 percent of the total net worth of U.S. households, according to aging expert Dr. Ken Dychtwald, author of *Age Power*.[8]

- More than 70 percent of Americans over age 65 will need some sort of home health care.[9]

- The number of employee caregivers is growing rapidly, and over the next 10 years is expected to increase to between 11 million and 15.6 million workers, or about 1 in 10 employees.[10]

- As many as 44 percent of middle-aged workers today are caring for both children and aging parents.[11]

- From 1993 to 1999, the number of long-term care (LTC) policies sold doubled from 3.4 million to more than 6.8 million, with 3,200 employers contributing about 25 percent to the 750,000 policies sold in 1999.[12]

- More than $1 billion worth of annual insurance benefits have been paid to tens of thousands of Americans receiving at-home and facility care.[13]

- Nearly two-thirds of those 65 and older either do not know, or have incorrect information about Medicare coverage for LTC.[14]

What Do These Numbers Mean?

Obviously, this country is aging – rapidly. Advances in medical science and the resulting longer life spans are well documented. No longer is it unusual for a person to live well into his 80's.

We are entering a new era for the elderly in this country. The image of a senior citizen as being frail, sick, and dependent on others is rapidly transforming into a more accurate picture of active, independent individuals who participate in many social and recreational activities, feel 15 years younger, may continue to work in some capacity, and have enough money set aside for the years ahead.

When someone told 89-year-old poet Dorothy Duncan that she had lived a full life, she responded tartly,' Don't you past-tense me!"[15] The elderly do not think of themselves as "old," something that agents should remember as they market products in the future. In 2002, a Michigan woman celebrated her 115th birthday with relatives at the nursing home where she lives. Her granddaughter, 53, noted the occasion by saying her grandmother had seen the invention of radio, television, and the space shuttle. The woman has lived in a nursing home since 1991 when she broke her hip.[16]

Esther Hemp, 102 of New Cumberland, PA. lives with her daughter and maintains a fairly active lifestyle. Though she needs help with basic activities like getting out of bed, Hemp is active in her local church and occasionally visits the senior citizens center. "I've got good health habits," she says. "I lead a clean life. I don't smoke and I have a positive attitude."[17]

Today's senior is different in so many ways. Longevity could mean more years in retirement, but don't tell that to many of the older workers who continue to contribute in important ways. Mildred LaPerche retired from nursing in 1989 – for one month. "Worst mistake I ever made," she says. But LaPerche, now 82, was able to go back to work at Baptist Health Systems of South Florida, a company that believes in hiring or keeping on skilled people even after they reach the traditional retirement age.[18] And so it goes. A 73-year-old drives a dump truck and a tour bus in Deland, Florida, while a 78-year-old former professional bowler works at an Orange City, Florida K-Mart, and an 84-year-old Pearl Harbor survivor continues to work at Publix Supermarket in Ormond Beach, Florida.[19]

The year 2001 marked the first time workers over the age of 40 outnumbered those under that age, according to the Bureau of Labor Statistics. Thirteen percent of U.S. workers today are over age 55, a number that will increase to 20 percent by 2015.[20]

Seniors are living better and they're living longer. General good health has kept many of them active, often postponing the inevitable health condition(s) that can slow them down and hasten the aging process. Some researchers say that the percentage of older Americans who are unable to perform everyday tasks and live on their own – a population that's already decreased by 25 percent from 1982 to 1999 – may continue to head downward.[21] Healthier lifestyles, a decrease in smokers, and better and more effective drugs are helping to contribute to the better health of the senior population.

But today's age 65 and older story is not only about good health and active workers. There are many fears that older Americans express, primarily having to do with rising out-of-pocket medical expenses and the potential to outlive one's financial assets.

Several years ago, a retired disability insurance agent contacted me to discuss health industry trends. Retired for 23 years, he was a wealth of information on Social Security and reminisced about the wage freezes during World War II and other issues that he dealt with while selling disability income insurance. Inevitably, though, our conversation turned to his own health and the cost of home health care he requires at age 84. The financial worry, attributed to the high cost of medical care, was of great concern to him. He feared that he would not outlive his wife and that his declining health would use up their money, leaving her in a desperate situation.

This is not an unusual story. AARP releases an annual report entitled "Beyond 50." It notes that good physical health is just one measure of health security or well-being. Other indicators are adequate health and long-term care insurance coverage; access to quality health care; protection against financially devastating health costs; and sufficient information for making sound health decisions. In the report's recent conclusion, it feared that many people over age 50 do *not* enjoy health security and are unlikely to in the future.[22]

The evidence continues to mount that medical costs are playing a major role in elderly insecurity. More than half the employers surveyed by Hewitt Associates in December 2002 indicated that they plan to raise premiums and increase co-payments for retirees over the next three years, including an increase in prescription drug co-payments. Nearly a quarter of these employers said they are likely to eliminate health coverage for future retirees.[23]

This increases the financial pressure on the senior trying to stretch retirement assets as far as possible. According to a report done by the Institute for Social Research at the University of Michigan, since 2000 retirees' portfolios have shrunk by about $678 billion dollars. This is critical, the report noted, as about 20 million older Americans rely on investment income in part to pay for living expenses.[24]

Washington continues to analyze two key senior financial programs – Medicare (health care for the elderly) and Medicaid (nursing home and long-term care services), without a long-term solution to the survival of either program. Medicare spent more than $15 billion dollars on nursing home and home health care in 2000, even though this program focuses largely on acute care – hospital and doctor bills.[25] Further, discussion on how to deter the rise in Social Security benefits in anticipation of the swift aging of our population has yet to be accomplished due to the tremendous backlash to be expected from the senior population, who not only count on benefit payments, but also feel a certain entitlement to these benefits. How easy will it be to change the Social Security program when the senior population doubles?

The children of our aging Americans are now starting in earnest to experience the crunch between the dwindling financial resources of their parents beset by medical issues and maintaining their own lifestyles. A care management company in Florida notes that a growing number of their clients have more parents to care for today than children, thanks to multiple marriages and dropping birthrates. One woman says she could potentially be responsible for seven older adults, while only having three stepdaughters.[26]

The Consequences of Aging

America is just beginning to see the effects of an aging population. On the one hand, it's wonderful that our children will know our parents. As a child, I only knew one of my grandparents and I still treasure her memory. She never missed listening to a Boston Red Sox baseball game on the radio. Her lifelong experiences taught me a lot and I was fortunate to have spent time with her.

It was also my first exposure to a nursing home, where my "Nana" spent the last couple of years of her life. Seeing people in poor health, unable to care, feed or dress themselves was very traumatic. Yet, this is to be expected of longer life spans. Simply because someone lives longer doesn't guarantee the quality of life. Our aging parents or relatives may live longer, but many will need our help both physically and financially.

The Society of Actuaries recently issued a report about health expectancy. The objective was not just to predict longevity, but to forecast how many of those years would be healthy ones. The results? A 65-year-old non-smoking female would live for another 24 years, on average. But only 18.3 years would be healthy, with the balance of 5.7 years labeled as unhealthy. For a male, age 65, non-smoker, the health expectancy was predicted as 16.6 healthy years and 4.9 unhealthy. The question is – how to define unhealthy? What will it mean in terms of today's rising out-of-pocket medical costs?[27]

The real aging crisis facing us isn't about numbers; it's about people. The demographics in this country are about to permanently change to the point where – in the not too distant future – one elderly American will be supported by only two working people. The United States has experienced a significant drop in the percentage of younger workers ages 25-34 since 1985.[28] It's not only about fewer people contributing to Social Security and Medicare programs. It's also about producing less goods and services for all – a coming calamity that will create a large demand outstripping supply, leading to certain price increases that threaten the lifestyle of everyone.

The dependency on the younger generation is creating difficulties of its own. The role reversal effect, aging parents now dependent on their children, has its own consequences. The two sides do not always share the same views of long-term care. In a recent survey, in the parent's view, 64 percent of parents with children over the age of 34 say they would not want to move in with their children in their later years if they needed care. By contrast, 44 percent of adult children believed their parents would want to move in with them if care was needed.[29]

As the population ages, more attention will be paid to diseases that generally affect the elderly. Alzheimer's disease will garner the "lion's share" of attention especially as the country watches how this illness affects Ronald Reagan and Charlton Heston. Alzheimer's is responsible for a significant number of people in nursing homes, the cost for which is paid by private money or, when that runs out, Medicaid. Many Americans today worry about the 125 million people today who live with chronic conditions – the type of health problem that often leads to a need for long-term care services. A recent Harris survey found that 72 percent of Americans say it is difficult for people living with chronic conditions to get necessary care from their health care providers. The survey also found that, on average, family caregivers provide care for their loved ones for 4.5 years, with the unpaid help of four friends or family members.[30]

The consequences of aging can be poor health, poor finances, and financial and emotional pressure on the next generation. As insurance agents and financial planners we must help our clients prepare for the possibility of living a longer life. We must assist them in planning for their retirement years by helping to ensure some measure of financial security. We can help create resources that won't leave them or future generations tapped-out if infirmity strikes.

The New Retirement

Future retirees will certainly be looking at a new type of retirement. Statistically, people who are 65 today will live, on average, four years longer than those who were 65 in 1960.[31] The trend is for people to retire younger than they did in 1960, so the period of years to fund in retirement is greater than ever.

In keeping with the vast changes in today's demographics, the new retirement is already happening, according to Dr. Ken Dychtwald. In a recent study of current retirees, the noted gerontologist identified four main types of retirees – the "four faces of retirement" – in an article published in 2002.[32]

The first group is the "Ageless Explorer," representing 27 percent of the new retirement. These retirees view retirement as an exciting new phase in their lives and would rather be too busy than risk being bored. They have attained the highest level of education and, on average, have saved for retirement for 24 years. Their average household income is $64,800 with an average net worth of $469,800.

Next up are the "Comfortably Contents, who make up about 19 percent of today's retirees. These are not the people still working, but instead living the more leisurely-paced lifestyle. They have saved, on average, for about 23 years, and have an average income of $61,200 and an average net worth of $367,500.

The other two clusters of retirees are not in as good a shape as their aforementioned counterparts. The "Live For Todays" (22 percent of retirees) spent their working years focused on the present rather than the future. They did not spend much time on retirement planning, saving, on average for about 18 years. Their average household income is $46,300 and average net worth estimated at $222,600. They are anxious about their financial situation, do not believe they have enough money for the extended years ahead, and will likely keep working to supplement their current level of savings. This group sounds amazingly close to a description of the Baby Boomers, a generation rapidly closing in on retirement.

Finally, there are the "Sick and Tireds," at 32 percent, the largest segment of the new retirement. They have less of everything – money, education, and even good health. They have saved, on average, for 16 years, with an average income of $31,900, and an average net worth of $161,200. Their "retirement" will be a difficult one.

What is interesting about these descriptions is that even the best off of today's retirees – the Ageless Explorers – are not that far off from economic difficulties should the need for long-term care services arise. There are plenty of examples of people spending $300,000 and more out-of-pocket for long-term care. With an average net worth of about $470,000, those assets could dwindle significantly and impact the remaining years of a healthy spouse's retirement.

Today's changing demographics has been noted by Michael Stein, CFP in his book "The Prosperous Retirement," as he suggests that retirement today differs from post-Depression retirement in six ways:[33]

-    Retirees may live longer and have more active lives in retirement;

-    Retirement may occur in phases;

-    The cost of a retirement lifestyle may be similar to that of a pre-retirement lifestyle;

-    Inflation may increase the need for income by two or three times during retirement;

-    Income sources for the new retirement will differ from those available to earlier retirees; and

-    Tax and estate planning and insurance are vital.

The new retirement is and will be filled with vibrant, motivated individuals, still interested in learning. A 10-week history course offered by the University of South Florida and held at the University Village Retirement Center in Tampa, Florida attracted 125 "students", five times the number expected.[34] A grant helped put the course together, but it demonstrates that the old stereotype of people spending all their retirement time on the golf course is no longer relevant.

As today's Boomers move closer towards retirement decision time, the question becomes what exactly will that phase of their lives look like? There is some pessimism among this group due to a decided lack of planning to this point. In a *Fortune* magazine study, some of the more revealing results indicate that 23 percent of Boomers believe they are not likely to receive any Social Security benefits whatsoever; 80 percent of Boomers expect to work in retirement and 46 percent of Americans believe that $1,000,000 is not enough to retire on.[35]

Boomers are also experiencing an erosion of assets due to long-term care expenses of their own parents. This has, in part, created some of the negativity as they watch the preceding generation retire in relative comfort only to see them lose much of what they had due to a medical circumstance where the safety net of Medicare and Medicare Supplements failed to provide sufficient financial assistance.

Generations

Our first concern should be our own family. Regardless of what stage our own lives are in, we will doubtless be touched by the aging of America in some way or another. Look around you. How old are your parents? Grandparents? Children? Yourself? Are you prepared in the event a long-term care situation arises similar to that of the Doan family depicted in Chapter 1?

Before we can do a proper job for our clients, we must first understand the consequences of aging in our own lives. When my father passed away in 1989, my mother quickly learned much about finances she didn't know before. Writing checks and balancing her accounts were new ground for her. She had read an article about long-term care insurance and decided she wanted to know more about it. She bought a policy for herself in 1990 and was satisfied that she had taken a large step towards protecting her finances from most long-term health problems that might arise. More important, to her, was that her children would not be forced to sacrifice financially or emotionally in the event of a long-term care need.

Analyze your own family situation first. Who is close to retirement? Are they financially ready? How is their health? Is there a role for long-term care insurance? This book will provide greater insights in the chapters that follow on who are the best candidates for this product. There may be an important sale for you within your own family circle.

Many insurance agents have sold disability income insurance to family members and others as income protection during the working years. Disability income coverage provides replacement of a portion of a person's earnings if he is unable to work due to an injury or illness. The purchase of this product provides financial security for these individuals and their families with continued income despite not being able to work.

These formerly ideal candidates for disability insurance are now ideal people to approach to discuss the consequences of aging. Advances in medical science are enabling them to live longer. Financial security is an issue and the threat of a long-term illness jeopardizing their retirement is a danger they won't easily ignore.

If you have any disability income clients that fit this description, a discussion of the consequences of aging is in order.

Many of these people are aging "baby boomers." This generation, approximately 30 percent of the nation's population, is poised to completely change the way we think about the elderly. Boomers have better lifestyle awareness, higher fitness levels, and more prudent considerations of both diet and health than any preceding generation.

This a large market of people numbering 77 million, who could use help with planning for the future.[36]

It won't be easy. After all, this is the group that embraced the song "My Generation" by The Who as its anthem with lyrics like "I hope I die before I get old." Boomers typically see themselves as 15 years younger than they actually are, which makes them great fun to party with, but it is a true challenge to have them admit they need to plan for a looming retirement.

This group, now turning age 55 in large numbers, is hardened by the burden of credit card debt, raising young children, and coping with aging parents all at the same time. Women today think nothing of having children at age 40 – the same age that their mothers had college age children. As a result, boomers will be facing college education costs of their children and possibly long-term care costs of their parents. Who could retire with those financial burdens?

Boomers are well educated, affluent, and the healthiest generation in our nation's history. They have redefined marriage, education, work, and family. They will eventually be part of "The New Retirement," and although it is too soon to predict exactly what that will look like, many of this generation could swell the ranks of Dr. Dychtwald's "Live For Todays."

This generation has not done much about long-term care, despite many personal experiences with it in their own families. The Center for Aging Research & Education in New York indicates that the high premiums associated with long-term care insurance, together with the lack of understanding and the lack of information available to them today on this issue, stop them from taking action on the purchase of this coverage. While 70 percent of Boomers believe that they need to be personally responsible for taking care of their own long-term care needs, very few have done anything about it.[37]

Boomers are presently dealing with another financial issue that has understandably sidetracked them from long-term care planning: the free-fall of their own retirement savings. In a Harris Interactive Survey, sponsored by Allstate Corporation, average retirement savings declined from nearly $120,000 in 2001 to $93,000 in 2002.[38] Market concerns dominate financial discussions today, and other planning elements are taking a back seat to these concerns.

The "X Generation" will have their own say about retirement. Surprisingly, unlike boomers, generation X'ers show sophistication about the intricacies of planning, saving, and investing for retirement. Not only are they not counting on Social Security, but they are also convinced that they will be on their own for health care costs, too. They have watched Boomers spend their money as fast as they can make it and know that ultimately this exacts a high price.

Long-term care insurance, especially in an employer-sponsored setting, has a growing appeal to generation X'ers. Now that the tax consequences have been resolved, sales will further increase with this group. They have read much about the aging of America and will continue to be inundated with information on the importance of planning ahead.

Generation Y may ultimately impact the financial consequences of aging. In each of the years from 1989 to 1993, U.S. births exceeded four million for the first time since the early 1960's. Today, there are around 57 million Americans under age 15 and more than 20 million between ages four and eight. They will reach the work force at about the same time the boomers start turning age 65, although it is still unknown as to the potential assistance this will lend toward the consequences of aging.[39]

Finally, September 11th may ultimately play a role in the planning process, as Americans re-evaluate their priorities in the wake of the terrorist attack. A post-September 11 survey indicated that 57 percent of consumers said that financial well-being was important to them, citing stress or concern about family security as the number one reason.[40] With long-term care taking such a heavy toll on families, consumer attitudes today may make it easier to stress the theme of wealth protection than it has been in some time.

Adult Lifestage Events

The insurance industry is catching on to the marketing potential of the "aging" of our country. Financial planning is critical in stretching the retirement dollar. A major reason for purchasing life insurance is to pay significant estate taxes. With the sophisticated life and annuity products on the market today, the insurance industry is also in a good position to serve the needs of aging America.

As noted in this chapter, there are many unique challenges ahead due to today's changing demographics that makes advanced planning critical. The "sandwich generation" is the term used for individuals who are typically female and who must raise children while caring for an aging relative. Delayed parenting has made this more of a reality and the financial setback accorded this type of arrangement can be devastating to the retirement hopes of the person caught in the middle.

More than one in three (37 percent) of Boomers will be financially responsible for children or parents during their own retirement years, and 7 percent will be financially responsible for both during this time frame.[41] This is one of the reasons Boomers are typically negative when it comes to retirement planning. For them, it seems like their lives are not theirs to control, and the insurance industry must create ways to make this burden easier to bear during the autumn of these people's lives.

This "sandwiched effect" has created a key adult lifestage event: caregiving. In one recent poll, 67 percent of employees called the effect of caring for an elderly parent "significant" on their family lives; 41 percent say their work is interrupted, and more than 10 percent say they have given up promotions or even their jobs to provide care.[42] With the bulk of our nation's women having joined the workforce, caregiving responsibilities represent an overwhelming burden in addition to working all week. The need for some type of insurance protection that can pay for someone else to do the caregiving while the family member is working has become critical.

Hispanic Boomers will be particularly affected by this lifestage event. A 2002 survey revealed that 53 percent of Hispanic Americans would be supporting children or elderly parents during retirement, and 19 percent said they would be responsible for *both* during their retirement years. Six percent of Hispanic Americans predicted that obligations to family members would be their biggest expense during retirement.[43]

For Boomers and the younger generations, planning ahead will be the key to success in dealing with the issues of aging. An HIAA report directed at younger potential buyers of long-term care insurance pointed out that 12.8 million Americans today need help with daily activities and 40 percent of them are working age adults. The report went on to indicate that 50 percent of all Americans will need long-term care services at some point in their lives and that by 2005, 12 million Americans over age 65 will need long-term care assistance.[44]

Insurance companies and agents, in striving to assist individuals plan financially and emotionally for the future, must be more aware of these types of trends.

The Business of Aging

Marketing to the elderly is the future for many industries. The demographic shift created by the baby boomers is tilting marketing angles towards an older population.

The secret to success here, though, is to understand that older individuals today (age 50 or older) does not think of themselves in those terms. How do you market to a John Glenn, who went back into space at age 77? Or to a Hale Irwin, currently rewriting the record books of the PGA's *Champions Tour*? Or an Alan Greenspan, who can, in his 70s, with a few words dictate a complete shift in the markets? These people typify the cliché "age is just a number."

These are just a few examples. Marketers must think more in terms of a new breed of older person, and their message should be one that positively reflects today's aging environment. Folks over 50 are being hailed as the new yuppies – about one-third of the U.S. population, but controlling three-fourths of its wealth.[45] While marketers concentrate on the younger buyer, they are missing the group that has the majority of discretionary income today. The 21st Century senior is different in many ways from seniors of previous generations, and those agents desiring to market long-term care insurance should be prepared for a more well-informed consumer.

This is also a wary bunch, and rightfully so. For years, seniors have been the targets of scams and inappropriate investments. Increasingly, many older investors are scouring financial publications, surfing the Internet, and pestering brokerage houses in an effort to achieve higher returns and quality investments. Agents can be sure long-term care insurance will be reviewed in much the same manner.

The Prospective Payment System

No discussion of today's changing demographics would be complete without a review of the impact of Medicare and its attempt to deal with a growing number of people over age 65.

The Medicare program, created in 1965, was conceived as part of John F. Kennedy's campaign platform for the 1960 presidential election and was implemented during the Johnson administration. Medicare was to provide older Americans with some form of guaranteed health care, thus preventing poorer older Americans from bankrupting themselves due to illness or injury.

The aging of our population has certainly taken Medicare to its breaking point. As more and more Americans qualified for "Part A" of Medicare at age 65, the resources set aside to fund the Medicare program began to deteriorate. Finally, in the early 1980's, faced with the increase in expenditures at an accelerating rate, Congress approved a prospective payment system designed to contain skyrocketing health care costs.

One feature of this system was the diagnostic-related groups (DRGs). Essentially, each medical condition treatable under Medicare was measured, on average, and a series of rules established identifying length and cost of each treatment. One outcome of the DRGs was to significantly curtail the amount of time spent in the hospital per condition with Medicare paying for only a stated number of days. If the hospital treated the patient in less than the time specified by Medicare, the institution would still be reimbursed for the number of days the DRG specified. If it took more time, the hospital was then expected to sustain the extra cost.

Most hospitals did not keep Medicare patients beyond the DRG-stated days. However, many patients were not well enough to leave the hospital. An interim stop-gap measure evolved whereby the patient would receive skilled, intermediate, or custodial nursing care in a different setting, usually in a nursing home facility. As a result, an awareness of the cost of a nursing home stay grew quickly among senior citizens. During the first 18 months following the introduction of Medicare's Prospective Payment System, nursing home admissions increased by 40 percent.[46]

Many of these medical situations were short term, but they did raise fears about the most significant loophole in the Medicare program – coverage for a long-term or chronic illness. According to the Center for Medicare and Medicaid Services, Medicare covers approximately 14 percent of the average nursing home bill.[47]

Most older people have at least one chronic condition and many have multiple conditions.

The costs to treat long-term chronic conditions can erode even the most substantial asset base. Traditionally, seniors have placed a lot of faith in Medicare, but their confidence in this government program has been eroded by their own nursing home experiences. The DRG program placed nursing homes center stage and created an even greater concern about the seniors' financial futures.

This has created an audience of seniors primed to talk with an insurance agent or financial planner who can help them prepare properly for retirement. These seniors have all heard that many people propose reforming Medicare by requiring seniors to spend more of their own money on medical bills. They also are increasingly aware of the costs of long-term care. Working with seniors in the long-term care market is one of the most exciting prospects for an agent in terms of potential.

The Ball Is In the Industry's Court

With today's changing demographics, the insurance industry has the chance to take the lead in assisting people with their financial goals and dreams. The government does not want the complete burden to fall on it – witness the recent reforms to the Medicare and Medicaid programs. Long-term care insurance and pre-retirement financial planning can play a key role in assuring people that they will not only survive their retirement years, but will have every opportunity to enjoy them as well. This work can also provide assurance for family members that their own lives are less likely to be disrupted without control.

In the future, this country will see a vast number of seniors in various stages of life – second or third careers and retirement. These individuals are determined to remain independent and active and are at the heart of the long-term care insurance market.

What these people primarily lack is coverage for those out-of-pocket long-term care expenses. This issue is not going away anytime soon, and the insurance industry has a terrific opportunity to step forward and help to fill in this vital financial gap.

Chapter Notes

1. "How Old Are We?", *Daytona Beach News Journal*, July 7, 2002, p. 3C.

2. Statistical Abstract of the United States: 2002, Tables 11 and 1308.

3. Genaro C. Armas, "Census Tracks Grandparent Caregivers," *Associated Press newswire*, July 7, 2002.

4. "Positive attitudes aid 100+ crowd," *Daytona Beach News Journal*, October 3, 2001, p. 3A.

5. Genaro C. Armas, "Number of Americans 100 or Older Rises," *Associated Press newswire*, October 3, 2001.

6. "HIAA Study Finds Long-Term Care Insurance Benefits Everyone," *HIU Magazine*, November 2002, p. 25.

7. John Knuble and Ed Auble, CLU, "LTC Insurance – A Product Whose Time Has Come," *Advisor Today*, June 2002, p. 47.

8. Lynn Vincent, "Breaking the Senior Barrier," *Advisor Today*, August 2001, p. 46.

9. "National Survey Identifies Myths and Misperceptions About Long-Term Care," *HIU Magazine*, November 2002, p. 27.

10. John Noble, "A New Role for LTC Insurance," *Advisor Today*, p. 52.

11. Sharon K. Moorhead, "Between A Rock and a Hard Place," *Florida Underwriter*, October 2002, p. 10.

12. Karen Lee, "HIAA research optimistic on LTCI market," *Employee Benefit News*, April 15, 2002, p. 15.

13. "LTC Milestone: Benefit payouts reach $1 billion mark," *BenefitNews.com Adviser*, January 22, 2003.

14. Chuck Jones, "Americans Still Unaware of LTC Costs," *Advisor Today*, August 2001, p. 35.

15. Barbara J. Lautzenheiser and Christine E. Delvaglio, "Senior Market Opportunities Abound," *National Underwriter*, Life & Health/Financial Services Edition, August 18, 1997, p. 8.

16. "World's Oldest Woman Has Birthday," *Associated Press newswire*, January 23, 2002.

17. Genaro C. Armas, "Number of Americans 100 or Older Rises," *Associated Press newswire*, October 3, 2001.

18. Francine Russo, "The Age of Experience," *Modern Maturity*, Nov/Dec. 2001, p. 94.

19. Morris Sullivan, "Groups honor older workers," *Daytona Beach News Journal*, May 24, 2002, p. 4C.

20. Francine Russo, "The Age of Experience," *Modern Maturity*, Nov./Dec. 2001, p. 94.

21. Susan Jacoby, "Living Better, Living Longer," *AARP Bulletin*, December 2002, p. 11.

22. Anne Pavuk Wright, "Health Beyond 50: Ouch!" *AARP Bulletin*, June 2002, p. 18.

23. Janelle Carter, "Retirees Face Increased Health Premiums," *Associated Press newswire*, December 9, 2002.

24. Melinda Logos, "As Portfolios Shrink, Retirees Warily Seek Work," *New York Times*, September 8, 2002.

25. *Statistical Abstract of the United States: 2002*, Table 125.

26. Jane Eisner, "Duty of caring for the elderly is falling on an unready nation," *Philadelphia Inquirer*, August 1, 2002.

27. Society of Actuaries, www.soa.org.

28. Francine Russo, "The Age of Experience," *Modern Maturity*, Nov./Dec. 2001, p. 94.

29. The Aging Dilemma, Zogby International Survey, *Advisor Today*, October 2002, p. 32.

30. "New Poll Reveals Americans' Concerns About Living With Chronic Conditions," *PR Newswire*, February 26, 2001.

31. "Americans Facing Retirement Crossroads," *Business Wire*, February 27, 2002.

32. Fred Brock, "The New Retirement Comes in Four Financial Flavors," *New York Times*, July 7, 2002.

33. "Retirement, the New Frontier," *Portfolio Edge*, published by First Union Securities, Inc., September 2001.

34. Pat Leisner, "USF Reaches Out to Seniors," *Associated Press*, February 20, 2002.

35. Christine Y. Chen, "Everything You Always Wanted To Know About Retirement But Were Afraid To Ask," *Fortune* magazine supplement, August 13, 2001.

36. Linda Koco, "Boomers Are Doing U-Turns On Aging, Retirement," *National Underwriter*, October 28, 2002, p. 4.

37. Kap Su Seol, "Baby Boomers Unprepared For Long-Term Care Needs, A New Study Suggests," *National Underwriter*, July 16, 2001, p. 40.

38. Trevor Thomas, "Boomers' Retirement Concerns Rose Sharply In Last Year," *National Underwriter*, August 26, 2002, p. 3.

39. Melinda Beck, "Next Population Bulge Shows its Might," *Wall Street Journal*, February 3, 1997, p. B-1.

40. "Study Finds American Baby Boomers and Gen Xers Care More About Their Money Than Their Mortality, But Priorities Are Shifting," *Business Wire*, January 15, 2002.

41. "Who is Your Target Market for 2002?" *LTC Sales and Marketing Insight*, published by Penn Treaty, January 2002.

42. Sharon K. Moorhead, "Between A Rock and a Hard Place," *Florida Underwriter*, October 2002, p. 10.

43. Marcella De Simone, "Hispanic Boomers Will Be Particularly 'Sandwiched,'" *National Underwriter*, November 25, 2002, p. 35.

44. John Noble, "A New Role For LTC Insurance," *Advisor Today*, February 2002, p. 52.

45. Michael McCarthy, "Some consumers want ads for a mature audience," *USA Today*, November 19, 2002, p. 1B.

46. Health Care Financing Administration data.

47. Center for Medicare and Medicaid Services data.

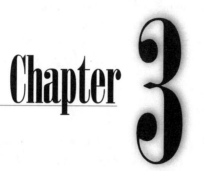

Chapter 3

The Emotional Burden of Aging

"What I look forward to is continued immaturity followed by death."

—Dave Barry

As insurance agents and financial planners we ask ourselves, what is long-term care? What exactly does long-term care cover? What do we hope to accomplish by addressing this need with our clients?

You will recall from Chapter 1, long-term care decisions involve both emotional and financial issues. While we are used to designing programs to assist our clients financially, the planning of long-term care also requires us to understand the emotional dynamics involved. Understanding the emotional implications of long-term care will help us better communicate the importance of advanced planning to our clients.

What types of situations could our clients face?

Long-Term Care Scenarios

Scenario #1

A 52-year-old New Jersey freelance writer can see the writing on the wall. His 85-year-old father who lives in Detroit is still in decent shape, but there is already trouble brewing among his siblings as to who will care for him should his health decline in the future. His sister also lives in Detroit and is terrified at the prospect of becoming the day-to-day caregiver for her father, picturing herself as the spinster who stays at home tending to a parent while the rest of the family goes out and has a life.[1]

Scenario #2

Long-distance caregiving can also take its toll. A New York woman cares for her 92-year-old mother, even though her parent lives in Florida. Every day she is immersed in a sea of mother-related activities – countless phone calls, a blitz of faxes and e-mails to the growing number of doctors and physiotherapists in charge of her care. She talks to pharmacists about the most economical, yet effective prescription treatment and struggles to understand Medicaid rules. In the midst of it all surfaces a troubling question for her: Who will be there for me?[2]

Scenario #3

A woman caring for her 80-year-old mother and her 3-year-old daughter calls her current role "extreme mothering" – the care and feeding of people on opposites sides of the life arc. As custodian for both, she makes their dinners, beds and doctor's appointments. After leaving work every day and arriving home at 5:00 PM, her second shift begins. Her life is a perpetual series of errands and tasks. Between her daughter's ear infections and her mother's occasional falls, the emergency room feels like a second home.[3]

Scenario #4

A man living in North Carolina moved his mother to a facility that accepted Medicaid. The nursing home was close to his house so he could visit every day and provide the kind of emotional support she needed. This arrangement seemed to go well for all involved until his niece in Florida intervened. She didn't want her great-aunt to be in a nursing home and if her uncle wouldn't take her into his own home, she would move her great-aunt to Florida to stay with her and her family.

So she moved her great-aunt to Florida. Even though he had no access to his mother, the son felt that she would be well taken care of in his niece's home rather than in the nursing home facility. It certainly had to be a better situation. Unfortunately, after two months, his niece realized she couldn't cope with the frail, elderly woman and arranged for her to move into a nursing home that was

Medicaid certified in a nearby Florida town. The result of this emotional tug-of-war was the ultimate placement of his mother in a facility that was a nine hour drive for him.

Scenario #5

A Missouri man remembers well the pain and burden of finding care for his elderly and mentally impaired father in the last and difficult years of his father's life. It was an emotionally trying experience for the retired TWA machinist and his spouse, one they don't want to see repeated for their own children. "We don't want to be burdens on our children and on our grandchildren," he said. For that reason, he and his wife sought out and purchased long-term care insurance.[4]

Role Reversal

Do these scenarios sound far-fetched? They are not. All of them are documented cases and are representative of thousands of similar situations across the country.

Very few people are prepared. The aging process carries with it an increased dependency, similar to that of a baby. Many elderly need assistance with eating, getting dressed and walking to name just a few activities. As seen with the example of "extreme mothering" noted above, the activities carried out with a child have equal applicability for the adult. It's just harder on the aging individual. A child has no expectations yet; an adult has already performed all these necessary functions capably for years and the loss of these simple abilities carries an emotional price.

The Boomers are living through what has been described by gerontologists as the first wave of longevity. Taking care of a dependent adult is becoming so commonplace an event, Boomers are building their own new homes with a separate wing for a dependent parent or other relative to stay when the time comes. It's not just the emotional concerns that must be faced, but the physical ones as well. Some of this comes down to the caregiver's choices, too. Those who care for a relative with dementia have less stress and better psychological well-being if they take advantage of adult day-care services, but fewer than 20 percent of caregivers do so.[5]

While the aging person copes with these adjustments, so too must their children. It is difficult to see your parents in a dependent role. After all, you were completely dependent on them as a child. This role reversal has a great impact on the lives of Americans everywhere. There is no rehearsal, no preparation. Longer life spans are something of a recent phenomenon and an aging parent or relative in his or her 80's is no longer the exception but the rule.

If you haven't been around your parents for some time, you may be surprised at the differences when you do see them again – changes that are not obvious from a regular phone call. The female baby boomer who has had a child at the age of 42 may look forward to bringing their new grandchild home to her parents only to discover that her parents don't have the patience for a young child any longer.

Various surveys taken over the last few years along with the personal experience of working with seniors have shown these to be most seniors' goals:

1.   Not being a burden on their families.

2.   Remaining physically and financially independent.

3.   Providing for their spouse.

These are not goals as much as they are fears, and the elderly are more determined than ever to live up to all three objectives. In Orange City, Florida, a fire destroyed the home of an 88-year-old woman and took the life of her 81-year-old male companion. A neighbor and her children took her in and have been looking after her ever since. Despite a deep depression over these events, the woman struggles to maintain her independence and is able to stay out of a facility thanks to the caring assistance of the people next door.[6]

The inability to remain independent, forcing a situation in which they are completely dependent on their families, can have drastic consequences for those unable to cope mentally with this lifestyle change. A large number of Americans over age 65 take their own lives each year, and sometimes these are people whose name you would otherwise associate with strength. Take the case of retired Admiral and World War II submarine hero Chester Nimitz, Jr.(son of the WW II Pacific fleet Commander) and his wife Joan. On January 2, 2002, they canceled their nighttime nurse and took an overdose of sleeping pills. Their suicide note says it all: "Our decision was made over a considerable period of time and was not carried out in acute desperation. Nor is it the expression of mental illness. We have consciously, rationally, deliberately, and of our own free will taken measures to end our lives today because of the physical limitations on our quality of life placed upon us by age, failing vision, osteoporosis, back pain and painful orthopedic problems.[7]

This fragile emotional state of the elderly places a substantial strain on the younger adult who is attempting to help. Individuals who put themselves in the role of caregiver may expect gratitude from the individuals they are taking care of and empathy from siblings who live a distance away. Very likely, they will receive neither. Along with her four siblings, a 53-year-old health care researcher from Maine, orchestrated the care of her 83-year-old mother after hip surgery. There was disagreement among the siblings about when their mom should be shifted into assisted living. "Some of us were looking for an action plan, that by such and such a date the house would be sold, etc., while some of us were look-ing for Mom to set the pace for herself." It wasn't easy, and the family had to work hard to reach an amiable decision for all involved.[8]

Try to imagine the fear that an aging person has in losing independence. Think about it. Many of us treasure the control we have of our own time and space. Now, in a caregiving situation, *both* caregiver and caretaker lose that con-trol. In life's role reversal that is the centerpiece of an aging America, the elderly need help doing all of the things they've done for themselves and their children must rearrange their own lives to care for their elderly relative. The emotional burden on both sides can further be magnified by any past resentments or fam-ily squabbles that are sure to surface with the responsibilities of caregiving.

Guilt is only one of the emotions that children will feel when trying to make the emotional decision of what to do about their parents. A nursing home place-ment is likely to leave a permanent emotional scar that no amount of visitation can heal. Trying to maintain the delicate balance within one's own household while making room for a new "boarder" is often a lost cause. Family members know they will lose some of the caregiver's attention and resent having to give up time and space to an elderly relative.

Long distance caregivers battle different problems. Guilt is still the primary feeling combined with the inadequacy one feels when a situation is out of con-trol. Hard as it is for the direct caregiver, the long distance caregiver will likely spend an inordinate amount of time on the phone to compensate for being away. The result is a similar loss of time for the caretaker's own immediate family. Sometimes it can work out. A 50-year-old New York man was con-cerned about his 80-year-old mother, who insisted on remaining in her Indianapolis home. On a recent visit, he dug around the neighborhood and encountered a charming couple living nearby. He convinced them to look in regularly on his mother and alert him to any problems they perceive. He con-sidered his situation lucky.[9]

These are problems that we must help our clients work through. A long-term care insurance product may help financially, but some of the emotional battering and the making of tough decisions will still be necessary. Recognizing these difficulties and playing a small, but important, role through advanced planning can make a world of difference when a long-term care situation arises.

The Sandwich Generation

For the first time in history, an entire generation may find themselves "sandwiched" between caring for growing children and aging parents. Nearly half of all Boomers age 45 to 55 have children at home and parents who are still living.[10]

Despite some societal progress, the role of caregiving will still fall to women. Because women traditionally have longer life spans, the person that requires care is also likely to be female. The combination of younger children and the fact that more females than ever before have joined the workforce is bound to create emotional fireworks in the future.

The numbers are overwhelmingly against the sandwiched Boomer. Older adults, age 65 and older, use 23 percent of ambulatory care visits and 48 percent of the hospital days. Twenty-six percent of older adults (65+) reported they were in fair or poor health in 1999, while people age 75 and over reported an average of three chronic condition problems at any one time and used more than 4.5 prescription drugs.[11] This simply compounds the caregiving problem.

How does one care for children, many of whom seem to be returning home after college due to a difficult job environment and a need for financial assistance, while dealing equally with a parent(s) who demands time simply for doctor visits and other medical-related errands?

The presence of younger children and aging parents are unique to the baby boomer generation. This group waited to have children and women giving birth in their 40's is quite common today. The unexpected consequence of this delayed parenting is that the raising of children is coincident to a need for assistance on the part of parents in their 70's and 80's.

Juggling a work schedule, having kids in school and day care and parents at home or in day care themselves (adult day care centers are a growing industry) requires an enormous amount of planning and organization. There will be days when you've promised an adult to take them shopping only to have to cancel because it conflicts with a PTA meeting. Or vice versa – you can't make it to your child's piano recital because your mother needs to go to the doctor's office.

"Caregivers today may be assisting not only their own children and parents but also grandchildren, nieces, nephews and even children of friends and neighbors," said the executive director of AARP in conjunction with the release of a report on the sandwich generation. Their study found that the burden of caregiving does not fall evenly across the board. The group most likely to be caring for parents or other older adults were those born outside the United States (43%) compared to 20 percent of people born in this country.[12]

The report showed that almost 75 percent of Asian-Americans expect children to care for elderly parents, versus 57 percent for Hispanics, 52 percent for African-Americans and 47 percent for whites. Asian Americans also cornered the market on guilt for not doing more to help their parents (72% feel this way) versus 67 percent of Hispanics, 54 percent of African-Americans, and 44 percent of whites.[13]

But what's a sandwich generation to do? The most traumatic decision to be made is deciding whether a parent will go into a nursing home or move in with you. There's no ducking the issue. It must be faced without regard to readiness. The key to a successful transition is to face the issues *before* something does happen.

It's easier said than done. When it comes to communicating about future planning and making decisions, neither child nor parent is exceptionally good at addressing the issues. Because both sides dread the possibility of an illness that is associated with aging, it's easier to avoid the subject than to talk about it.

Communication

Planning ahead of time requires good communication between parent and adult. There is no better time to do it than when everyone is healthy and putting the plans into action seems a long way off. Talking about long-term care will elicit parent's wishes in this regard. The child may be surprised when parents say they'd prefer a nursing home facility to being dependent on their children. Without a discussion of long-term care needs a parent would not ordinarily volunteer this information.

The ideal situation would be to have a parent taken care of by a home health care nurse or aide in his or her own home. Leaving parents in familiar surroundings rather than disrupting them with a move to an institution or another family member's home is a preferred arrangement for all concerned. If it can be done financially, it is likely to be the first choice. Medicare may or may not cover the expense, but a long-term care insurance policy today would handle the majority of the costs.

Keep in mind that a person has to qualify for the policy and, as such, must apply for it before the necessity for long-term care services arises. Unless there are early discussions about planning for this possibility, long-term care insurance is unlikely to be an option considered. In Chapter 1 of this book, the lack of advanced preparation meant Mrs. Doan didn't have, among other things, a long-term care insurance policy to provide a possible solution in the event of a long-term illness.

In addition to insurance, there are a variety of resources available to seniors which can be of help during a time of need. It's much easier to learn about these resources in advance of needing them. A listing can be compiled and kept in a safe place for consultation purposes when a long-term care plan of action is put into effect. (A listing of resources appears in Chapter 21, "The Agent's Checklist.")

Those "sandwiched" between children and a dependent adult need to realistically assess their abilities to handle both should it be needed. For someone who works, it would be impossible to do it all. Much as one may want to take on the entire burden, the "Superwoman" label will wear thin before too long. Communicating in advance about what can be done practically will be critical to organizing a plan that will actually work.

There will be arguments. Discussing parents' future situations only serves notice as to one's own eventual needs. Unless prior communication is done about possible long-term care situations, the entire family will be placed in the position of having to make rash decisions at a most difficult and emotional time. Decisions made under these circumstances are usually not the best decisions.

The agent and financial planner should know this. The same considerations – emotional and financial – used when planning in the event of a death should also be used in planning for long-term care. Advanced planning is what our jobs are all about.

Emotional Assistance

A person should not feel he or she is battling this alone. In the scenarios outlined at the beginning of this chapter, individuals were either suddenly thrust into the caregiving role without adequate time to prepare or looking at the future with dread as to their own potential for being a caregiving burden to someone else.

No matter what happens, there is no substitute for planning for this long-term care contingency ahead of time. However, since this preparation may not happen, when dealt the caregiving hand the best thing to do is: get some help! Save your own emotional well-being if possible. The more help one gets, the more likely the avoidance of the inevitable burnout that "extreme mothering" creates. Working a 9 to 5 job and then coming home to work another few hours leaves little time for one's own self, and this neglect will ultimately prove costly – emotionally, physically and psychologically – for the caregiver. Life spans of caregivers have been dramatically affected –negatively – as a result.

In addition to family, friends and neighbors, there are medical case managers who can help ease the emotional burden of caregiving. They are licensed pro-fessionals and include social workers, nurses, gerontologists and others who can provide an assessment of the long-term care situation and develop a plan to meet the needs of the person needing assistance. It may be easier for an unbiased third party to come in and help bridge the communication gap between the par-ent and child.

These managers can handle every aspect of an aging adult's care from inter-viewing and hiring household help, paying the bills and managing the financial accounts, arranging transportation as needed and calling on community resources that might otherwise be unknown to the children. They are meant to be a liaison between the family and the dependent adult and the help one can get from the medical and social community at large. You can find experienced geri-atric case managers through the National Association of Professional Geriatric Case Managers at caremanager.org.

The responsibilities and costs associated with the geriatric case manager can be discussed as part of the advanced preparations the family makes for such sit-uations. If there is any distance between children and parents, the subject (and how to pay for it) should be addressed.

While it may be unusual for the insurance agent or financial planner to become involved in the caregiving process of a client, there will be times when this assistance will be welcomed. Most caregivers welcome the help, even if it's just staying and visiting with the dependent adult while the primary caregiver does other errands. Caregivers and their dependents are, unfortunately, often deserted after a time by friends and family and even regular phone calls and offers of help (cook a meal, take them out) will help ease the emotional trauma both are enduring.

Even though there may be initial cooperation from all parties in the beginning of the caregiving process, do not assume that this harmony will continue when the actual time arrives. It is common for an older person to deny that assistance is necessary even though it seems obvious to everyone else. There may be some resistance in implementing these plans.

A third party can be of great emotional assistance here. Whether it's a case manager or a doctor or a social worker, nurse, insurance agent or friend, enlisting help should be part of the planning process.

Planning

It all comes down to planning. As an insurance agent and financial planner, your role in long-term care planning with a family involves both emotional and financial planning. Often the emotional issues dictate the financial choices that are made.

Above all, the agent should remember that there is the likelihood of the same situation happening in one's own family. There is a need to plan your actions and those of aging parents and relatives in the event a long-term care situation arises.

A member of the National Association of Health Underwriters recently shared his story with other members. His father, in the beginning stages of Alzheimer's, was cared for by his mother for some years. When his mom passed away, the caregiving burden would fall to the children. They started with a sitter for him 10 hours a day, 7 days a week, but it became too costly and the toll that the other hours in the day took on the family caregivers led them to ultimately have the father admitted to a nursing home. His father's income was sufficient to fund the nursing home charges, although not enough to pay for his life insurance and Medicare Supplement. Having another choice other than facility admission or paying out-of-pocket for home care would have made a world of difference to this family and helped them focus on easing their own emotional strain of seeing a parent transform before their own eyes.

The emotional aspect of what to do with one's own parents will be followed by the financial situation and consequences of each action. As a plan is formed, it is important to note the financial impact of each decision. It can create its own emotional burdens on family members. What a difference an understanding and well-prepared insurance agent can make.

Chapter Notes

1. Karen Houppert, "Looking After Yourself," *My Generation* (Nov./Dec. 2002), p. 45.

2. Barbara Gordon, "Who Will Be There For Me?" *My Generation* (May/June 2002), p. 62.

3. Elizabeth Cohen, "The Life and Times of An Extreme Mom," *Newsweek*, March 4, 2002.

4. Paul Wenske, "Check Out Long-Term Care Policies," *Orlando Sentinel*, November 21, 2001, p. B6.

5. Karen Houppert, "Looking After Yourself," *My Generation* (Nov./Dec. 2002), p. 47.

6. Mark Harper, "Growing Old, Growing Up," *Daytona Beach News Journal*, July 28, 2002, p. 1A.

7. Sara Rimer, "Admiral Maintains Command until the End," *Daytona Beach News Journal*, January 13, 2002, p. 5A.

8. Karen Houppert, "Looking After Yourself," *My Generation* (Nov./Dec. 2002), pp. 45-46.

9. Barbara Gordon, "Who Will be Me for Me?" *My Generation* (May/June 2002), pp. 63-64.

10. Chris Elia, "In the Middle," *My Generation* (Sept./Oct. 2001), p. 88.

11. Christine Tassone Kovner, et al., "Who Cares for Older Adults?" *Health Affairs* (September/October 2002), pp. 79-80.

12. Randy Schmid, "Baby Boom Generation Feeling Squeeze," *Associated Press*, July 11, 2001.

13. Chris Elia, "In the Middle," *My Generation* (September/October 2002), p. 88.

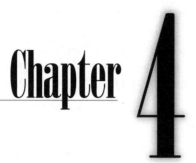

Chapter 4

The Financial Strain of Aging

"I couldn't be out of money. I still have checks."

– Gracie Allen

No one expects to outlive his or her money. Yet that is exactly what's happening to many Americans around the country. Take central Floridian Elsie Ryan, for example.[1]

Elsie's husband passed away in 1978 when she was 80 years old. "We weren't millionaire-wealthy," she says but she had a decent trust fund that she figured would last the rest of her life. At 97, she was living in a nursing home in Orlando.

The nursing home cost Elsie over $33,000 a year and after a few years in the nursing home, the trust fund was depleted. The nursing home personnel assisted Elsie in applying for Medicaid, the joint state-federal program for those living at or below poverty level.

Her mind still sharp, Elsie has endured a hip replacement, is crippled with arthritis, no longer has the use of her right leg, and is legally blind. "I've lived much too long," she says. Her trust fund was a lot of money seventeen years ago, but longevity of life and nursing home costs have created a situation that has forced her to become dependent on welfare.

The Financial Black Hole

It's not just Wall Street that has people financially down today. Granted, the nearly 3-year tumble for the stock market has eroded paper assets substantially. But add in a lengthy illness or injury, and many people are in serious danger of outliving their income.

Let's say you retired at age 67 with a retirement income of $40,000 a year. You have money in the bank, no debts and nothing but a comfortable lifestyle ahead. But then…

Your spouse is diagnosed with Alzheimer's and is in the early stages of the disease. While you had anticipated days filled with relaxation, your days are now filled with taking care of your spouse, trips to the doctor and pharmacy, general housekeeping, and preparing meals. You can no longer leave your spouse alone, so every trip is a joint trip.

You realize you can't cope with it alone and you hire a home health aide. The aide is there during the day while you have night duty, but even that is getting to be too much of an emotional strain for you. Your finances are almost exhausted because the cost for the home health aide is $100 per day.

The only alternative left is a nursing home, and even at a reasonable rate it will likely run $125 a day or more than $45,000 a year. The $75,000 in savings will be exhausted in less than two years. Although your spouse's condition is slowly deteriorating, it is more than likely he or she will live longer than two years. While the welfare program Medicaid has some built-in asset and income protections for the spouse, the retirement you were so looking forward to has been sidelined by the financial (and emotional) realities of long-term care.

In 2001, Americans spent $98.9 billion on nursing home care and $33.2 billion on home care.[2] One in 10 Americans older than age 65 and almost half of those age 85 and older who live in the community require assistance with their everyday activities.[3] The average daily rate for nursing home care in 2002 was $168 per day for a private room and $143 per day for a semi-private room. The average hourly rate for home care is $37 per hour for a Licensed Practical Nurse and $18 per hour for a home health aide.[4]

What do you do when you are suddenly faced with an additional expense of $25,000 to $60,000 per year? How does this affect your retirement? What about your children or heirs?

These questions should be asked by an insurance agent and financial planner when assisting individuals with their retirement and estate planning. If they are not addressed early on, the alternatives are limited and the decisions that must be made will inevitably be unsatisfactory and potentially financially devastating.

The New Retirement, Part 2

As the number of people heading into retirement mount, their financial preparedness is still a dominant question mark. There is likely a significant difference in what people have set aside for these golden years and what they will actually need. Only about 25 percent of people entering their retirement years have a net worth in excess of $300,000. Only 10 percent of households with people ages 50-59 have a net worth in excess of $725,000, and about the same percentage of households with people ages 60-69 have over $1 million.[5]

The general make-up of income sources for the retiree has changed dramatically, too. Gone are the days when the majority of people worked primarily for one employer and had a sizable defined benefit pension to draw from to supplement Social Security. Today's new retiree has multiple sources, and far more of it is tied up in investments. It is estimated that retirees who rank in the top 20 percent in earnings during their careers typically have more than one-third of their assets tied up in the stock market, and another 20 percent in pension funds. Their asset base is shrinking due to the stock market's plunge, and some who have fully retired are returning to work for the money. Those who are in the bottom 20 percent of earnings are less likely to have to return to work because 80 percent of their money comes from the (for now) more dependable Social Security trust funds.[6]

Now, factor in medical spending during retirement. Many people do not, by the way, when they plan the amount of money they will need to live on after giving up that regular paycheck. But the amount of spending on health care costs increases dramatically with old age (typically during retirement). The over-age 65 population made 25 percent of all visits to doctor's offices in 1999. That same year, they sought care from nonfederal short-stay hospitals at a rate of 2,256.8 days per 1,000 population nearly triple that of the next closest age group. Of the 7.6 million people who received formal home care services in 1999, 69 percent were age 65 or older, and almost 90 percent of nursing home residents in 1999 were over the age of 65.[7]

The most costly medical conditions in the United States were almost all afflictions older adults must deal with on a chronic basis. According to the 1996

Medical Expenditure Panel Survey data, these are, in order from most to least expensive, the top 10 financially draining medical conditions:[8]

1.	Ischemic heart disease	$21.5 billion
2.	Motor vehicle accidents	$21.2 billion
3.	Acute respiratory infection	$17.9 billion
4.	Arthropathies	$15.9 billion
5.	Hypertension	$14.8 billion
6.	Back problems	$12.2 billion
7.	Mood disorders	$10.2 billion
8.	Diabetes	$10.1 billion
9.	Cerebrovascular disease	$8.3 billion
10.	Cardiac dysrythmias	$7.2 billion

Aside from higher medical costs, there are millions of Americans already unprepared for a lengthy, *healthy* retirement. What would long-term care expenses do to that picture? Nursing home and other long-term care costs certainly contribute to higher medical expenses among the senior population. As the body ages and begins to weaken, the recovery period is longer and results in higher costs for medical services provided.

What are some long-term care costs? Looking first at nursing homes, Figure 4.1 is a 2002 survey of the daily costs of a nursing home facility stay, by region.[9]

FIGURE 4.1

Nursing Home Costs by State

REGION	AVERAGE DAILY COSTS	
	Semi-Private	Private
Anchorage AK	$321	$331
Birmingham, AL	109	121
Little Rock, AK	99	118
Phoenix, AZ	131	162
Los Angeles, CA	124	174
San Francisco, CA	147	250
Denver, CO	130	141
Hartford, CT	214	233
Washington, DC	193	203
Wilmington, DE	142	161
Jacksonville, FL	122	137
Miami, FL	137	194
Atlanta, GA	115	130
Honolulu, HI	173	221

FIGURE 4.1 (continued)

REGION	AVERAGE DAILY COSTS	
	Semi-Private	Private
Des Moines, IA	103	116
Boise, ID	135	147
Chicago, IL	124	140
Indianapolis, IN	114	163
Wichita, KS	109	119
Louisville, KY	114	125
New Orleans, LA	89	95
Boston, MA	207	244
Baltimore, MD	151	159
Brunswick, ME	164	183
Detroit, MI	119	126
Minneapolis, MN	130	168
St. Louis, MO	110	148
Jackson, MS	100	126
Billings, MT	123	135
Charlotte, NC	135	148
Fargo, ND	156	156
Omaha, NE	134	207
Manchester, NH	173	188
Cherry Hill, NJ	188	206
Albuquerque, NM	126	154
Las Vegas, NV	129	199
New York, NY	269	274
Columbus, OH	145	159
Oklahoma City, OK	97	125
Portland, OR	122	144
Pittsburgh, PA	154	164
Providence, RI	170	181
Charleston, SC	112	126
Dell Rapids, SD	112	116
Nashville, TN	113	127
Dallas, TX	102	143
Salt Lake City, UT	112	149
Richmond, VA	127	141
Rutland, VT	186	201
Seattle, WA	169	204
Milwaukee, WI	165	163
Martinsburg, WV	154	163
Worland, WY	113	126

These costs, as you can see, range widely with each state. It is important to keep in mind that while these are average daily costs of a nursing home for a specific area, where your client actually intends to seek long-term care services will ultimately be the measurement used to determine the cost of a nursing home facility.

In California, for example, the daily average varies between Los Angeles ($122/day for semi-private room), San Diego ($136/day), and San Francisco ($147/day). A stay in a nursing home in a smaller city would likely be less than some of these larger city averages.

It is easy to see how someone like Elsie Ryan can run out of money even if she was reasonably financially set when her retirement began. It's why Medicaid remains the largest third party payer of funds for long-term care.

The "New Retirement" means confronting some uglier realities than in days gone by. Bruce Springsteen, in his 1990s hit "Youngstown," sang about the plight of steel workers working in the blast furnaces and being left to their own devices when their companies up and left. He could have anticipated the current controversy at Bethlehem Steel in Pennsylvania. For the many workers who stuck it out "handling molten slag and inhaling steel dust", there was some gold to be found at the end of the career, namely a decent pension and a lifetime of nearly free health care for the worker and family.

In February 2003, Bethlehem Steel announced it was seeking bankruptcy court approval to terminate life and health benefits for more than 95,000 retired workers and their dependents effective March 31, 2003. While Medicare will help some of those over age 65, many are reeling from this news, facing prescription drug costs for asthma and lung-related problems. Long-term care needs lurk over the horizon and the retirement all of these people looked forward to is now tinged in the kind of hazy darkness in which they spent their entire working environment.[10]

This type of news is more commonplace then we would all like to believe. Folks need help not just in retirement with these health cost issues, but long before they reach the age when they stop working. The financial aspect of long-term care is vital; when combined with the emotional dangers, it's an absolute must to plan ahead.

So where does one pick up local long-term care cost data? Information on nursing home costs in your state can be found by contacting one of the state resource numbers listed in Chapter 21, "The Agent's Checklist." The information you can turn up while conducting some research can be substantial. To obtain the latest long-term care cost data for Central Florida, I located the website for the Agency for Health Care Administration in Tallahassee and I found listings of the nursing home facilities for the entire state.

One listing in Seminole County was for the Life Care Center of Altamonte Springs. In addition to the address and phone number, the information listed:[11]

Owner - For profit
Licensed Beds - 240 total, 182 semi-private and 3 private rooms
Payment Forms Accepted: Medicare, Medicaid, Private, Insurance/HMO and
    Worker's Compensation.
Overall Inspection Ratings: Rated Overall, for Quality of Care, Quality of life,
    Administration, Nutrition and
Hydration of patients, restraints and abuse, pressure ulcers and others
Daily Semi-Private room rate - $135.
Special Services were available for: Alzheimer's, respite care, dialysis,
    pet services, tracheotomy, 24 hour onsite
RN coverage.
Languages spoken: Spanish, French, Creole

That same source also has a listing for the Village on the Green facility, also in Seminole County (Longwood, Florida). Their data:

Owner: Non-profit
Licensed beds: 60; 58 semi-private and 2 private rooms
Payment Forms Accepted: Medicare, insurance, HMO
Overall inspection ratings: Overall, quality of care, quality of life,
    administration, nutrition and hydration of
Patients, etc.
Daily semi-private room rate: $125
Special services were available for: Alzheimer's, respite care and pet therapy
Languages spoken: Spanish, Italian

This information not only outlines cost, it can help eliminate some of the potential facilities someone would be interested in for a dependent adult with its ratings. Explanations of the ratings are given for each facility.

Reality Bites

Compounding the problems already outlined here is the remarkable difference between belief and reality for most Americans. There have been many reports and surveys clearly illustrating that the public perception of the cost of long-term care is far removed from the actual data.

The AARP report "The Costs of Long-Term Care: Perceptions vs. Reality" shows a "disturbing lack of knowledge regarding the costs associated with long-term care." The survey indicated the average monthly cost of a nursing home in California is $4,654. Only 21 percent of Californians age 45 or older came close to naming that figure. An astounding 66 percent pleaded pure ignorance – they had no idea as to the amount of the average monthly nursing home cost.[12] Sadly, unless agents and financial planners do their jobs properly, many of those polled for this report will not discover the real cost until they have to start paying out of pocket for a stay for themselves or another family member.

Many consumers are also confused by Medicare's coverage of long-term care. In yet another survey, 39 percent of U.S residents over age 65 still think that Medicare or Medicare Supplement insurance covers long nursing home stays, and 24 percent are confident that it does. Adding to this confusion has been the release of nursing home comparison data by the Centers for Medicare and Medicaid Services, leading to the expectation that Medicare provides more extensive coverage than it does.[13] (More on this in subsequent chapters.)

Boomers are not much better at their financial guesswork as they move rapidly closer to retirement age in large numbers. They are confident, to be sure, but somewhat shaky with the math. In an Allstate Financial "Retirement Reality Check," 78 percent of Boomers believed they were prepared to meet the financial aspects of retirement and 69 percent said they were confident they knew how much money they needed to save in order to maintain the retirement lifestyle they want.[14] On average, those surveyed said they would need $30,000 per year for basic living expenses during retirement. Without questioning the amount, to generate $30,000 annually Boomers would need to save about $1 million, factoring in an 8 percent return and an average 4 percent inflation. What those surveyed have actually saved to date is about $120,000 – only 12 percent of what they will need for a 20-year retirement.

Boomers have more problems than just underestimating retirement needs (and completely overlooking long-term care needs). With personal finances, things for them can be very complicated. There are an overwhelmingly large number of remarried Boomers. Many of these Boomers have financial obligations to previous spouses, are putting children through college, and are looking after and perhaps supporting elderly parents. Often, the new spouse has a different level of wealth and and a varied viewpoint about spending and saving. Financial planners are helping to lead these individuals in a discussion about finances before it turns into conflict.[15]

Many of these same individuals are torn between paying for their children's college education and saving for retirement. Financial planners advise to put the money away for their own futures, noting that there are many sources to turn to for financing an education. But if you are short on your own retirement funds, you could be out of luck.[16]

Long-term care is also starting to affect employer costs. It's not that younger employees (or even older ones) are starting to personally require long-term care services in large numbers. It's more their responsibility for taking care of a dependent adult that is starting to cost the employer money. The estimated cost to employers today for productivity losses from employees with caregiving responsibilities is $29 billion dollars.[17]

As these costs are felt, the market for employer-sponsored long-term care insurance has been steadily increasing especially in light of the tax clarification of the employer-sponsored long-term care product in the Health Insurance Portability and Accountability Act of 1996.

And it's not just employers feeling the financial crunch. On average, individuals providing care for a family member will lose $566,000 in wages, $25,000 in Social Security, and $67,000 in pension contributions.[18] Long-term care cuts a wide financial swath and agents and financial planners need to emphasize that with each and every family meber of a prospect for this type of coverage.

Long-Term Care is More Than Just a Nursing Home

Nursing homes are not the only contributor to the high costs of long-term care. Only a small percentage of those needing long-term care services actually receive their care in a nursing home.

Today, more than ever, advances in medical science have permitted medical technology to be transported right into one's own living room. Nurses and aides can provide the same type of care that one would receive in a nursing home. Since many people prefer the convenience and familiarity of their own surroundings, the majority of long-term care services are provided in this fashion.

Typically, the costs are not as high as for those staying in a nursing home unless 24-hour care is needed. As Karen Parker learned in the introduction to this book, full-time home health care can cost more than $300 a day.

The average cost of a home health aide visit is substantially less than a daily nursing home rate, if the visit is for a brief period of time such as one to two hours. Those patients requiring skilled nursing care will incur higher costs than patients needing more basic help. A nurse's aide can assist an individual at home with the basic activities of daily living (ADLs). Alzheimer's patients and those with severe arthritis are usually in need of this kind of assistance. The simple tasks of bathing and dressing are particularly difficult to do if you have any type of infirmity. The home health aide can also assist in essential household chores and even grocery shop for the homebound patient.

Adult day care centers, serving the same purpose as day care centers for children, are becoming more common today. Couples who are working and have a dependent adult staying with them use these facilities, much as they use day care centers for dependent children. The average daily costs run about 30-50% of nursing home rates. Adult day care centers are further explored in Chapter 5, "Defining Long-Term Care Services."

Assisted living facilities are also growing in popularity. Assisted living facilities offer full-time adult day care with apartment-type living and aides on staff to assist with ADLs. (In addition to bathing and dressing, these can include eating, mobility or transferring positions and continence.) The cost of the average assisted living facility runs about 30-60 percent of daily nursing home rates. More information can be found in Chapter 5, "Defining Long-Term Care Services."

Is Self-Insurance an Option?

Today's 50 and over population has fewer options than the youth of America. Social Security and Medicare are focal points of their retirement planning. There is not much room for the additional expenses of long-term care. The necessity of a nursing home stay or other long-term care need can financially ruin a retired couple in a relatively short period of time.

Today's seniors are conservative with their investments and are afraid to do anything aggressive for fear of losing their "nest egg." They deal with premium increases to their Medicare Supplements each year as Medicare raises deductibles and co-payments annually. They were cautiously optimistic about Medicare+Choice, which gave them more choices for their health care needs, including HMOs that had traditionally provided greater benefits for long-term care needs than the standard medical plan. But these managed care entities found they could not support the cost of long-term care services either and many of these plans have picked up and moved on, leaving seniors to return to the regular Medicare program with its abbreviated coverage for long-term care.

The great majority of Americans are either consciously or unknowingly self-insuring their long-term care risk at this point. Is this the wisest choice? Let's look at an example.

When talking to an individual or couple about their future potential long-term care needs, it is important to quantify the risk. If we are looking at a couple, age 50, and their present local area skilled nursing facility cost is $150 per day, the future financial risk is calculable. Ask the couple when they think they might need LTC assistance; you can bet it's a long way off. For this example, assume 30 years (age 80) is that point in time. Also ask them about inflation. Certainly they will believe medical costs go up. Often they will agree that a 5 percent compounded increase is acceptable for the example, and perhaps even conservative.

In present day dollars, $150 per day for a 5-year claim equals $273,750. Thirty years from now, at a 5 percent compounded rate, the daily benefit needed will be $648/day, totaling over a million dollars ($1,183,132) for a 5-year claim. If inflation did not compound, the 5 percent simple increase would take the daily benefit to $375/day, or a 5-year claim at age 80, or nearly $700,000. And that's just for one of them.

Do people have even $273,750 available for LTC services, let alone anywhere from $700,000 to over a $1,000,000? How much money would need to be put aside each year to achieve that amount in 30 years? Most people have not done the math to see what the risk would be in the future. If they assume they can take the chance that they can handle it themselves, there is a good chance they do not know the numbers.

What about insuring the risk? This 50-year-old couple could buy a 5-year benefit plan, $150/day in coverage, first day coverage, with a 5 percent compounded inflation rider for about $2,800 in annual premium. With no rate increases, that's $84,000 in premium for the 30 years to buy over $2 million in coverage between the two of them at age 80. Could they invest that $84,000 and come up with those numbers in 30 years? What if a need happened earlier? The full policy benefits would be there. There may not have been enough time to invest the money to create a comparable resource. Who wants to guess what investments will do these days?

Self-insuring has its own issues aside from the numbers. Since it is highly unlikely the money would be available, assets would need to be liquidated. Could this couple obtain the price their assets are worth if they are forced to sell? Would there be fees from the person who sells the assets? Would there be capital gains taxes? Is it not simpler to put an affordable amount of money aside each year and insure the risk rather than assume it? There are far too many unknowns to take the chance.

There's also the health issue. Long-term care insurance will be underwritten and as long as people remain healthy, the coverage will be obtainable, although the price will be higher. How long can the 50-year-old couple wait to act on this future need and protect their assets?

In 1999, a 63-year-old healthy real estate investor was doing well. He owned land and a couple of motels. But in 2000, he was diagnosed with multiple systems atrophy, a rare disorder that slowly will rob him of his ability to care for himself and even to speak. Six months prior to the diagnosis, the investor and his wife acted on some advice and purchased long-term care insurance, never dreaming that it would be needed so soon. He is still able to run his business from his home, but needs daily care from a nurse. The policy has been covering those expenses. His wife said, "This disease came completely out of the blue. Long-term care insurance made all the difference."[19]

Where Do the Elderly Turn for Help?

The obvious answer is their children. When financial help is necessary, what else can they do? That answer is Medicaid. (See Chapter 7, "Government Programs.") However, the repercussions from this under-funded government program are not widely understood by those who encourage their parents to qualify for Medicaid benefits.

Medicaid is only available to those who spend down their income and assets, running through the inheritance money in short order. And if the loss of this projected revenue is not enough, there are some states that allow nursing homes to use a child's assets to pay for the long-term care costs of a parent. This is a shock to the adult child who may see funds for his or her children's education and own retirement used to pay for a parent's nursing home stay. What is the financial responsibility of an adult child for his or her parents? To what length can the state go to attach a child's assets to help pay for long-term care costs for his or her parents?

It may take several years to arrive at answers. Public funds are diminishing and the reluctance to pay more taxes may result in other alternatives such as requiring an adult child to participate in paying the cost of a parent or relative's long-term care.

Adult children are already feeling the financial pinch of caregiving. This country's base caregiver is a working woman under age 65, who has no college degree. She has been caring for a disabled elderly relative for more than two years. There is no private long-term care insurance. This information, from the MetLife Mature Market Institute, also reinforced the strength of long-term care insurance. The 2001 study found that daughters, daughters-in-law, and other relatives responsible for caring for disabled elderly individuals were almost 50 percent more likely to hold jobs if the recipients of care had private long-term care insurance.[20]

Thus, lack of planning on the part of parents can have a substantial negative impact not only on their own finances, but on their childrens' as well.

Planning Ahead

While it is difficult for family members to discuss these issues, talk they must. *Fortune* magazine listed the eight biggest mistakes parents might be making right now with their finances.[21] These were:

1. There is no will, it is unsigned, or nobody knows where it is.

2. The parents have not drawn up a financial or medical power of attorney.

3. The trust the parents set up is not properly safeguarded.

4. The trust is outdated.

5. Fearful that a long illness in a nursing home might eat up everything, parents have put assets in their children's name.

6. To elude creditors, Dad has put everything in Mom's name.

7. Parents are giving away as much as they can or should.

8. Parents automatically hand over control of their money to the kids.

These issues will be addressed at various places throughout this book.

The insurance agent and financial planner can be a key conduit in facilitating important financial conversations between parents and children. These discussions must take place to enable long-term care needs to best be met.

The numbers in this chapter give you familiar ground with which to approach existing and potential clients about the importance of planning ahead. The financial impact of long-term care is already felt by millions of Americans. Countless more await a similar fate unless some advanced preparation is done.

Chapter Notes

1. "Her Money Ran Out Long Before She Has," *Orlando Sentinel*, August 6, 1995, p. A-1.
2. "Latest Update on LTC Insurance and Characteristics," *LTC Bullet*, provided by the Center for LTC Financing, February, 2003.
3. General LTC Statistics, Source: LTCConnection.com, February 2003.
4. Source: MetLife Mature Market Institute 2002 study.
5. Marcella de Simone, "Cash Management Will Be Increasingly Necessary For Retirees," *National Underwriter*, November 25, 2002, p. 44.
6. Melinda Ligos, "Retirees forced to return to work," *Daytona Beach News Journal*, September 8, 2002, p. 2A.
7. Christine Tassone Kovner et al,"Who Cares For Older Adults?" *Health Affairs*, Sept./Oct. 2002, p. 80.
8. Benjamin G. Druss, et al, "The Most Expensive Medical Conditions in America," *Health Affairs*, July/August 2002, p. 107.
9. Source: MetLife Mature Market Institute 2002 study.
10. David Caruso, "Benefits in Peril for Bethlehem Retirees," *Associated Press*, February 9, 2003.
11. Source: Agency for Health Care Administration.
12. "Most Americans Unprepared for Long-Term Care Costs," *PR Newswire*, December 11, 2001.
13. Allison Bell, "Older Seniors Confused About Medicare Nursing Home Benefits," *National Underwriter*, July 23, 2001, p. 31.
14. "Allstate Financial 'Retirement Reality Check' Reveals Financial Crisis For Baby Boomers Heading Into Retirement," *PR Newswire*, November 27, 2001.
15. Joyce M. Rosenberg, "Boomer Couples Can Encounter Financial Headaches," *Los Angeles Times*, November 4, 2001, p. C3.
16. Diane Harris, "Whom To Bank On?" *My Generation*, AARP magazine, p. 24.
17. Source: General LTC Statistics, LTCConnection.com, February 2003.
18. Source: General LTC Statistics, LTCConnection.com, February 2003.
19. Paul Wenske, "Check out long-term care policies," *Orlando Sentinel*, November 21, 2001 p. B6.
20. Allison Bell, "Study Finds That LTC Insurance Keeps Workers Working," *National Underwriter*, July 30, 2001 p. 47.
21. Susan E. Kuhn, "Dealing with your Parent's Finances," *Fortune*, September 30, 1996, pp. 274-275.

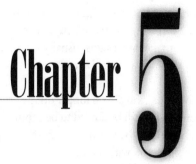

Chapter 5

Defining Long-Term Care Services

"A hospital is no place to be sick."

— Samuel Goldwyn

What long-term care services might an individual need? It was mentioned in Chapter 4, "The Financial Strain of Aging," that long-term care goes well beyond the need for nursing home care. In reality, more people access long-term care services *outside* of a nursing home setting.

It is important to understand exactly what constitutes long-term care. As an insurance agent or consumer, you must understand exactly what a long-term care insurance policy will cover. This should include an intimate understanding of the various types of long-term care services.

Levels of Health Care

The type of care accessed is generally based on the severity of the health problem. The health care service administered is divided by the length of time a patient is monitored. The type of long-term care, whether it is maintenance, ADL assistance, or therapy, can be provided in a variety of settings.

Intensive care is for the most serious of medical situations where a patient is monitored at all times. A person may be placed in intensive care following surgery and be monitored for any negative signs, usually on a 24-hour basis. A hospital is the most common facility for intensive care.

Acute care is for those individuals who are no longer on the critical list and do not need 24-hour care, but there may still be a need to be monitored periodically to warrant remaining in a hospital-type setting. In a 24-hour period, medical personnel may spend up to eight hours with a patient.

Skilled care is another decrease in the monitoring level of acute care. Skilled care may be needed up to half the time necessary at the acute care level. It is intended for people who have uncontrolled, unstable, or chronic conditions requiring intensive care or for people who are recovering from a condition that initially required hospitalization. This type of care can be administered in the home, an assisted living facility, a nursing home, or a hospital.

Intermediate care is similar to skilled care except that it is provided on a periodic basis. It is designed for people with chronic conditions who are, at present, unable to live independently, and stresses rehabilitation therapy that enables individuals to either return home or regain and retain as many activities of daily living as possible. The changing of a bandage every eight hours, for example, is considered intermittent treatment. Skilled medical personnel would deliver or monitor this type of care.

Custodial care involves assisting individuals in activities of daily living (ADLs). These ADLs include, but are not limited to, bathing, dressing, eating, and walking. This type of care is usually performed by a trained nurse's aide. As people get older, this type of care is common. Spinal cord injuries may also require this type of care.

Sub-acute care is provided by nursing facilities that specialize in treating patients who require extensive physiological monitoring, intravenous therapy or postoperative care, intensive rehabilitation or other medically complex interventions.

Intensive care and acute care are short-term in nature and are often covered by comprehensive major medical insurance. HMOs and PPOs and other managed care programs also provide benefits for this type of care.

Skilled, intermediate, and custodial care are considered long-term levels of care. The objectives of these types of care are to prevent a patient's health from deteriorating any further. This "maintenance" care is often not covered to any degree in a comprehensive major medical insurance policy, nor by the elderly person's primary medical program, Medicare.

Sub-acute care is a form of long-term care, but is typically of short duration. This may or may not be covered by the usual major medical coverage or Medicare program.

The lack of coverage available for skilled, intermediate, and custodial care (and, to some extent, sub-acute care) has left the door open for the emergence of long-term care insurance. As the population continues to age, the chance that more individuals will have a need for this form of medical treatment increases dramatically.

Care for the elderly is still burdened with risk. It is easy for a long-term care situation to escalate into an acute or intensive care need. For example, a 92-year-old woman with severe arthritis and bad circulation was on long-term care maintenance when she developed a foot ulcer. She had two medical alternatives – amputation, a "simple" procedure with a high degree of success but resulting in the loss of her foot, or an operation where healthy blood vessels are grafted in an attempt to save her foot.

Doctors make difficult choices for elderly patients, an oppressive situation compounded by having to deal with well-intentioned family members. Whichever alternative was selected, there was only a limited chance of walking normally. Her family, of course, wanted the foot saved. The 92-year-old woman had little say in the matter.

During the operation she suffered a heart attack. She was taken to intensive care and placed on a respirator. The grafting on her foot soon became infected and was treated with antibiotics, which triggered debilitating diarrhea. The long hours of anesthesia also led to prolonged post-operation mental confusion. The surgery only worsened the woman's already declining health and she still had the foot ulcer. The only other alternative was amputation.[1]

Long-Term Care Services

Skilled Nursing Care

Skilled nursing care is care provided on a regular basis by licensed medical professionals such as registered nurses or professional therapists, working under the order or direct supervision of a physician. Some people need skilled care for only a short period of time following an illness.

In Chapter 2, "Today's Changing Demographics," Medicare's prospective payment system illustrated this type of skilled care. The person was not sick enough for acute care, but was still in need of skilled care and some monitoring. The recognition of skilled care became widespread as more and more Medicare patients were discharged from the hospital only to go into another type of facility, such as a nursing home to receive skilled care.

A disability requiring skilled care is not as uncommon as someone would think for a supposed healthier society. In 2000, the Census Bureau revisited their periodic study of Americans with disabilities, focusing on the year 1997. Overall, 19.7 percent of the population was cited as having a disability, 12.3 percent were severely disabled, and over 10 million people who are disabled required assistance. Over half of those requiring assistance were over age 65 (53 percent). This means that 47 percent of the disabled population requiring assistance is under the age of 65.[2]

A person in need of skilled nursing care other than on an acute basis often receives a treatment plan. This program details the specifics of the treatment needed, both in description and frequency.

Today, retirement communities include independent living and personal and health care assistance. Many of these communities are also adding a skilled nursing facility to their "campus" to create a full continuum of care. Individuals start out living independently, progress to home care, then to assisted living care, and finally to skilled nursing facility care as their condition progressively worsens.

Intermediate Nursing Care

Intermediate nursing care is provided patients in stable conditions who require daily medical assistance on a less frequent basis than skilled nursing care. The type of care to be administered is ordered by a physician and normally carried out under the supervision of a registered nurse. While intermediate nursing care is less specialized than skilled care, it is often administered over longer periods of time.

With skilled care, you are often working towards a stated goal. In a long-term care scenario, that objective is not always full recovery. More likely, it may be to bring the patient to a level where the care needed is only intermediate, allowing more independence from supervised medical scrutiny. Intermediate care could be as simple as giving medication to a group in physical therapy once a day. Intermediate nursing care is generally in the patient's home, although you will also find examples of it in various facility settings.

Custodial Care

Custodial care provides assistance with everyday activities of daily living (ADLs). While less intensive and complicated than skilled or intermediate care, the individual providing it must have some training in order to become proficient at assisting someone in necessary daily activities. Even a family member who might provide this assistance at home would be wise to seek training in ADLs. This training can usually be obtained for a small fee.

Custodial care may also be called personal care. It is usually defined by the actual ADLs that require help – bathing, dressing, eating, walking, getting in and out of bed, continence, and taking medication are the more commonly defined ADLs.

ADLs originated more than 30 years ago from *The Index of Independence in Daily Activities.* Daily activities are defined by a person's ability to perform normal functions. This book also linked the ability to achieve the normal function with a person's behavioral level.

There is a unique correlation between the stages of childhood and the stages of growing older. A friend of mine is fond of asking consumers before she begins a long-term care seminar if any of them have personally experienced long-term care. A couple of hands might go up, and then she tells them that all of their hands should be raised. Everyone experiences long-term care when they are born. A newborn infant is entirely dependent on another individual. When it happens in adulthood, it is called long-term care.

The lack of independence and inability to function is the same during childhood as it is in the elderly stage of life. Children generally learn and perform the following functions independently in this order:

- eating – first with hands and then with utensils;

- walking – first crawling and then culminating with baby's first steps;

- using the toilet; and

- bathing.

As people age, the inability to perform normal functions follows the adage "last learned – first lost":

- needs assistance to bathe;

- needs assistance in performing the task of going to the toilet, including getting undressed;

- mobility becomes more and more difficult for an elderly person slowed by arthritis and other ailments; and

- eating – inability to hold a utensil or feed themselves.

According to a recent study, there are now about 12 million adults who require personal assistance with ADLs (contrasted with over 10 million in the Census Bureau review of 1997 adults). About 13 percent of those reside in a nursing facility. Of the remainder who live in the community, a quarter of them are severely impaired, needing personal assistance with three or more ADLs.[3]

The definition of each of these activities of daily living is more complex than someone might think. The majority of long-term care insurance policies measure eligibility for benefits on the basis of the ability to perform, or not perform, the usual ADLs. The following definitions are important:

Bathing – washing oneself in a bathtub or a shower, including getting in and out of the bathtub or shower, or giving oneself a sponge bath, constitutes an independence from any assistance.

Bathing is the most problematic ADL for an elderly person. A lack of balance or an unsteady gait may necessitate assistance in getting in and out of a bathtub or shower. A wet surface combined with the fragility of an older person can be a hazardous combination. It is generally the most common ADL for which people need help.

Dressing – the ability to get clothes from the closet or drawer and dress one's self, or to attach a brace or prosthesis without any assistance. These activities require a certain dexterity of the hands and motor coordination. It is easy to take for granted the simple tasks of buttoning a shirt or tying a shoelace. And it is even more difficult to perform these tasks with decreased motor skills, or even arthritis of the hands.

Toileting – the act of going to and from the bathroom, getting on and off the toilet, and performing the necessary hygiene associated with going to the toilet without assistance. The location of the bathroom will have some impact on a person's ability to perform this daily activity. If access is difficult, assistance may be required.

Bathing and getting dressed are activities easily lost or made more difficult for an older person. It is not unusual to require assistance as one gets older and it does not necessarily mean the individual is severely disabled and in need of significant assistance. The need for toileting assistance, though, may well be the benchmark by which doctors measure the need for ongoing long-term care services. Toileting is the critical point in the typical ADL hierarchy. Lack of independence in performing this function is the warning sign for further future loss and eventual total dependence, and often results in the need for around-the-clock care.

Mobility (also called transferring positions) – the process of walking without the assistance of a mechanical device (from cane to wheelchair) and moving from a bed to a chair without assistance. A considerable amount of strength in the arms and legs is necessary to adequately perform this function.

Continence – refers to one's ability to control bowel and bladder function voluntarily and to maintain a reasonable level of personal hygiene. This is independent from the physical ability to use the toilet and may involve the mental capacity of an individual to recognize the need to use the bathroom.

Eating – means the process of getting food from the plate into one's mouth without assistance. It requires the coordination of at least one of the hands. A person can use a straw or a modified utensil and still remain independent.

Administering medication is an activity of daily living and requiring assistance in taking the prescribed amount at the designated time and in the proper manner is a loss of independence.

It has taken several decades of gerontological and health research to place these ADL measurements into universal, standardized categories. Once the need arises, medical assistance is often next prescribed. This medical assistance is often in the form of long-term care. The loss of independence in performing these ADLs is often irrecoverable at an advanced age. Unless a person has had a specific trauma that renders him temporarily unable to perform some of these functions, the loss may be permanent. Thus, the individual may require assistance for the rest of his life.

The concept of medical assistance does not necessarily mean "hands-on." *Standby assistance* can still constitute the loss of an ADL. If the patient's condition warrants a nurse or nurse's aide close by to supervise the performance of an ADL in the event the individual cannot successfully perform it, this may still be considered an ADL loss. This type of care oversight has taken on added importance with the passage of the Health Insurance Portability and Accountability Act of 1996 (HIPAA). A more detailed discussion of HIPAA can be found in Chapter 13.

Figure 5.1 lists ADL losses in two separate settings: skilled nursing and assisted living facilities:

FIGURE 5.1	**Percentage of Nursing Home Residents Age 65 Or Older With Specific ADL Loss[4]**											
Age	Dependent Mobility			Incontinent			Dependent Eating			Loss of All Three		
	1985	1995	1999	1985	1995	1999	1985	1995	1999	1985	1995	1999
65 or older	75.7	79.0	80.3	55.0	63.8	65.7	40.9	44.9	47.3	32.5	36.5	36.9
65 to 74	61.2	73.0	73.9	42.9	61.9	58.5	33.5	43.8	43.1	25.7	35.8	31.7
75 to 84	70.5	76.5	77.8	55.1	62.5	64.2	39.4	45.2	46.6	30.6	35.3	35.4
85 and up	83.3	82.4	83.8	58.1	65.3	65.3	43.9	45.0	49.0	35.6	37.5	39.4

Source: Administration on Aging

FIGURE 5.1 (continued)

Percentage Distribution of Assisted Living Residents who need Help with ADLs[5]

Activities of Daily Living	% of Residents Needing no help	% of Residents Needing some help	% of Residents need significant help
Bathing	28%	42%	30%
Dressing	43%	33%	24%
Transferring	64%	19%	17%
Toileting	58%	22%	19%
Eating	77%	13%	10%

Source: National Center for Assisted Living

These statistics are used by actuaries to compute long-term care morbidity rates and benefit eligibility when pricing a long-term care insurance policy. Bathing and dressing are the overwhelming loss leaders in ADLs. The inability to perform these functions qualifies a person for long-term care insurance reimbursement.

The table below illustrates the number of people needing assistance with these activities of daily living. The need for assistance in personal care will grow dramatically in correlation to the increasing number of people living longer lives.

Age	1980	1990	2000	2010	30 yr % change
65-74	737,139	869,412	863,487	996,042	35.1%
75-84	735,990	945,052	1,142,015	1,159,308	57.5%
85 +	535,386	779,486	1,106,664	1,462,926	173.2%
TOTAL	2,008,515	2,593,949	3,112,166	3,618,276	80.1%

Source: U.S. Census Bureau Projections multiplied by Table rates provided by the Supplement on Aging Survey

Between 1980 and 2010, the increase in the number of people needing long-term care assistance is projected to be a phenomenal 173.2 percent among the 85-and-older crowd. This type of care is usually associated with assistance in performing activities of daily living.

Instrumental Activities of Daily Living: These are the type of actions that are essential to leading an independent life in a community. Common IADLs are: managing money, doing housework, taking medications, shopping, preparing meals, and using the telephone. A loss of one or more of these IADLs is typically a precursor to losing ADLs, a more serious consequence of disability and dependence.

A 1998 study of people over age 65 needing help with IADLs from 1982 to 1994 found the greatest need for help to be with heavy work, getting around outside, traveling, and grocery shopping.[6]

Further, a 2001 survey of assisted living residents demonstrated the following IADL needs:[7]

Percentage Distribution of Assisted Living Residents who need IADL assistance

Instrumental Activity Of Daily Living	% of Residents who need no help	% of Residents who need some help	% of Residents who need significant help
Telephoning	51%	22%	27%
Shopping	17%	30%	53%
Meal Preparation	7%	14%	80%
Housework	7%	20%	73%
Money Management	22%	19%	59%
Traveling	12%	22%	66%

Source: National Center for Assisted Living

It is interesting to see that the more current Assisted Living IADL results almost mirrors the lengthy study noted above done from 1982 through 1994 in terms of the most regular types of assistance necessary.

Custodial care is the most common type of long-term care assistance needed. It is provided to people needing help with ADLs and IADLs. This type of care will become even more prevalent in the future, and with this care will come the need for additional funding. Long-term care insurance can fill this gap.

Care at Home

All of the long-term care services mentioned above can be performed within the familiar confines of the patient's home. Physicians often recommend care at home as it provides an important foundation to the emotional well-being of the person in need of care. Care at home, if it can be provided, is important to all ages but particularly to the elderly.

There was not a large need for home care prior to 1984. But concurrent with the advent of Medicare's prospective payment system, the rules changed. No longer was it economically feasible for hospitals to keep patients indefinitely until they recovered. Now when a patient is discharged, quite often medical treatment accompanies this person to the next destination.

Often, that destination is home. Surveys of community residents show a strong aversion to a nursing home. In one recent study of people over age 70 who were seriously ill, 29 percent said they would rather die than enter a nursing facility.[8] For most people today, home is obviously a preferred site for care.

Some of this attraction is founded on living arrangements. People living alone are more likely to face an institutionalization, simply because they are unable to easily bring in a caregiver for assistance. Today, 55 percent of non-institutionalized persons live with a spouse. This is especially true of men (73 percent of those over age 65 living with a spouse).[9] Thus, the transition to home care is much easier when there is someone present to help with the basics.

Long-term care in the home is associated with the following positive factors:[10]

- control of one's lifestyle, including the designated times for daily activities and social life;

- being within one's own environment;

- emotional and physical security;

- independence;

- privacy and the maintaining of one's own space;

- memories, magnified by being in the presence of personal history;

- source of financial security; and

- extension of one's self-expression.

All of these positive factors can have a profound effect on a person's health. Older home care consumers value interpersonal qualities such as the caregiver liking them, caring about them, and being compatible with them (which is more likely in a spousal relationship). They also value reliability, task competence, and adequacy in the amount of care and help received.[11] Thus, if care can be delivered in the home, it is often preferred by the person receiving long-term care.

Advances in medical science bode well for the future of home health care. Most care, from custodial care (assistance with ADLs) to the highly skilled care performed by a registered nurse, can be provided at home. For example, assume a stroke or an accident renders a person temporarily incapacitated and in need of hospitalization. Both bed rest and assistance with household chores and common ADLs are needed. Where better to obtain the needed bed rest than that person's own bed? A home health aide or family member can perform the rest of the assistance that is necessary.

Care in the home can be divided into two categories: home health care and home care. Home health care may include skilled nursing care, physical and speech therapy, lab services, and intermediate care. Home care is a supportive service which includes assistance with the previously defined ADLs and IADLs.

These services are provided by home health care agencies which may be independent or affiliated with a nursing home or hospital. Private duty nurses operating independently can perform many skilled care functions for the individual patient at home. Chapter 6, "Elder Care Services: Growth and Pressure," takes a detailed look at the growth of this market, and the assorted problems created by this expansion.

Home health care and home care have been incorporated into most long-term care insurance policies. It is often where long-term care begins, and while it may eventually progress to some type of facility care, it allows a dependent adult to maintain independence and dignity much longer. With Medicare tightening its rules and reimbursement levels for this type of medical service, it further underscores the potential importance of long-term care coverage.

Other Long-Term Care Services

Adult day care centers, also known as adult day care services, have been providing a form of respite care for caregivers for more than twenty years. According to the National Adult Day Services Association (NADSA), there were only 300 such centers nationwide in 1978. By the mid-1980s there were 2,100 centers and today there are more than 4,000 centers nationwide.[12]

An adult day care center is similar to a child day care center. Today, many working adult caregivers find these facilities to be critical to their continued caregiving support of a dependent adult. Money must still be made and, like a dependent child must be dropped of at a day care center, a dependent adult must be dropped off. Many Boomers today face the prospect of doing both every day.

A dependent adult in a day care center is supervised, fed, administered medication and, in some cases, receives skilled care. Adult day care is not designed to replace the nursing home environment where a significant amount of skilled care is required, but it is a perfect place for adults who cannot stay home alone and function on their own during the course of the day.

It helps that some adult day care centers provide activities with speakers, music, and even field trips. Many dependent adults may have diminished physical capabilities but are still sharp mentally, and this type of stimulation is both healthy and helpful. Good health is often a byproduct of performing some regular activities.

Respite care is a service where temporary professional care is employed to give the caregiver some time off. With so many adults today providing care for a dependent parent or relative, the need for a break can be as often as once a week to run errands or perhaps to take a vacation.

Home health care agencies are a common source for providing personnel such as a nurse, home health aide, or personal care attendant who can be retained depending on the level of need for the patient for short periods of time.

Call centers are becoming the norm in today's managed care health environment. A Medicare HMO, for example, may often have a toll-free phone number staffed by nursing personnel to answer medical questions posed by its members. The elderly, in particular, seem to have a need for this support, and these helplines stay busy. In addition, company employees may also receive advice and guidance on long-term care issues, including insurance, through a similar arrangement. Employers, concerned with caregiving issues that beset their employees today, have been more amenable about setting up this type of resource where the employee can secure answers regarding medical and caregiving issues. This type of information support can be helpful.

Alzheimer's disease is now the eighth leading cause of death in the USA with 44,507 lives lost to the disease in 1999, according to the Centers for Disease Control and Prevention.[13] Prior to death, however, is a lengthy illness as the disease takes a horrific effect on the patient, family members, and caregivers. In 1994, former President Ronald Reagan shared the news with the country that he was suffering from the effects of Alzheimer's. In 2002, it was Charlton Heston, Hollywood's "Biblical Giant", and Pauline Phillips, writer of the "Dear Abby" column who told us they were dealing with the early stages of this disease.

Experts say that without a cure, an estimated 14 million Americans will have Alzheimer's by 2050, up from 4 million today.[14] While many family members tough it out at home caregiving, there are specific facilities that cater to the Alzheimer's patient that may be a better, albeit more financially burdensome, alternative.

Yet, even as the need for this type of care looms larger in front of us, public funding is running short to provide the necessary services. In Florida, budget woes had lawmakers looking to trim more than $10 million from their statewide elder services program. Among the potential casualties: the Alzheimer's Disease Initiative, which provides respite care to relieve full-time caregivers.[15] These types of struggles are examined in full in Chapter 6.

Geriatric services are also becoming commonplace as the health care industry prepares for America's aging future. Companies like Geriatric Services of America work with insurance companies, Medicare, AARP, third-party administrators, pharmaceutical suppliers, home health care agencies, and visiting nursing associations to provide special expertise in dealing with the elderly. Much of this support is in regard to long-term care.

This may not be able to make up for primary care delivered by geriatric-specialized physicians. The Alliance for Aging Research recently reported that the United States currently needs 20,000 physician-geriatricians to care adequately for the U.S. population of 35 million seniors. Of the 650,000 licensed physicians practicing in the United States, fewer than 9,000 physicians have met the qualifying criteria in geriatrics.[16]

Perhaps it is the lack of this type of physician that has created a need for geriatric care managers. A man traveling to Chicago on business decided to look in on his wife's 90-year-old aunt and 88-year-old uncle. While the couple was still ambulatory and proud of their independence, he found no food in the house and the formerly fastidious couple was no longer taking care of themselves or their home. The solution was to hire a geriatric care manager who could plan and organize care for these adults.[17] Especially in the case of long-distance caregiving, this care manager can mean the difference between staying at one's home or the dreaded alternative of institutionalization.

Improvement in medical technology will likely keep people alive much longer than ever before as the nation goes into the new millennium. Long-term care services will continue to evolve, but there will be cost — necessitating the need for some form of long-term care insurance coverage.

The various types of long-term care discussed in this chapter are the primary long-term care services provided today. Remembering the various definitions and the context of these services will be important for you when analyzing a long-term care insurance policy. The type of care, the eligibility requirements for benefits, and specific types of assistance are all tied into the care provided in a long-term care setting.

Chapter Notes

1. Judy Foreman, "Assessing Medical Needs for the Elderly," *Daytona Beach News-Journal*, 1995.
2. Source: U.S. Census Bureau, 2000.
3. Martin Bayne, "Useful Prescription," Mr. LTC Website, February 2003.
4. Administration on Aging, *Profile of Older Americans 2000*, released in 2002.
5. Source: National Center for Assisted Living, March 2001.
6. K.G. Manton, et al, "The Dynamics of Dimensions of Age-Related Disability: 1982 to 1994 in the U.S. Elderly Population," *Journal of Gerontology*, 1998, vol 53A, no. 1, B59 – B70.
7. Source: National Center for Assisted Living, March 2001.
8. Robert L. and Rosalie A. Kane, "What Older People Want From Long-Term Care, and How They Get It," *Health Affairs*, November/December 2001, p. 114.
9. Source: Administration on Aging, *Profile of Older Americans 2000*, released in 2002.
10. "Home: What Does it Mean?," *The Sandwich Generation* (Issue 1, 1995) p. 12.

11. Robert L. and Rosalie A. Kane, "What Older People Want From Long-Term Care, and How They Can Get It," *Health Affairs*, November/December 2001, p. 114.

12. Source: National Adult Day Services Association.

13. Jane J. Eves, "Remembrance," *Health Insurance Underwriter*, February 2002, p. 25.

14. Peggy Eastman, "Keeping Alzheimer's At Bay," *AARP Bulletin*, March 2002, p. 14.

15. Donna Callea, "Aging with dignity might be harder," *Daytona Beach News Journal*, October 21, 2001, p. 10A.

16. Stephen A. Moses, "The Unnecessary Tragedy of Long-Terrn Care," *LTC Bullet* from the Center for Long-Term Care Financing.

17. Linda Greider, "Care managers emerge as new force in helping," *AARP Bulletin*, December 2001, p. 9.

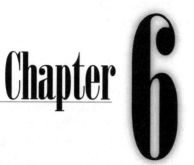

Chapter 6

Elder Care Services: Growth and Pressure

"It's no longer a question of staying healthy. It's a question of finding a sickness you like.."

–Jackie Mason

Statistics show that nearly one in four adults currently cares for an elderly loved one, and caregiver numbers are growing annually. Baby boomers represent the average caregiver (54 percent are under age 45, according to the Kaiser Foundation), while Gen Xers increasingly find themselves pressed into service.[1]

But how easy is it to work caregiving into everyday life? When both husband and wife work, the burden of caring for elderly parents at home is overwhelming. Moreover, a recent study indicated that members of racial and ethnic minority groups are more squeezed between caring for parents and children than whites, with women in low income brackets feeling particularly beset by caregiving pressures.[2]

The future? Many adults are able to rely on a spouse for caregiving needs, keeping the burden away from children and even further away from a housing need. But today's Boomer leads prior generations in yet another category that may affect future long-term care needs. The percentage of Boomers who have never married is 12.6 percent, significantly higher than in prior generations: 5.2

percent of those 55-64, and 3.9 percent of those 65+.[3] When you factor in the high divorce rate of this generation, the lack of an easily available informal caregiver will force people to look elsewhere for caregiving assistance, including institutions.

When caring for an older relative or parent in one's own home is too difficult, it remains for the adult children to make other arrangements for their loved ones to receive the long-term care needed. These alternative choices have resulted in a rising tide in the growth of elder care services nationwide. As the population continues to age, it is clear that this upward spiral will continue or even accelerate.

The setting in which long-term care services are rendered has become an important factor in determining eligibility for benefits under a long-term care insurance policy. Long-term care used to consist largely of nursing homes for the elderly, involving custodial patients too dependent to live alone, but too healthy to stay in a hospital. The government began to fund nursing home benefits on a grand scale in the 1960s under the then-new Medicare program. This funding led to rapid nursing home construction. But when providers took advantage of the funding pipeline, the government capped nursing home construction and reimbursement rates. When quality of care began to decline, government further squeezed nursing homes by mandating higher care standards without offering financial help.[4] This has created intense pressure on the types of housing that could ease the caregiving burden.

Due to nursing home difficulties, both in perception and reality, long-term care insurance policies had to become more refined, and the variety of long-term care settings acceptable to insurers broadened considerably. Considering that many new types of facilities for long-term care are now available and less costly than a nursing home, it makes sense to encourage individuals to elect a more inexpensive environment.

This chapter will examine the variety of places where an individual can receive long-term care, from the original standard, the nursing home, to one's own home and assisted living facilities. In addition, each section will address an equally important issue that agents and consumers need to be aware of in their search for the proper LTC setting. The LTC delivery system is severely hampered today by financial concerns and staffing shortages; problems that will affect how people receive their LTC care in the future. Geriatric physicians are in low supply, when only 9,000 of a needed 20,000 doctors are certified in this important specialty and that number is expected to drop to as few as 6,100 in 2004.[5] In 2001, Jacksonville, Florida found itself with a nursing home shortage of 300 Certified Nursing Assistants and 77 additional nurses for the 51 nursing homes in its surrounding environs, due to legislatively-passed staffing requirements.[6]

This is merely the tip of the iceberg and continued staffing and financial problems for long-term care related institutions could create a setting where supply rapidly outstrips demand, setting prices at levels well ahead of the policy benefits of a LTC plan, never mind the out-of-pocket costs for those who do not opt for the insurance method of financing this risk.

The Nursing Home

From the introduction in this book, it was obvious how both Mrs. Doan and her daughter, Karen Parker, felt about nursing homes. For many, the term *nursing home* has a negative connotation.

Compounding this public relations problem are the continued controversies that haunt these skilled facilities. A 2002 study on nursing homes, prepared for the Department of Health and Human Services, found that the vast majority of the nation's nearly 17,000 nursing homes have too few workers to care properly for residents, putting them at risk for health problems like bedsores, blood-borne infections, dehydration, malnutrition and pneumonia.[7] This kind of information has sent legislatures scrambling to pass something to protect these residents. In Florida, on January 1, 2003, nursing homes in the state were required to increase staffing to levels so that each resident receives at least 2.6 hours of nurse aide care daily.[8]

The nursing home as a medical setting has been changing for the last several years. Today, their residents are either on a fast-track recovery, having been discharged from the hospital but not well enough to go home yet, or they are the neediest of the long-term care patients, where the nursing home is probably their last move.

This change in type of resident coincides with a recent avalanche of bad publicity. In Georgia, a nursing home was cited for allowing a 93-year-old woman's ear to become infested with maggots. Another home in the same city was cited for serious deficiencies related to flies and poor treatment of the resident.[9] This is just one city, one state. These situations do not help the public image of the nursing home.

It has also led to a decline in nursing home patients and facilities, which has been falling steadily since 1998 when the industry peaked with 1.51 million residents in 17,259 facilities. In 2001, the number of certified nursing homes had slipped below 17,000 (to 16,675) and on an average day cared for 1,469,001 residents.[10]

The question then becomes, why would anyone consider placing an individual in a nursing home? Certainly the percentage of people over age 65 who live in a nursing home at any given time has been dropping and for most families, like Mrs. Doan's, it is the last resort when long-term care services are needed. The rate of nursing home residence for people over age 65 (per 1,000) had declined from 54.0 to 43.3 from 1985 to 1999.[11] However, there are times when a nursing home is the only possible option for an individual and family.

For some, a nursing home may still be the best situation. If there is no one to care for them elsewhere, a nursing home represents a place where they will receive some attention, be close to medical services, and be able to socialize with others. In some cases, a person will receive reimbursement for the cost of care provided from Medicare, insurance, or Medicaid.

The key is to find the right nursing home for a parent or aging relative. This is not easily done. Help from state and local ombudsmen (individuals who resolve complaints on behalf of nursing home residents) rarely draw negative reviews concerning a nursing home.

In November 2002, consumers could access quality indicator information on the nearly 17,000 nursing homes across the country as rated by the Centers for Medicare and Medicaid Services (CMS). This data was available through the government web site (medicare.gov) or through an "800" toll-free number. Several states had been part of a pilot program that started in early 2002 and the nationwide expansion meant that people across the country could now review this information as part of the process of selecting a nursing home.

Full-page advertisements ran in the daily newspapers with a chart comparing nursing homes on three quality indicators:[12]

Facility	City	% of residents with pressure sores	% of residents with loss of ability in basic tasks	% of long-term stay residents with pain
Florida state average		10%	15%	10%
Avante at Leesburg	Leesburg	5%	12%	19%
Health Central Park	Winter Garden	4%	13%	10%
Mariner Health – Conway Lakes	Orlando	16%	46%	21%
Palm Garden	Orlando	14%	21%	6%
Tandem Health Care	Kissimmee	13%	15%	6%

As of November 13, 2002

The success of this program will largely depend on what you can make of the data. If a facility has a high percentage of residents with a loss of basic task ability, shouldn't there be a higher percentage of patients in pain? Or with bedsores, since it would be unlikely the residents would move around much, unless a staff member was able to move and treat them to prevent this situation.

The quality measures can be helpful and they enable nursing homes to compare (and improve) with other facilities in their area. But they shouldn't be the only factors in selecting a home. An analyst with AARP's Public Policy Institute advises that the data is still no substitute for visiting a facility in person and talking with staff as well as families and residents.[13] The Ohio Health Care Association added that the CMS measures say more about the type of patients a facility serves than its quality of care and that nursing facility services are very complex and the CMS ads grossly oversimplify the equation.[14] Finally, the General Accounting Office (GAO) had serious concerns about the potential for public confusion by the quality information published. CMS acknowledged that further work would have to be done to refine the initiative, but believed enough in its indicators as sufficiently valid to move forward with its ads.[15]

This leaves the final say for finding the right nursing home to the individual family. And why not? If you are looking for a home, you wouldn't leave it up to someone else to make the choice for you.

As an insurance agent, you will often be asked to recommend a benefit amount (usually a daily benefit) for a policy and, in order to give proper counsel, it will be necessary for you to visit some of the nursing homes in your area to determine which facilities would be acceptable. The CMS ads could steer you away from facilities way off the charts for quality. It will also be necessary for you to average the costs among the more favorable facilities. This will give you the information and opportunity to endorse those facilities to potential clients.

Recommending a nursing home facility requires a visit. An insurance agent informally researching nursing homes in his community would be wise to ask a friend in the nursing field to accompany him for an "unofficial inspection." Nurses often spot problems well before most others and can help avoid a facility that looks good on the surface but may harbor problems internally. It is important to view several facilities rather than to rely solely on one recommendation.

Where would a person begin researching nursing homes? In Florida, for example, the Agency for Health Care Administration can provide a list of nursing home facilities by county. (See Chapter 4, "The Financial Strain of Aging.") The list contains useful information about nursing homes – the number of beds, whether they accept Medicare or Medicaid reimbursement, the special services offered and similar data. It also offers the address and phone number of the facilities and will help you map out, geographically, unofficial inspections of the facilities. This material is now available to be downloaded from the Agency's web site, and this is true in many states across the country, ensuring the information is relatively up to date.

For example, a listing for Palm Garden (also in the CMS ad above) shows that the facility has 100 beds, accepts Medicare, Medicaid, private pay, insurance, and hospice patients and runs near full capacity, meaning a bed may be scarce.[16]

Most facilities will be glad to give you a tour if someone is available, especially if you've indicated that you have a parent or relative who may be a potential resident. Upon inspection, there will be obvious signs to look for such as smell, lighting and cleanliness. If, for example, there's an undesirable smell, this is an indication that the staff does a less than acceptable job of keeping the residents and facility clean. Look also for a facility that is bright, with plenty of windows and light. The darker the building, the more depressing it is likely to be for a resident.

A copy of the nursing home's latest inspection report should be requested. Federal law requires this report to be public record and you have the right to ask for and receive a copy. If a copy is not provided, the questions to ask are why would they not release the inspection report and what does the facility have to hide?

Another key area to explore would be the nursing home's contract. The contract typically is about 20 to 30 pages long and should be reviewed by an attorney before the elderly adult (or person with a durable power of attorney) signs it. An insurance agent can assist clients with this procedure. There are a growing number of attorneys specializing in elder law and, though a fee will be charged, it is well worth the expense.

There are a number of clauses that should be examined carefully, among them:[17]

1. Requiring a large lump sum payment up front – Homes can ask for a month or two's security deposit which must be returned when the patient leaves or dies, but cannot require a lump sum payment as a condition for admission.

2. Requiring a spouse or child to agree to pay as a private pay patient as a condition for admission – This is a violation of Federal law.

3. Holding a spouse or adult child liable for payment of a patient's bills if a patient defaults or runs out of money and is not eligible for either Medicare and Medicaid – Again, Federal law clearly prohibits this type of contract language.

4. Requiring a patient to turn over control of assets before entering a facility as a condition of acceptance – A spouse or other family member can maintain control of the patient's assets and use them to pay the individual's bills.

5. Requiring a patient or sponsor to designate the nursing home as the payee for the patient's Social Security checks or other income or assets as a condition of acceptance.

6. Charging additional amounts not detailed in the contract – If not detailed, these additional services must be considered part of the daily benefit charge.

7. Transferring a patient from one room to another without proper notification to the family, including solicitation of permission from the patient or family.

As noted in Chapter 4, the average nursing home cost is over $60,000 annually. Nursing home coverage is typically incorporated in a long-term care insurance policy. Since the average American cannot afford this type of care for very long, a long-term care insurance policy represents an invaluable source of funds for these services.

Even though nursing home residency is expected to increase, nursing homes are taking on a new type of patient – those in need of *subacute care.* This service mirrors what hospitals are doing today by providing skilled nursing and rehabilitative care to patients. These people have been discharged from the hospital but are not well enough to go home.

This is a fallout from the managed care shakeup in the health care industry which stepped up pressure to cut medical costs and discharge people earlier, giving nursing homes another revenue source for those individuals considered too healthy to stay in the hospital but not well enough to go home. Since the nursing home can receive four or five times the dollar reimbursement to provide subacute care than what would be received for a nursing home resident, there is a flurry of activity to make way for more subacute patients.

This also has an effect on the number of beds available in a nursing home. In particular, low-profit elderly patients on Medicaid are often the first to have to give up their beds if it's a choice between a subacute patient or the Medicaid resident. Subacute care will increase the popularity of other, lower-cost elder care living choices in the future.

Nursing homes will continue to exist and the insurance agent will play a key role in helping to advise elderly clients on options available. Insurance agents who follow some of the suggestions made in this chapter will provide a great service to their clients and families.

This is no guarantee that once a good facility is chosen, it will operate indefinitely. The difference in the names, make-up and amount of nursing facilities just over the last five years signifies an incredible amount of change. One of the best local residences in the Daytona Beach area, the Holiday Care Center, was one of the gems of the local nursing home facilities. Many Medicaid patients ended up here, a better than average choice for those who no longer have an option financially. But in 2002, the Center closed its doors due to the owner's own health problems. She sold the property and family members had to start the process of selecting a home for their loved one all over again.[18]

It's not only health problems causing turnover in this industry. Financial failures, due to a shortfall in covering costs of low payments from both Medicare and Medicaid, increasing liability premiums and legislatively-enforced staffing requirements, are besieging the industry on a regular basis. There is a substantial amount of mergers and buy-outs in this industry, too, and name changes and closings are often part of the changing face of this section of the long-term care industry.

It has reached the point where the founder of a nationwide nursing home chain stepped down as CEO to focus on a lobbying effort to the federal government to better fund long-term care. His primary concern was more Medicare provider cutbacks that, on top of the annual deficit due to low Medicaid reimbursements, might cause permanent harm to the long-term care industry.[19] Nursing homes probably won't go away, but the nature and make-up of the facility is in a constant state of flux today.

As the population continues to age, nursing homes and other facilities will have to do a better job of attracting and retaining quality nursing personnel. It is imperative that insurance agents keep up on what's happening in the elder care industry in their locale. Clients are counting on this kind of information and, if one can speak knowledgeably of the local long-term care industry, it will add favorably to the agent's credibility.

Hospitals

In today's health care environment, hospitals must do something to keep their beds occupied at full capacity. Managed care systems are extracting patients from the hospital at a quicker pace only to have the patient go to another facility. Hospitals are asking why not address all of the care and services needed for patients under one roof?

For this reason, some hospitals have taken the initiative and converted wings of their facilities into *extended care* beds in order to provide the same type of subacute care that nursing homes are gearing up to provide.

Caring for the elderly is more than a case of a doctor or nurse listening to symptoms and complaints from the patient. A doctor must "read" the individual who is not capable of asking for the services he or she needs. The elderly patient may often be confused or mentally incapacitated and hospital personnel must be trained specifically to deal with this type of situation. Older people often start out in the hospital, as evidenced by 2000 statistics showing that over age 65 individuals had about four times the number of days of hospitalization (1.8 days) than did those under age 65 (0.4 days). The average length of hospital stay was 6.4 days for those over age 65, a decrease of 6 days since 1964, and a signal to hospitals that providing further nursing care of another type is critical to their financial survival.[20]

But if a hospital is to be an alternative facility for care of the elderly patient, nursing personnel trained in elderly care should be provided. The idea of "switching" beds from acute care to subacute care to long-term care makes sense and could be an important revenue source for hospitals in the future.

Home Is Where the Care Is

Family members play a vital role in the health care process, especially for a patient who is not able to communicate well or has difficulty absorbing information. There are so many decisions to be made that coherent minds are needed to understand the care choices available and select the best and most appropriate of these.

In today's "continuum of care" health system, there may be a highly-detailed plan drawn up, involving several levels of care and different facilities available to provide treatment. If an individual begins the odyssey through the health care system in the hospital, a key individual to seek out is the discharge planner. (In the introduction, Karen Parker received help from Mrs. Becker, the hospital's discharge planner and social worker.)

The discharge planner, working in conjunction with the patient's physician, can make a full assessment of health care needs and draw up a plan of care dedicated to the patient's recovery, improvement, or maintenance of the present condition. Most often, the end result is to work towards getting or keeping the patient home. Care still may be necessary, but if it can be done at home, all the better. Given the option, it is not surprising that most choose their own home for treatment.

There is usually a psychological edge to recovering at home. Maintaining some type of routine is much easier in familiar surroundings. Remember that the retention of independence is vitally important to the elderly individual. Being at home keeps one in a familiar environment and closer to family and friends who are often in the best position to provide much needed emotional support. Recent medical scientific advances have reduced bulky equipment to portable size for easier access in the home. Home health care services help prevent the need for hospitalization for the chronically ill patient typically in need of long-term care services with the help of the new equipment.

No wonder the fastest growing type of health care in the 1980's was home health care. If you look at any forecast for the top jobs in the future (not limited to health care), home health personnel are high on the list. The continued shift toward receiving care at home has outpaced the supply of trained professionals who can provide this care. With fewer potential family members to provide care-giving in the future, the future of the industry will likely rest on how well-staffed home health agencies will be to meet the growing demand.

Home care covers a variety of services, skills and equipment. The different types of care that can be provided at home, to name a few, are skilled nursing care, physical, speech or respiratory therapy, medical equipment and supplies, occupational counseling, chore services (light housekeeping, laundry and cook-ing), companion services, respite care, physician services, hospice care, social services, transportation services, meal delivery, nutritional counseling and everyday assistance with activities of daily living (ADLs).

It is almost always less expensive to have the care provided at home rather than at a hospital or nursing facility, unless the need is for highly skilled or around-the-clock care. The MetLife Mature Market Institute published a nationwide list of home health care average charges in 2002.[21] The average cost of a home health aide ranged from a low of $12/hour to a high of $27/hour, with a national average of $18/hour. An LPN (Licensed Practical Nurse) could run from a low of $22/hour to a high of $96/hour, with a nationwide average of $37/hour. Quite often, the home health agency has a minimum charge (often four hours) that must be paid regardless of the amount of time actually spent with the homebound patient.

Medicare is concerned about the growing costs associated with home health care. (See Chapter 7, "Government Programs.") In an effort to bring the same cost controls to home health care that have been adopted for hospitals and physicians, a new cost containment program has been introduced that address-es all outpatient-type costs, including home health charges. Home health rates have been modified again since, and these cutbacks created a downturn in the number of home health agencies in general and the ones that would continue to accept Medicare reimbursement.

Another problem Medicare faces is home health care fraud. There have been a number of well-documented cases that have resulted in billions of dollars being paid out to scam artists. Because the administration of Medicare has so many loopholes, fraud is not difficult to perpetrate. During the 1990s, the head of HCFA (now CMS) went on record as saying that Medicare unquestionably pays substantially more than anyone else for the same type of home health care services. The Clinton Administration attempted to tighten the reins on this type of wasted spending as one means of protecting the long-term solvency of the Medicare home health care program. Since home is where most people prefer care, the Medicare budget remains strained due to the costs of home health care coverage.

Home modifications has become a cottage industry, primarily due to renovations in anticipation of aging needs. Couples like Alan and Julie Stewart converted their kitchen cabinets into drawers to hold pots and pans, widened doorways and eliminated all stairs in the house. They age-proofed it – for themselves. In their 80s, it's their chance to "age in place" and retain their independence for as long as possible.[22]

Experts are calling it the "home of the future." Wider hallways, nonslip floors, bathroom grab bars and adjustable shower seats are among the features. Susan and Mel Womble spent $180,000 to remove steps at the front door, widen hallways and doorways, install grab bars in the shower, build a caretaker's apartment in the basement and even lower sinks and stoves for easy and comfortable reach, all in anticipation of Mel's future health concerns after being diagnosed with Huntington's disease, a genetic disorder that gradually reduces a person's ability to walk, talk and reason.[23]

The National Home Builder's Association estimates residential remodeling to be a $180 billion industry today. Harvard's Joint Center for Housing Studies projected that Boomers will account for the creation of 12 million new households as a result of empty nests and anticipated aging needs.[24]

As Americans are living longer, the preference for home care is easily seen through this remodeling. People with modified homes will have the greatest chance of being discharged back to home following a medical event. Moreover, part of the remodeling boom has been to make homes safer for older adults. More than 7 million Americans suffered disabling injuries at home in 2000. The majority of falls afflicted people age 65 years of age or older. Since 80 percent of all Americans age 55 and over own their homes, look for continued home modifications to help people remain in their comfortable, familiar environment longer and avoid (if possible) the nursing facility stay.[25]

The home care market is a strong one that appeals to most everyone and likely will continue to take an ever-growing percentage share of the long-term care tab being paid today. If elderly parents and their adult children have their say, home care will be the primary method of dispersing long-term care for the future.

Assisted Living Facilities

Beyond nursing home and home care environments, there are an assorted number of boardinghouse-type residences that cater specifically to those needing long-term care. These centers are commonly known as assisted living facilities (ALFs), adult congregate living facilities (ACLFs), personal care homes, extended congregate care residences, continuing care retirement communities (CCRCs), Elder Cottage Housing Opportunity (ECHO) homes and others.

Essentially, these facilities provide room and board as well as offer additional services. They are primarily intended to provide shelter for individuals that can no longer take care of their own home or who may need assistance with the normal activities of daily living.

Assisted Living Facilities: The assisted living facility as a site for administering long-term care services is on the rise. That said, because assisted living facilities are called by any number of names (including some noted above), a single definition of assisted living facilities is difficult to come by. These facilities provide a way for older adults to continue to maintain an independent lifestyle with some assistance and support. These individuals are not in need of skilled care, but assistance with Activities of Daily Living (ADLs) and Instrumental Activities of Daily Living (IADLs). The primary characteristics of an assisted living facility setting are: security and independence, privacy and companionship, and physical and social well-being, according to the National Center for Assisted Living (NCAL). Residents live in a congregate residential setting that generally provides personal services, 24-hour supervision and assistance, activities and health-related services, designed to:

-       minimize the need to relocate;

-       accommodate individual residents' changing needs and preferences;

- maximize residents' dignity, autonomy, privacy, independence, choice, and safety; and

- encourage family and community involvement.

Assisted living services can be provided in freestanding facilities, on a campus with skilled nursing facilities or hospitals, as components of continuing care retirement communities, or at independent housing complexes.[26]

A recent analysis by the National Center for Assisted Living indicates that there are approximately 33,000 assisted living residences housing 800,000 people around the country. The average ALF has 30 beds and 23 residents. They typically charge an average monthly fee of $1,873 that includes rent and most additional fees. About 15 percent of ALFs charge more than $2,500, while 19 percent charge less than $1,000.[27]

In the 2002 MetLife Mature Market Institute's study of Assisted Living Facility costs, they found the average charge to be $2,159/month, with the lowest monthly average in Jackson, MS at $592/month and the highest being in New York City at $3,697/month. The study also found that 19 percent of facilities charged an extra fee for assistance with ADLs above and beyond the base level of care provided. Some of the ALFs (12.3 percent) had separate units for specialized care for people with Alzheimer's disease or related conditions. Monthly fees for special care units ranged from $1,450 to $6,800/month.[28]

The average age of residents in these ALFs in 2000 was 80. Over two-thirds of the residents are female and, on average, residents needed help with 2.25 ADLs. A full 93 percent of ALF residents needed or accepted help with housework, while 86 percent needed or accepted help with their daily medication (IADLs). The majority of residents came directly from their homes (46 percent), followed by a transfer or move from another ALF (20 percent), transfer from a hospital (14 percent), or transfer from a nursing facility (10 percent). At the other end of the spectrum, 61 percent of residents either transfer out to a nursing home (likely for more comprehensive care) or die.[29]

During the 3rd quarter of 2000, the average occupancy rate for assisted living was 88.7 percent[30] and continued to decline from that point forward each quarter until 2nd quarter 2002. This was due largely to overbuilding, but as less construction activity took place, bed utilization started to stabilize. In the 2nd quarter 2002, occupancy actually increased slightly from 84.0 to 84.5 percent. Net move-in rates per facilities open less than 2 years was 1.9 per month, a cause for some optimism as it has stayed steady over a couple of quarters, but the National Investment Center for the Seniors Housing and Care Industries (NIC) indicated that a net move-in rate of 1.9 per month is not likely generating enough cash to avoid the necessity of tapping into existing equity for cash flow purposes.[31]

Marriott Corporation has started a chain of assisted living facilities. Marriott obviously recognizes the potential growth for assisted living facilities for the aging population. They figure if they can check in people to a regular hotel, what's the difference in checking in unhealthier people for a longer period of time? These residences are among the more popular in the cities where they are located.

Affordability may become a primary issue here. While averaging 60 percent less than skilled nursing facilities, the cost is still beyond the reach of many elderly. Over nineteen million seniors in the United States (nearly 55 percent of the senior population) have annual incomes of less than $15,000, while another 7.5 million seniors (22 percent) have incomes less than $25,000. These seniors will probably require significant financial assistance from family members or the government to afford assisted living.[32]

Long-term care insurance policies are beginning to recognize these alternative living arrangements. Due to financial considerations, a nursing home (where insurance eligibility is common) may not be feasible or circumstances may prevent the use of one's own home or the use of a family member's home, yet, the need for long-term care assistance remains.

Caution, however, should be exercised in evaluating this type of housing. While nursing homes have set minimum standards to follow, the laws governing the licensing and regulation of assisted living facilities vary widely. In some states it's not clear whether there are laws that govern assisted living facilities. Oregon passed the first licensing law aimed at assisted living in 1989. By the end of the century, more than 60 percent of states had followed with similar legislation.[33] While states remain concerned about oversight, they are still encouraging the growth of these types of lower-cost facilities that can accommodate many of the state's residents as an alternative to skilled nursing institutionalization.

Assisted living facilities are also facing the same liability issues (and subsequent large insurance premium increases) that skilled nursing facilities are battling. A woman living in the Alzheimer's wing of an ALF fell and broke her hip. A subsequent lawsuit claimed that this wing of the facility was run by a convicted felon who received only a few hours of video training and was placed on the floor caring for some 15-20 residents, and resulted in a jury award in 2002 of

$1.5 million for negligence.[34] Staffing, liability and reimbursement issues will mirror the problems of the skilled nursing home industry going forward, and agents and consumers should be aware and on the lookout for the type of problems this generates.

Each assisted living facility differs in the degree of its success in helping individuals remain relatively independent. For this reason, any recommendations you as an insurance agent might make should only be done after careful personal inspection of any facility. Treat this research as you would if you were looking for a nursing home for your relative. Many adults will opt for this type of housing in lieu of a nursing home environment, and the quality of local assisted living facilities as well as the average cost will be good information to have.

Continuing Care Retirement Communities (CCRCs): These major developments contain both independent and assisted living space. Residents contract with the community for a living unit and any other care services that are needed. A person can start out in an independent unit and, as his or her health declines, move to the assisted living units that provide long-term care services. Many of these communities have built a nursing home on-site for the purpose of 24-hour care. A resident can contract for additional services as his needs change without having to leave the community. This type of care is expensive and requires an admission fee which can range from $30,000 to $150,000 or higher. The monthly fee can run from $750 to $3,000 or higher. A contract is also required for the purposes of securing a long-term commitment.

Adult Congregate Living Facilities (ACLFs): These facilities are designed more for the middle to lower income groups. They offer communal apartment-type living with at least one meal served in a central dining room. There are social and recreational activities organized for residents and general housekeeping is provided. Aides are available to assist with activities of daily living and in some cases skilled care is provided. There is no admission fee, instead a monthly charge ranging from $1,000 and up is assessed. Public funds might defray some of the cost if a resident qualifies for a congregate living facility. A number of ACLFs around the country have attracted negative publicity, so it pays to inspect the premises before making any recommendations. Since it is communal living, talking to residents during your visit may elicit far more information than you can find elsewhere.

Extended Congregate Care Facilities: This type of care falls somewhere between an adult congregate care facility which generally provides custodial care and a nursing home which provides all types of long-term care services. For those that need more than custodial care, but are not in need of long-term care services, this type of housing may be a wise selection. It is similar to an ACLF in living arrangement, but has more medical services available. The fees will run slightly higher than an ACLF, and some extended congregate care facilities accept Medicaid reimbursement.

Senior Residential Care Homes: These are facilities that provide a room, meals and supervision, but no nursing services. Services vary but may include dietary and housekeeping services, monitoring of prescription medication, social and recreational opportunities, and assistance with activities of daily living.

Elder Cottage Housing Opportunity (ECHO): This type of housing is made up of small, self-contained mobile units that can be placed in the yards of a single-family home. They are specifically designed for older and disabled persons and the construction allows for mobility within the unit. This type of housing allows a person to be near family and friends without actually living under the same roof. They are economical with a one-bedroom unit costing under $25,000. Two-bedroom units are also available. Whether the adult child can provide this type of housing for his or her parents depends upon the community's zoning laws and utility connections. Many zoning codes do not allow ECHO housing while others only allow a variance for people over 55 years of age.

Alzheimer's Facilities: There are stand-alone housing units dedicated exclusively to Alzheimer's patients. With the high profile illness affecting individuals like former President Reagan and Charlton Heston, the awareness level of this disease has never been higher. With the Alzheimer's Association projecting the annual cost of the illness to be $375 billion alone by 2050, work is being done to find a cure.[35] There have been more breakthroughs of some significance in the research into this disease than in any other recently. In the meantime, publicity continues as AARP recently featured an interview with author Amy Tan, whose mother succumbed to Alzheimer's disease three years ago.[36] There's even an Alzheimer's Store, selling popular items like "Aerobics of the Mind" memory cards, clocks that feature the day and date in large figures to eliminate the need to constantly ask that question, and The Memory Phone whereby people can select the number they wish to dial by pushing a picture of the person they want to call.[37]

The aging trend and housing has even affected the church. In Illinois, the Sisters of St. Joseph of the Third Order of St. Francis looked toward the future and saw that in less than fifteen years, about 30 nuns would be trying to support the 230 or more that no longer work. They do own land, though, and have proposed building a senior housing project for lay people, the income from which will be used to support its three retirement homes for their nuns. The nun population has declined from 179,000 in 1965 to 78,000 in 2001, meaning fewer new nuns coming to the order to help support an aging group that is beginning to retire in large numbers.[38] Sound familiar?

The differences in price, services offered and accommodations make it difficult to generalize about assisted living facilities. It is an increasingly popular option for many elderly or for those in need of long-term care assistance. As such, the insurance agent or financial planner working in the long-term care market should be familiar with the various options in the community. Some suggestions in looking for a nursing home are applicable here: avoid unlicensed facilities, request a copy of the latest inspection report, have an attorney review the contract and obtain a list of rules and regulations.

Long-term care insurance policies will adapt and generally work with most types of services and facilities. Since some of these facilities are lower in cost, there may eventually be incentives within the long-term care insurance contract encouraging these cost effective living arrangements. At the very least, insurers' "Alternate Plan of Care" is intended to recognize that future services and settings that haven't been invented yet could quickly come to market. The intent of this policy provision is to ensure that the policy would be able to cover it even if not specifically named within the contract.

The following list is meant to assist the agent in helping clients (and families) ask the right questions in choosing senior housing.[39]

1. Take the initiative. The burden is on the person/family looking for the housing to research with the tools at hand to try and find the best place possible.

2. Decide what type of home is best for the dependent adult. Assisted living, for example, is not an option for people whose illnesses are so debilitating that they're unable to leave their beds.

3. Weigh the finances. Assisted living facilities are less expensive than nursing homes, but some nursing homes might have an assisted living option. Generally, Medicare does not cover ALFs and pays for only a small portion of skilled nursing facility care.

4. Check the ratings. ALFs will vary in their state licensing requirements although the majority of states today have licensing laws for them. Nursing facilities are required by federal law to make available to visitors the annual state and federal survey of their facility. This will detail the facility's track record in, among other things, cleanliness, administration of medicine, nursing care, and the nutritional quality of food. And now there's always the CMS quality indicators for all nursing facilities.

5. When checking a nursing home, look for warning signs. Items such as "Tags" and "Deficiencies" on the surveys reflect problems. Some things to look for include the incidence of bedsores among residents, use of restraints, frequency of falls, all of which can indicate low staffing levels.

6. Ask questions. Who owns the nursing home? What is the staff-to-patient ratio? How does the home recruit and maintain good staff people? What improvements are they working on? Have they raised their prices lately? How much and how frequently?

7. Be a careful observer. Watch the residents. What is their general appearance? How about the staff? Are they friendly, stressed or what? Look for uncollected garbage from the rooms, dust dirt, linens, etc. Ask to see the menu for the dining room. Where do the residents eat breakfast? Is it served in a bed or on a tray or, like most good homes, are the residents up and out to the dining area?

8. Be thorough. Try to avoid making a decision before actually visiting a residence. A geriatric manager can help speed the process up if you can afford to hire one.

Choosing a home health agency:[40]

1. Is the company a licensed home care provider?

2. Are the companies' employees bonded and insured?

3. Does the company conduct criminal background checks prior to hiring employees?

4. Who is responsible for paying workers' compensation if an employee is injured while in the home, you or the agency?

5. What orientation is given prior to sending a new employee into a home? Are return demonstrations given to verify skills and ensure that new employees can perform all requested tasks?

6. What is the level of supervision? How often are employees supervised to ensure they are performing competently? How often will a supervisor visit a client's home while care is being provided?

7. Are you given a list of the services and their costs, plus a written estimate of monthly charges prior to starting services?

8. Are the client's rights explained in detail to you and/or your family member?

9. What will happen if you don't like the assigned caregiver? Whom do you tell and what should you expect?

10. Are you given emergency agency contact information for after regular business hours? How quickly will someone call you back?

Chapter Notes

1. Kelly M. Blassingame, "Eldercare benefits expand as number of caregivers rises," *Employee Benefit News*, September 15, 2002, p. 73.

2. Alan Dessoff, " Caregiving burdens hit low-income and minority boomers the hardest," *AARP Bulletin* (September, 2001), p. 6.

3. MetLife Mature Market Institute: "American Baby Boomers in 2003 – A Demographic Profile" (February, 2003).

4. Ron Panko, "Hope for a Healthy Marketplace," *Best's Review* (April, 2002), p. 75.

5. Janelle Carter, "Shortage Noted in Geriatric Doctors," *Associated Press*, May 5, 2002.

6. Sarah Skidmore, "Long-term care centers need nursing assistants," *Florida Times Union*, August 11, 2001, p. A1.

7. Carole Fleck, "Nursing home care is found wanting," *AARP Bulletin* (April, 2002), p. 16.

8. "Long-Term Care Battle Not Over," *AARP Bulletin* (December, 2002), p. 9.

9. Carrie Teegardin, "After prodding, state agency cites Jonesboro nursing home," *Atlanta Journal-Constitution*, November 19, 2002, p. A18.

10. LTC Bullet, Center for Long-Term Care Financing, October 4, 2002.

11. Source: Federal Interagency Forum on Aging-Related Statistics, "Older Americans 2000," published 2001.

12. "Data on quality of nursing homes available to consumers," *Orlando Sentinel*, November 13, 2002, p. C1.

13. Carole Fleck, "Sizing Up Nursing Homes," *AARP Bulletin* (January, 2003), p. 15.

14. "Ohio Health Care Association Official Says Nursing Facility Quality Information Could Mislead Public," *PR Newswire*, April 24, 2002.

15. Source: GAO Report: "Nursing Homes: Public Reporting of Quality Indicators Has Merit, but National Implementation is Premature" (October, 2002).

16. Source: Agency for Health Care Administration, Florida web site.

17. "What You Need to Know about Those Illegal Clauses," *The Sandwich Generation* (Spring, 1996), p. 21.

18. Donna Callea, "Nursing home's shutdown magnifies others' ratings," *Daytona Beach News Journal*, April 28, 2002, p. 1A.

19. Josh Goldstein, "Genesis Health Ventures CEO resigns," *Philadelphia Inquirer*, May 29, 2002.

20. Source: Administration on Aging: Profile of Older Americans: 2002, "Health, Health Care and Disability."

21. Source: MetLife Mature Market Institute, "Survey on Nursing Home and Home Care Costs 2002."

22. Jennifer Hamilton, "Aging Homeowners Are Staying Put," *Associated Press*, June 26, 2002.

23. Janelle Carter, "Boomers Age, Housing Needs Change," *Associated Press*, March 31, 2002.

24. Jennifer Hamilton, "Aging Homeowners Are Staying Put," *Associated Press*, June 26, 2002.

25. Janelle Carter, "Senior Friendly," *Daytona Beach News-Journal*, April 28, 2002, p. 1F.

26. "Assisted Living: Independence, Choice and Dignity," National Center for Assisted Living, 2001.

27. "Assisted Living Facility Profile, 2000," National Center for Assisted Living.

28. Source: MetLife Mature Market Institute, "Survey on Assisted Living Facility Costs 2002."

29. "Assisted Living Resident Profile, 2000," National Center for Assisted Living.

30. "LTC Occupancy Rates Stabilizing, NIC Survey Says," *Provider* (February, 2002), p. 9.

31. "Average Occupancy Rates Up Slightly for Assisted Living and Skilled Nursing," *Business Wire*, October 7, 2002.

32. Source: Joint Center for Housing Studies, Harvard University, "Affordable Assisted Living: Surveying the Possibilities" (January, 2003).

33. Anjetta McQueen, "Report Looks at Frail Elderly Care," *Associated Press*, August 12, 2001.

34. "Manassas Nursing Home Forced To Pay $1.5 Million in Negligence Suit," *PR Newswire*, April 2, 2002.

35. "Alzheimer's frightening rise," *USA Today*, editorial, 2002.

36. "Secure in our memories," *AARP – The Magazine* (March/April, 2003), p. 16.

37. Phil Galewitz, "Alzheimer's Store helps holiday shoppers," *Daytona Beach News-Journal*, December 15, 2002, p. 2A.

38. Don Babwin, "Nuns get into senior housing," *Associated Press*, 2002.

39. Dimitra Kesseneies, "Selecting Senior Housing," *My Generation* (November-December, 2002).

40. Source: Kelly Home Care Services, "Buyers Guide, 2002."

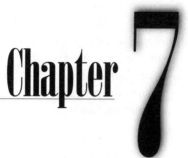

Chapter 7

Government Programs

"A government that robs Peter to pay Paul can always depend on the support of Paul."

– George Bernard Shaw

"If a free society cannot help the many who are poor, it cannot save the few who are rich."

– John F. Kennedy

What's a government health program to do? The expenditures continue to climb for both Medicare and Medicaid and, as the population continues to age, we are constantly reminded about the increasing cost pressures that will drive both of these programs into bankruptcy. Certainly, the odds appear against these programs' survival and unless some changes are made, Medicare and Medicaid may not be there as a safety net for future beneficiaries.

Already, in January 2003, the General Accounting Office (GAO) said that Social Security must be changed from its present structure or the government-run retirement system will need an extra $3.4 trillion over the next 75 years to meet the demands of retiring baby boomers. Without some kind of reform, the GAO said, American workers will face benefit cuts, tax increases, a higher retirement age or a combination of those steps to run the system.[1] Certainly, the Medicare and Medicaid systems are destined to hit the financial wall before that.

The Health Insurance Portability and Accountability Act of 1996 (HIPAA) hoped to make some strides in helping out these government plans. Tax clarification of long-term care insurance was a subtle message to the under-age-65 crowd to look to private long-term care insurance for future potential needs. It was thought that if the incentives were sufficient to motivate people to protect themselves with private long-term care insurance, rather than rely on Medicare, or more significantly, Medicaid, some of the fastest growing health care costs in these programs may be harnessed.

According to a study by LifePlans, Inc., the 4.5 million private U.S. long-term care insurance policies already in place could save Medicare and Medicaid about $30 billion. The researchers found that private LTC coverage saved an average of $1,668 in out-of-pocket expenditures per month for insureds who used home care and $2,458 per month for insureds who needed nursing home care. Private LTC coverage reduced the probability that an insured would become poor enough to qualify for Medicaid nursing home assistance to 3 percent, from 9 percent. The researchers' estimates of future savings was $23 billion for Medicaid ($5,032 per insured) and $7 billion for Medicare ($1,609 per insured).[2]

Up until now, the assumption most commonly made about long-term care costs by the elderly is that it isn't a problem. If you ask the average senior citizen how will he pay for his costs associated with his long-term care needs, the reply heard often is "Medicare and my Medicare supplement." Thirty-nine percent of U.S. residents over age 65 think that Medicare or Medicare supplemental insurance might cover long nursing home stays, and 24 percent are confident that it does. Further, women are more likely than men to believe Medicare might cover long-term institutional care and people over age 85 are more likely to hold that belief than those under age 85.[3] Unfortunately, this illustrates how little people understand the purpose of Medicare and Medicare supplements.

It's Medicaid, not Medicare, that is the federal government program that funds most long-term care costs today. While Medicaid pays about 48.1 percent of the cost of nursing home care nationally, the program covers 70 percent of nursing home residents and pays something toward the cost of nearly 80 percent of all patient days.[4] Many people confuse Medicare and Medicaid. This chapter will define these programs, the coverages provided, the qualifications required for reimbursement, and discuss how the country's national and local budget woes, and easy qualification for these programs are affecting the future of both these government benefits and the sale of private long-term care insurance.

Here are two important points in understanding these programs:

1.   *Medicare* currently covers about 14 percent of the total long-term care expenditures.[5] Recent legislation has continued to cut into what Medicare does cover. In its 2003 guidebook "Medicare and You," the Centers for Medicare and Medicaid Services (CMS) flatly states on page 60: "Generally, Medicare does not pay for long-term care." The next paragraph then references another CMS publication "Choosing Long-Term Care: A Guide For People With Medicare", Publication No. 02223, that details what to look for in private LTC insurance.

2.   *Medicaid* is a welfare program that is based on poverty-level qualifications, not age eligibility. Medicaid pays the costs of long-term care only after individuals have exhausted their personal assets, including their income. Do not be misled by the word "exhausted." It is not that difficult to qualify for Medicaid benefits as evidenced by the statistic that over 2 million Americans with incomes greater than $75,000 are on Medicaid according to a 2002 U.S. Census Bureau Report.[6] Because of this qualification, one of the major sources of revenue for providers of long-term care is the joint federal-state funded program, Medicaid.

With this understanding, it will be easy to communicate to your client the differences in these two programs. As an agent, you must identify potential sources of available funds that an individual might draw upon for the financing of his long-term care needs. Medicare and Medicaid are two such sources.

Medicare

In 1960, John F. Kennedy, a presidential candidate, presented a program as part of the Democratic platform that would help elderly Americans pay for health care expenses without having to go into bankruptcy. Even though there were far fewer seniors in 1960 than there are today, a greater percentage of the elderly lived close to the poverty line. Some analysts feel that by using the approach of a federally funded program to subsidize health care costs, Kennedy used the senior vote to propel himself into the White House by a narrow margin.

President Kennedy did not live to see this idea come to fruition. That was left to his successor, Lyndon Johnson, who witnessed the birth of Medicare in 1965 as an amendment to the 1935 Social Security Act. As one solution to the problem of the elderly in poverty, this program has helped to reduce the percentage of elderly who are below the poverty level to 10.1 percent.[7] The Medicare program design was based on an acute care oriented medical model which reimbursed people age 65 and over for hospital and physician services.[8] The acute care model was designed to reimburse acute-type expenses, such as those often associated with hospital stays. It was never intended to reimburse disability-based stays, which utilize more long-term care services. Thus, from the beginning, the idea that Medicare cover long-term care expenses was never intended.

Also eligible, without regard to age, were qualified disabled individuals (under Social Security's definition), and those suffering permanent kidney failure. Medicare is administered by the Centers for Medicare and Medicaid Services (CMS).

There are three parts to Medicare – Part A, Part B, and Part C.

Part A benefits cover institutional care including inpatient hospital care, limited skilled nursing home care, some home health care expenses, and hospice care. Part A is financed almost exclusively by payroll (FICA) taxes (1.45 percent of all income earned). There is no additional premium cost to those eligible for Medicare coverage.

Part B is a supplemental and optional program. Coverage includes physician services, outpatient hospital care, physical therapy, and other miscellaneous medical expenses. Twenty-five percent of the premium is paid by the Medicare beneficiary and 75 percent from taxpayer general revenues. In 2003, the monthly premium for Part B is $58.70. This premium is usually deducted from the Social Security benefit check being paid to the Medicare-eligible individual. The individual over age 65 does not have to elect Part B coverage and has an option of enrolling in the program within the first 90 days of each year.

Part C is known as Medicare+Choice. Beginning in November 1999, Medicare beneficiaries had the choice between the traditional Medicare fee-for-service program and the Medicare+Choice program. Medicare+Choice offers beneficiaries a number of health delivery models, including HMOs, preferred provider organizations (PPOs), provider sponsored organizations (PSOs), Medical Savings Accounts (MSAs), and private fee-for-service Medicare. While this program initially had a large number of provider options, the number of Medicare+Choice plans dwindles each year.

Medicare and Long-Term Care

This chapter is intended to discuss Medicare only as it relates to coverage of long-term care expenses. As an insurance agent and financial planner, your knowledge of the long-term care aspect of the Medicare program is vital to properly designing and communicating a solution to your client's or prospect's long-term care needs.

Medicare is the most misunderstood government program in identifying what is actually covered for long-term care services. As noted earlier, the Medicare program was primarily designed for acute medical care needs. But the health problems the elderly are faced with today are related to the inability to perform activities of daily living (ADLs). This treatment model is primarily a disability model, not an acute medical care model.[9] The expectation level for comprehensive long-term care coverage under Medicare should not be high since Medicare is not designed to cover chronic care conditions.

Medicare Part A addresses two primary areas of long-term care – nursing home and home health care.

Nursing Home Coverage

Skilled care in a nursing home environment is the only type of care that Medicare will cover. It can be either skilled nursing care or skilled rehabilitation care. Individuals needing intermediate care or custodial care (assistance with activities of daily living) are not covered and will not receive any financial assistance from Medicare.

To be eligible for reimbursement for skilled care in a nursing home facility, the patient must meet five requirements:

1.   A consecutive three-day hospital stay (not including day of discharge) must precede entry into a skilled nursing home facility (providing the nursing home admission occurs within 30 days of hospital discharge) and the same medical cause must exist for both hospital and skilled nursing facility admission.

2.   The care needed by the patient must be skilled nursing or skilled rehabilitation services.

3.   The skilled nursing home facility must be certified by Medicare.

4.   A physician must certify the need for this skilled care on a daily basis.

5.   The beneficiary's condition must be improving.

All five of these requirements must be met in order to become eligible for coverage for skilled nursing or rehabilitative care received in a skilled facility. Unless all of these requirements are met, Medicare will not pay the claim.

If all of the requirements have been met, up to 100 days of skilled nursing care benefits are provided. However, it is not as simple as it may seem. Here is what Medicare will pay for skilled nursing care in a certified facility in 2003:

Days	Amount
1 - 20	up to 100% of approved amount
21 - 100	all but $105 per day
101 +	nothing

Medicare's "approved amount" for the first 20 days is based on a set rate schedule for a geographical area. If a nursing home charges more than the approved amount, the patient is responsible for the difference in the rates. However, the nursing home facility, certified by Medicare, is likely to accept the Medicare rate. Thus, for the majority of cases, the full rate (for a semi-private room) will be reimbursed by Medicare for the first 20 days.

The second benefit phase, days 21 through 100, requires the patient to pay the first $105 per day in 2003. As you can see, Medicare's financial responsibility diminishes significantly. According to the MetLife Mature Market Institute, in 2002 the average semi-private rate for a nursing home in the U.S. was $143/day.[10] So a person staying in a nursing home facility that charged the average rate of $143/day would pay the first $105/day, while Medicare paid the $38/day balance during this period.

The sizable co-payment required for days 21 through 100 reduces the payout from Medicare. If the patient has a Medicare supplement that covers the skilled nursing facility co-payment, the patient could be reimbursed this $105 a day from the supplemental policy.

After 100 days, the patient is responsible for the entire cost. Neither Medicare or a Medicare supplement will cover skilled nursing care after this period.

A better description of Medicare's skilled nursing care coverage under Part A of Medicare might be:

"Under Medicare, one might receive benefits for up to 20 days for *certified* skilled care rendered in a skilled nursing facility if one meets certain conditions. One might also receive a small amount of money during the next 80 days of skilled care provided in a *certified* skilled nursing facility."

The CMS publication "*Medicare and You*" defines skilled nursing facility care as semiprivate room, meals, skilled nursing and rehabilitative services, and other services and supples (after a related 3-day hospital stay).

It is important to note that many skilled nursing facilities specifically do not accept Medicare patients. This becomes an important question to research or ask the management of the facility that is being considered so that the resident is assured eligibility for Medicare reimbursement.

An example might clarify the extent of Medicare's skilled nursing care coverage. Assuming that a Medicare patient met all of the previous requirements to be eligible for Medicare reimbursement for a skilled nursing facility stay, how much would Medicare cover for a 180-day stay at $120 a day in a skilled facility?

DAYS	MEDICARE DAILY COVERAGE	TOTAL	PATIENT DAILY FISCAL RESPONSIBILITY	TOTAL
1- 20	$120/day	$2,400.00	-0-	-0-
21- 100	15/day	1,200.00	$105	$8,400
101-180	-0-	-0-	120.00	$9,600
		$3,600 (17%)		$18,000 (83%)

The coverage for a skilled nursing home facility stay is limited. The gaps in this coverage are:

1.   A $105 daily co-payment beyond the initial 20 days of treatment.

2.   No coverage for skilled care beyond 100 days.

3.   Patient is responsible for any charges above the Medicare approved amount in the first 20 days.

4.   No coverage for intermediate or custodial care.

5.   No coverage if the three-day hospital stay requirement is not satisfied or if the patient is not transferred to a skilled nursing facility on a timely basis (within 30 days of the hospital stay).

From the mid-1980s through 1997, Medicare's spending for skilled nursing facility (SNF) care rose at an average annual rate of 30 percent. In the Balanced Budget Act of 1997, a SNF prospective payment system (PPS) was put in place, just as Medicare has for hospital stays. In the PPS system, SNFs receive a fixed payment that covers almost all services provided during each day of a Medicare-covered stay. Congress subsequently modified the PPS with several temporary payment increases. In 2000, Medicare SNF expenditures were about $13 billion for services provided to 1.4 million Medicare patients, two-thirds of whom received care in freestanding SNFs (the balance in hospital-based SNFs). On any given day, about 10 percent of freestanding SNF residents were Medicare beneficiaries. Under the PPS method of reimbursement, most freestanding SNFs payments substantially exceeded the costs of caring for Medicare patients, according to a GAO report.[11] Despite political and provider pressure, expect that to change in the near future.

As noted earlier in the book, CMS has embarked on a mission to inform Medicare beneficiaries of quality indicators for SNFs, primarily to avoid situations like the one Anna Spinelli confronted. She was forced to move her relatives several times trying to find a quality home, due to incidents of poor care. In one case, she went to see her brother-in-law on Christmas Eve. He looked like he had not been cleaned since the day before when she was there, with wet sheets and an unshaven appearance confirming her thoughts.[12] Skilled nursing facilities remain the long-term care delivery service of last resort.

Home Health Care

Long-term care services usually involve custodial care. If custodial care is administered, Medicare can pay the claim as long as it is in a home setting.

Medicare will pay the costs of medically necessary home health visits. There are requirements needed to be satisfied before Medicare will approve a claim:

1. Part-time or intermittent home health care is covered. Medicare will not pay for 24-hour care.

   Medicare defines intermittent care as skilled nursing care provided on fewer than seven days each week, or less than eight hours each day (combined) for 21 days or less (with extensions in exceptional circumstances when the need for additional care is finite and predictable). Individuals requiring daily skilled nursing care at home, even if not on a full-time basis, may have difficulties with their claim.

2. The patient must be house-bound. This is defined as a medical condition restricting the ability to leave the house except with assistance. The patient is also considered house-bound if it is medically inadvisable to leave the house.

3. The patient must be under a physician's care and the physician must certify the need for the home health care.

4. The home health care agency providing the services must be certified by Medicare.

5. The beneficiary's condition must be improving.

Unlike skilled nursing care provided in a certified skilled nursing facility, home health care reimbursements do not have co-payments. The only exception is the need for durable medical equipment (wheelchairs, hospital beds, etc.). In this case, Medicare pays 80 percent of the cost.

Covered services include:

- part-time or intermittent skilled nursing care

- physical therapy,

- speech-language therapy,

- occupational therapy,

- medical social services under the direction of a physician (for example, counseling for emotional problems),

- medical supplies,

- part-time or intermittent services of a home health aide, and

- durable medical equipment,

Medically necessary use of durable medical equipment, such as wheelchairs, oxygen equipment, artificial limbs, braces, ostomy supplies, and hospital beds, is covered at 80 percent. The patient must pay for 20 percent of the cost. A bathroom grab-bar, for example, is not covered because it is not medical in nature. Neither are elevators or lift devices since people who are not sick or injured use them. Medicare adheres to its requirements and the slightest infraction can result in non-payment of a claim.

Medicare specifically does not cover:

- full-time nursing care,

- meals delivered to the home,

- prescription drugs,

- twenty percent of the cost of durable medical equipment or charges in excess of the Medicare-approved amount for such equipment, and

- homemaker services that are primarily needed to assist in meeting personal care or housekeeping needs.

The home health care benefits under Medicare are intended for part-time, medically necessary care that is associated with a skilled need. Thus, while custodial care is covered, it's important to note that if it's 100 percent custodial care without any skilled care needed, the claim runs the risk of being denied.

While coverage for nursing care is very limited, Medicare's reimbursements for home care, despite the aforementioned requirements and payment cutbacks, soared in the last part of the 20th Century. After rising rapidly for most of the 1990s, total home health spending finally fell 37 percent in 1998. An increase in year 2000 spending (from 1999) brought the home health care tab up to $9 billion. The average number of persons served by Medicare home health agencies was 95 per 1,000 Medicare enrollees and the average number of home health visits was 51.[13]

Under provisions of the Balanced Budget Act of 1997, more than $16 billion in home health services were scheduled to be deleted from projected Medicare expenditures over a five-year period (1998-2002).[14] Essentially, Medicare did not change home health care eligibility rules as much as altering the way home health agencies are reimbursed. Instead of being paid visit by visit virtually without cost controls, a new annual limit was imposed on home health care agencies. The limits are based on the number and average cost of patients served in the past. Home health agencies, with an eye to their budgets, began cutting back on home care services. Some agencies filed for bankruptcy due to the reimbursement change. And there were concerns on the part of many states that this might place pressure on the Medicaid program because seniors close to the poverty line would switch to Medicaid if denied Medicare benefits for home care. If this happened consistently, the government would only be reshuffling the money, passing along more liability to states through the Medicaid program.

There is a delicate balance between quality care and budgets, as managed care has illustrated. The government can't be faulted for making its most recent policy decisions with an eye on the upcoming large volumes of new Medicare beneficiaries.

Even so, in 2002 the White House quietly authorized Medicare coverage for the treatment of Alzheimer's disease. This policy change meant that Medicare beneficiaries could not be denied reimbursement for the costs of mental health services, hospice care or home health care because they have Alzheimer's. This change was made based on new studies showing that people with Alzheimer's can often benefit from psychotherapy, physical and occupational therapy, enabling people to live longer on their own.[15]

This change is somewhat misleading since the Medicare beneficiary will still have to meet the several normal requirements as already outlined above. This does not create any new benefits; it simply means that if the individual with Alzheimer's still meets the normal definitions (and in the later stages of this disease, one might) to qualify for home health care (or possibly skilled nursing facility care), benefits cannot be denied strictly on the basis of this disease.[16]

Medicare's contribution to overall long-term care costs is currently minimal and there is every expectation that it will continue to promote funding alternatives to salvage the program for future beneficiaries and cover what its creators initially intended – acute care. This coverage leaves some significant gaps, creating rising out-of-pocket health costs for beneficiaries. The estimated average annual out-of-pocket costs per Medicare beneficiary grew from $2,308 in 1998 to $3,054 in 2002 and were projected to hit $3,383. *And*, these out-of-pocket costs do not reflect people's expenses incurred for long-term custodial care services.[17] The requirements needed to receive benefits from Medicare eliminate many of the standard long-term care claims that would otherwise be filed. Long-term care insurance was designed to cover these types of claims.

The Balanced Budget Act of 1997

When Congress passed the Balanced Budget Act of 1997 (BBA), it was clear there would be an impact on Medicare. As noted above, a new method of reimbursing home health care agencies has already led to cutbacks in long-term care provided. In addition, the Act places heavy emphasis on encouraging Medicare beneficiaries to choose managed care health plans.

The new Medicare+Choice plans give seniors the option to select an alternative method of receiving health care other than the traditional Medicare program. Choices include Health Maintenance Organizations (HMOs), Preferred Provider Organization (PPOs), Point-of-Service (POS) plans and Provider-sponsored organizations (PSOs). It was thought that there would be some more coverage for long-term care services than might be available in the traditional fee-for-service Medicare plan.

In the Medicare select program (the precursor to Medicare+Choice), which gave Medicare beneficiaries a choice of enrolling in an HMO, long-term care coverage had typically been more extensive than in the traditional Medicare program. This has changed over time, as Medicare HMOs experienced more intensive claims in this area than expected.. The result has been a pullback in the number of these Medicare+Choice plans, and a curtailing of some of the "extra" benefits like more expansive LTC coverage. These new plans might eliminate the need for a Medicare supplement.

Mainly, the BBA created a downsizing of provider fees that generated controversy and change. In each year since passage, the BBA has been tweaked to either reverse cutbacks or freeze them. The latest round came in 2003 when Congress passed the Omnibus Appropriations Bill, part of which contained a temporary solution to stop the continuing cutbacks in provider fees, due to hit March 1, 2003.[18] A portion of these cuts was due to an error in calculating the Medicare physician payments in 1998 and 1999, including underestimating the gross domestic product (GDP) and leaving out the cost of medical care for one million seniors.[19]

A federal judge also intervened on behalf of Medicare beneficiaries to force CMS to mail seniors information on private health plans that particispate in Medicare+Choice earlier than CMS routinely did, so that these individuals could make up their mind about participating in a Choice plan or returning to (or staying with) the tradiitonal Medicare plan.[20] All told, the BBA Medicare changes have been far from smooth sailing and have served to point out how vulnerable seniors still are to out-of-pocket costs from this government program.

Medicare Supplements

Do Medicare supplements help?

Some. But these policies, so familiar to seniors, only fill in the gaps of those services Medicare designates to be paid. Supplements don't add much to those gaps Medicare has left behind.

For example, for a patient receiving skilled nursing care in a skilled facility, Medicare will pay the first 20 days up to its approved amount. A co-payment of $105 (in 2003) for the next 80 days is required from the patient, with Medicare paying the difference. The Medicare supplement that includes coverage for the SNF co-payment will pick up this $105 co-payment.

However, after 100 days, neither Medicare nor a Medicare supplement will pay anything. Supplements are *not* designed to add extra benefits to what Medicare already pays, but to supplement the existing benefit.

Medicare supplement policies are sold in ten standard, but specific plans, labeled A through J. Not every insurance company selling Medicare supplements offers ten plans. Some insurance companies do not offer the same number of plans in every state.

Neither plan A or plan B offers coverage for the co-payment of $105 for the skilled nursing facility. Plans C through J, however, do cover co-payments. If your client has Medicare supplement plan A or plan B, the lack of co-payment coverage should be identified.

Medicare supplement plans D, G, I, and J assist with home care benefits. Here, the coverage, labeled at-home recovery benefits, pays up to $1,600 per year for short-term, at-home assistance with activities of daily living for those recovering from illness, injury or surgery. The assistance must be in the form of Medicare-covered home health care services and must be ordered by a physician.

There may be limits on the number of visits and dollar amounts. For example, some plans pay up to $40 a visit for up to seven visits a week for a period of up to eight weeks *after* Medicare-covered home health care benefits cease. A supplement will not duplicate Medicare coverage. However, insurers have the option of offering expanded benefits under these plans.

Costs do increase for this supplemental coverage each year due to the expansion in coverage because of Medicare's changing deductibles and co-payments. The premium increase is not uniform for each plan. In 2002, the percentage change in average Medicare Supplement premium was as follows: Plan A: 9.91%; Plan B: 5.97%; Plan C: 7.35%; Plan D: 3.90%; Plan E: 4.36%; Plan F: 5.18%; Plan G: 2.38%; Plan H: 3.18%; Plan I: -.21%; Plan J: -21.24%.[21] These increases were the lowest in several years.

The majority of seniors believe that Medicare or a Medicare supplement will pay for long-term care costs. As an agent it is your responsibility to explain the gaps in these coverages. There is an increasing skepticism with which the elderly view Medicare in light of the Balanced Budget Act of 1997, and the heated discussions on Capitol Hill that revolve around the Medicare Program. Discussing Medicare and what is covered is important to your client.

Medicare: The Political Hot Potato

There has been much speculation about what Congress will and will not do to the Medicare program. Crucial to these discussions is long-term care, since it is potentially the greatest financial problem the elderly will face given Medicare's current lack of comprehensive coverage for long-term care services.

Discussions in Congress have not centered on how to add more benefits to Medicare. Instead, talk of requiring home health care co-payments was part of one balanced budget proposal that was eventually dropped. A number of health care analysts believe that there will eventually be home health care co-payments as part of the Medicare program.

As noted earlier, the federal government is "experimenting" with managed care in the form of Part C: Medicare+Choice. This program allows the elderly to enroll in a Health Maintenance Organization (HMO) instead of the regular

Medicare program. Some of the early plans offered somewhat more long-term care coverage – both for skilled nursing and home health care than the current Medicare program. Seniors, though traditionally unwilling to give up their choice of physicians in a managed care setting in exchange for greater benefits, did enroll in Part C due to better coverage for prescription drugs in addition to long-term care. But it was a short-lived benefit expansion as many of the Medicare HMOs didn't financially survive a year or two out of the gate, and many seniors were forced to return to the traditional Medicare program.

On several occasions, the Clinton Administration pushed for lowering the Medicare eligibility age to 55 with a buy-in deal that requires a monthly premium ($400 was proposed) for those aged 55-64 who wish to take advantage of this option. They were onto something here. The latest report regarding the uninsured in America had the age 55-64 bracket as the most without private health insurance after children under 18.

The Medicare program lately seems to please no one. A report by the Health and Human Services Inspector General found numerous problems, including that patients have to jump through too many hoops to file complaints; that the system rarely holds doctors or hospitals responsible for their actions; and that responses to complaining patients are limited, leaving them frustrated and unsatisfied.[22]

Whatever changes to Medicare loom ahead in the future, long-term care coverage will remain a significant gap for those 65 and over eligible for Medicare. Medicare and Medicare supplements, while a consideration in long-term care planning, do not reimburse enough of the costs to be considered as reasonable financial assistance if the need for long-term care arises.

The Center for Medicare and Medicaid Services (CMS) has developed online training modules on the Medicare program. You can find this information at http://www.cms.gov/partnerships.

Medicare Disclosure

For those individuals that own a Medicare supplement policy and wish to buy a long-term care insurance policy (or any other type of health insurance that offers coverage for long-term care services), a disclosure form is required by the Social Security Amendments of 1994. The form, adopted by the National Association of Insurance Commissioners in 1995, and by most states, is generally disclosed in the Outline of Coverage form that must be delivered to the individual applicant, and generally looks, as follows:

FIGURE 7.1

Important Notice to Persons on Medicare.

This is not Medicare Supplement Insurance.

Some health care services paid for by Medicare may also trigger the payment of benefits under this policy.

Federal law requires us (insurer) to inform you that in certain situations this insurance may pay for some care also covered by Medicare.

- This insurance provides benefits primarily for covered nursing home services.

- In some situations Medicare pays for short periods of skilled nursing home care and hospice care.

- This insurance does not pay your Medicare deductibles or coinsurance and is not a substitute for Medicare Supplement insurance.

Neither Medicare nor Medicare Supplement insurance provides benefits for most long-term care expenses.

Before You Buy This Insurance

- Check the coverage in all health insurance policies you already have.

- For more information about long-term care insurance, review the Shopper's Guide to Long-Term Care Insurance, available from the insurance company.

- For more information about Medicare and Medicare Supplement insurance, review the Guide to Health Insurance for People with Medicare, available from the insurance company.

For help in understanding your health insurance, contact your state insurance department or state senior insurance counseling program.

The intent of this is to avoid scandals such as the one that plagued insurers and insurance agents several years ago when elderly individuals purchased several Medicare supplement policies that duplicated benefits. Many state insurance departments have been carefully regulating and monitoring the sale and marketing of long-term care insurance to avoid any future problems.

The Medicare Catastrophic Act of 1989

On January 1, 1989, the Medicare Catastrophic Act was passed. This legislation, propelled through Congress by Democrats Dan Rostenkowski and Pete Stark, altered both Medicare and Medicaid.

The changes to Medicare primarily concentrated on long-term care benefits. Skilled nursing or rehabilitative care was extended to 150 days and home health care benefits were increased. Although altering the co-payment structure for these services, the new law failed to provide custodial care coverage in a skilled facility.

To fund this benefit expansion, a tax was levied on senior citizens and was based on their taxable income. Wealthier seniors were going to pay the bulk of these new taxes.

The backlash was tremendous. The vocal elderly let their Congressional representatives know exactly what they thought of this bill, resulting in its repeal which, although not unprecedented, was certainly a rare occurrence.

The changes to Medicare were in effect for one year. On January 1, 1990, Medicare benefits returned to previous levels where they remain today. Critical changes to Medicaid, however, (covered later in this chapter) were not repealed and remain of vital importance today.

Congress received a taste of what can happen when Medicare benefits are altered and the changes are perceived to be negative, or as in this case, where taxes are involved in paying for these benefits. Though this political body is asserting itself more in the latest round of Medicare discussions, Americans are discovering that they have strength at the ballot box and their voices will be heard once again when the discussions are complete and legislation is passed.

Medicaid

Medicaid is a different program entirely. Other than the fact that both Medicare and Medicaid are government programs financed by taxes, there is little relationship between the two. Medicare is a health care program for Social Security-eligible seniors who automatically qualify for benefits when they reach age 65. Medicaid is a joint federal-state plan that pays health care expenses for low-income individuals. There is a significant difference in eligibility requirements:

> *Medicare* – Individuals become eligible by reaching age 65 (Part A) and paying a monthly premium (Part B (optional)).

> *Medicaid* – Individuals become eligible by having income and assets at or below poverty level (amounts vary by state).

Medicaid is a welfare assistance program for low-income individuals. Many low-income elderly have come to rely on Medicaid to pay for long-term care costs. Funded with state and federal money, it provided health care to 32 million low-income individuals in 2001, including 3.2 million elderly.[23] For these elderly, Medicaid pays for nursing home costs, home health care and prescription drugs, the major out-of-pocket expenses for this age group. Established in the 1960's, Medicaid is funded by state and federal funds, with varying subsidies going to states from the federal government (from 50 to 87% depending on wealth of the state). Congress has paid close attention to Medicaid in recent years, because it must account for only roughly more than half of the funding of any new program involving Medicaid. This led to complaints from the individual states about unfunded mandates. Unfunded mandates require local governments to find the dollars to support federal legislation. Congressional legislation passed in 1995 at the federal level was intended to prevent this from happening in the future.

While there are some federal guidelines concerning Medicaid, every state designs its own program. This creates a diversity of eligibility and plan benefits from state to state. Services covered under the Medicaid program include:

- inpatient hospital care,

- inpatient skilled nursing facility care,

- home health care,

- physician services,

- outpatient hospital services,

- transportation costs to medical facilities,

- laboratory services,

- x-ray services, and

- Medicare deductibles, co-payments, coinsurance and premiums.

Steps in qualifying and applying for Medicaid are:

1. The individual needs long-term care and receives it from a nursing home, at someone's home or in an assisted living facility.

2. The patient files for Medicare benefits in the event Medicare will reimburse some of the cost.

3. If private insurance coverage exists, the patient must file a claim with the insurance company.

4. The patient begins spending and then exhausts all of his money, or utilizes any number of methods to qualify.

5. The patient then files a claim for Medicaid benefits.

How common is this scenario? Today, primary funding of the costs for long-term care services are paid for by either the individual in need of care or by Medicaid.

Medicaid is available to any American who can satisfy the eligibility requirement of low-income and little or no assets. This eligibility requirement differs for single persons and married persons thanks to the previously noted Medicare Catastrophic Act of 1989. Each state has its own income and asset eligibility guidelines.

Generally, a person's assets must be at or near poverty level to qualify. Many states set the poverty level at $1,500-$3,000 of assets. The Medicare Catastrophic Act of 1989 also affected Medicaid by installing safeguards for the spouse of the person requiring long-term care services. Prior to the Medicare Catastrophic Act, the at-home spouse was included in the eligibility requirement of low-income in order for the person requiring assistance to qualify for Medicaid. This often left the healthier individual in a near-bankruptcy situation. The Medicare Catastrophic Act established the minimum monthly income and shelter allowance for the at-home spouse to prevent bankruptcy.

While Medicaid requires individuals to exhaust their income and assets, a few items are exempt from this financial free-fall:

1. The house (while spouse is living), regardless of value.

2. One automobile.

3. Household and personal belongings.

4. Wedding and engagement rings.

5. Life insurance cash value if face amount is $2,500 or less.

6. Prepaid burial plots and funeral expenses.

For the at-home spouse the monthly income and shelter allowance can go as high as $4,000 per month. The community spouse is also allowed to retain one-half of the couple's assets up to $90,660 (in 2003), varying by state and indexed by inflation.

For the single individual, the need for long-term care services precludes the necessity of retaining assets above $2-3,000. The nursing home resident is also permitted a personal needs allowance that is extremely low and also varies by state. There are a number of states, including Florida and Texas, where one cannot qualify for Medicaid nursing home assistance at all if income generally exceeds 300 percent of the federal poverty level ($1,656/month in 2003).

These numbers magnify the importance of planning ahead. To lose the bulk of one's assets and income due to the need for long-term care services can be devastating. However, since the majority of people aren't planning ahead for the long-term care contingency, many of these individuals are finding Medicaid at the end of the financial road. This has placed a heavier burden on government, which passes that encumbrance on to taxpayers.

Medicaid is the most significant payer of long-term care costs in this country. This government program pays the bills for 80 percent of Georgia's nursing home residents.[24] In Florida, projected 2002-03 budgetary expenditures for Medicaid show that 19.04% of the total Medicaid spending spending in the state is allocated to nursing home costs, and an additional 7.48% projected for home and community services.[25]

Budget-Busting

States are currently busting the bank when it comes to the outflow of Medicaid dollars. While Medicaid spending grew at the relatively modest average annual rate of 5.5 percent between fiscal year 1996 and 1999, it grew by 9 percent in fiscal year 2000 and by an estimated 11 percent in fiscal year 2001.[26] Cash-strapped states searching for ways to trim their budget in light of the recent economic downturn have naturally turned their eyes to the Medicaid program. A recent study by Families USA noted that every state except Alabama was doing some form of cost containment in the Medicaid program.[27]

Medicaid is the second largest item in most state budgets, after elementary and secondary education. In state after state, declining tax revenues have pushed soaring costs for Medicaid to the crisis point.[28] Tighter eligibility requirements (Oklahoma requires stricter income tests for its Medicaid program and has disqualified "medically needy" individuals due only to large medical bills) and the imposition of co-payments on services are the paths being followed by states in the wake of their financial woes.

Long-term care reimbursements are a large enough part of Medicaid spending to command attention. Following the tobacco settlement case, eighteen states allocated some of their tobacco settlement funds specifically to long-term care programs, including home and community-based care designed to keep elderly in their homes.[29]

States are working on co-opting some of their financial problems onto long-term care providers. Medicaid is by far the lowest payer of nursing home costs in the country. A nursing home owner in a St. Louis suburb says he is losing more than $20/day on each of the 115 or so Medicaid patients at his facility. The medical staff and the housekeepers, the liver lunches and the scrambled eggs on request, the balloon volleyball games, the pet therapy, the concerts of patriotic music – all cost him close to $107/day. Medicaid reimburses him $86, with a governor's proposal to slash another 9 percent off in the coming year.[30]

There is a growing nursing home trend to cost shift in nursing homes from Medicaid patients to private paying ones because the state had maximized their Medicaid budget and the daily benefit amount was not sufficient to sustain the cost of care, creating cash shortfalls for providers.[31] This follows years of a similar practice in hospitals.

Beginning in 1995, some 34 states and the District of Columbia began implementing user fee programs on nursing home beds in an attempt to shore up Medicaid shortfalls. This "bed tax" applies to all non-Medicare beds and is intended to provide a relief to the state's Medicaid budget by producing additional revenue. Naturally, only private-pay or insured patients are footing this extra surcharge.[32] Medicaid problems are simply driving up the costs of nursing home care for non-Medicaid patients.

The Home and Community Care Option

Medicaid has traditionally funded long-term care services for a qualified individual only if they will reside in a nursing facility. With the ever-increasing opportunities to keep people at home longer due to advances in medical technology, it would seem natural that a budget-strapped program would look to generally lower home and community-based care as a lower cost alternative of providing LTC services. Until recently, though, this shift in services did not occur.

In June 1999, the Supreme Court ruled in *L.C. and E.W. vs. Olmstead* that it is a violation of the Americans with Disabilities Act for states to discriminate against people with disabilities by providing services in institutions when the individual could be served more appropriately in a community-based setting. As a result, states are now required to provide community-based services for people with disabilities if treatment professionals determine that it is appropriate, the affected individuals do not object to such placement, and the state has the available resources to provide community-based services.[33]

In Florida, this led to the establishment of a new state office charged with providing more community-based services and alternatives to nursing homes and who will coordinate the efforts of multiple agencies engaged in long-term care.[34] CMS announced that states can receive federal payments for certain one-time expenses associated with helping Medicaid beneficiaries move from institutional to community settings.[35]

States can fund home and community-based care in three ways:

1. In addition to home health services covered under Medicaid, states can offer optional Medicaid services, including personal care for assistance with activities of daily living.

2. States may obtain waivers from the federal government, allowing them to design home and community-based programs for specific target populations to pay for services not traditionally covered by Medicaid.

3. States may fund home and community-based programs through their general revenues.

Medicaid spending for institutional services accounted for about 71 percent of all Medicaid LTC spending in FY 2001, while spending for community-based long-term care services (HCBS waivers, personal care and home health services) accounted for 29 percent of Medicaid long-term care spending.[36]

Expect this trend to continue into the future as Medicaid will continue to undergo transformation in order to stay afloat.

The Transfer Game

To determine eligibility, Medicaid reviews the income and assets of the applicant and his or her spouse. The types of assets that Medicaid looks at, and which must be disposed of if a person applies for Medicaid assistance, are a second car, vacation home, investment properties, savings and certificates of deposit, bonds, IRAs, and other retirement vehicles.

It is possible to transfer some of these assets to another person. Transferred properties are not considered assets when qualifying for Medicaid. Although Medicaid was not designed to aid the wealthy, a substantial number of Americans have been making arrangements to transfer their assets to avoid spending their own money.

It's so easy to do this that the temptation for wealthier people (and their attorneys) to become "poor" on paper is too great to pass up. During the early 1990s, when the economy seemed destined for life support and state budgets were fiscally flatlining, Congress began paying attention to revenues and tried to close some of the loopholes that make this transfer game possible. OBRA '93 mandated estate recoveries, HIPAA imposed financial and criminal penalties on the people that make the transfers, and the BBA '97 directed these penalties against the planners that moved the assets instead.

A relative lack of enforcement of these legislative discouragements, followed by several years of robust economic times did not accomplish the intended goal – keeping Medicaid as a safety net for those that were truly poor. Today, it is still easy to qualify for Medicaid. As Stephen Moses of the Center for Long-term Care Financing puts it, "Medicaid does not require a low income, merely that the individual have a cash flow problem. In most states, one can have any amount of income and qualify for nursing home benefits as long as the income is insufficient to pay all of one's medical expenses, including private nursing home care. In other states, people whose income exceeds the 2003 limit of $1,656 can place excess income into a vehicle called a Miller Trust to become immediately eligible for Medicaid benefits."[37]

Is it any wonder that 2,080,000 people with incomes of $75,000 or more are on the Medicaid dole?[38]

In addition to an ease in income for qualifying, assets have never been much of an obstacle to Medicaid eligibility for most Americans. Over half of the net worth of the median elderly household is in a home. Under Medicaid, as previously noted, the home and its continguous property are exempt from spend down regardless of value. One business including the capital and cash flow of unlimited value is also exempt. Ditto for one automobile, with no limit on value if it's used at least occasionally for the elder's benefit. Add in pre-paid burial costs and term insurance in any amount plus household furnishings that have a limited value that is rarely if ever enforced, and there is a lot of room to maneuver even before consulting the elder law attorney.[39]

Gypsies, Tramps, and Thieves

Attorneys specializing in elder law often use an elaborate plan called reconfiguration. This involves transferring assets to someone else, typically a child. The object of the transfer game is to see how many assets could be legally moved and how fast Medicaid eligibility was achieved once the senior client became ill. In so doing, the client steps up his eligibility for Medicaid assistance by avoiding spending those assets. Legally, the client no longer has assets.

With the passage of OBRA '93, regular transfers of assets must occur 36 months prior to applying for Medicaid and transfers out of a trust must occur 60 months prior to applying for Medicaid. These transfers go on regularly as people scramble to save these assets from spending on LTC and other medical expenses. Why pay for care yourself if the government is willing to do it for you?

A newspaper columnist took exception to this transfer practice in a recent article, noting that these "senior advisors" capitalize on the myth that eldercare should be free and promising to save well-to-do people (as one mailer used puts it) from Medicaid's 'greedy henchmen.' The writer goes on to point out that Medicaid's 'greedy henchmen' are you and I, the taxpayers. Ultimately it is public money that picks up the costs for people who are able to effect their transfers and hasten their Medicaid eligibility.[40]

Who really wins in that scenario? Not the states, especially as the 21st Century has dawned with a return to our economic dark ages and forced them back into crackdown mode to try and preserve Medicaid for its intended beneficiaries. Not the taxpayers who finally must be willing to finance the increasing budgets needed for Medicaid services. And, oddly enough, not the person who qualifies artificially for Medicaid, either. There have been some unexpected outcomes for those who have played the transfer game. Many people who transferred their assets found themselves in the unwanted position of having to ask their children or relatives for money. Many nursing facilities and home health care agencies do not accept Medicaid assignment so individuals who otherwise would have had the choice of a nursing home facility or home health care agency were limited to facilities that accepted Medicaid. The nursing home facilities that did accept Medicaid patients often crowded them three to four in a room. In short, the final results from the transfer were financially acceptable (especially to heirs) but emotionally difficult for the individual and close family members.

Bizarre happenings rule the day with Medicaid. In New York, a sick husband or wife can transfer all of their assets to a spouse, who then can refuse to pay for their care. In that case, Medicaid steps in and picks up the tab.[41] It's not as if some states haven't tried to discourage this practice. OBRA '93 mandated that individual states had to enact, by 1995, legislation concerning estate recovery. As a result, Estate Recovery or Lien Recovery Acts have been enacted in all states. The estate recovery programs direct the recovery of transferred assets of a Medicaid beneficiary in an amount equal to that spent under Medicaid to provide long-term care services. For example, let's say Mrs. Barnes qualified for Medicaid after transferring her assets and the cost to the state and federal government to take care of her until her death was $35,000. The Estate Recovery Act allows the government to recover the $35,000 (as long as her spouse is no longer living) from wherever the assets were transferred.

In their zeal to recover some of these transferred assets, innocents get caught up in this deplorable game. In West Virginia, a woman who legitimately spent her savings down to pay for long-term care, went on Medicaid when the money ran out. She died in 1997, leaving her blue bungalow home overlooking the city of Clarksburg to her niece. A year after her aunt's death, the niece received a bill from Medicaid for $51,000 for the Medicaid costs of her aunt's care. The niece's choice was to pay the $51,000 or sell the house to raise the money. A schoolteacher, the woman had neither the ability to pay the $51,000 or another place to live.[42]

For those desiring to transfer assets, this must be done 36 or 60 months prior to applying for Medicaid. OBRA '93 also penalized those who transferred assets during this period. The ineligibility period is extended based on both the amount transferred and the cost of the average daily nursing home rate in one's geographical area.

For example, let's say our Mrs. Barnes transferred assets of $250,000 and then applied for Medicaid within the 36 month eligibility period. Since the local average monthly nursing home rate is $5,000, this transfer and subsequent application will disqualify the individual for 50 months ($250,000 divided by $5,000) instead of 36 months.

But advisors and lawyers have figured this out as well. The penalty period is measured from the date of the actual asset transfer. So, in making the transfer, the attorney calculates the penalty period and applies immediately after that. Eligibility for Medicaid is immediate and the transferred assets have been preserved. The state of Connecticut is trying to help close that loophole by applying the penalty period from the date of Medicaid application, not the asset transfer date.[43]

The Health Insurance Portability and Accountability Act of 1996 raised the ante on the transfer game even more. HIPAA made asset transfers, in certain cases, a federal crime if the transfer was done in an attempt to qualify for Medicaid. There are many in government who feel the Medicaid program can survive if benefits are confined to aiding only those who are truly needy. There is little patience with the individual who has achieved the poverty level on paper.

There are three conditions that raise the red flag:

1. Assets are transferred to someone other than a spouse.

2. The transfer is done willingly and purposefully to qualify for Medicaid.

3. The transfer triggers an "ineligibility" period (see reference to 36 and 60 months above).

The penalty was possible jail time and/or a fine levied for the person whose assets were transferred. This had the unintended effect of scaring the wits out of senior citizens. So the Balanced Budget Act of 1997 attempted to right this wrong by exonerating the person whose assets are transferred and instead directed the jail and/or fine at the planner who assists in the transfer. While this has had an initial chilling effect on elder law attorneys, Congress is full of people of this profession and the enforcement of this law was negligible at best. The transfer game survived.

Medicaid was intended to be a true welfare program, not an artificial one. People who do not wish to spend their own assets have legally avoided doing so and are now siphoning dollars away from the legitimate poor who need care. The Medicaid program is simply running out of money. An attempt by the government to reduce costs by cutting back reimbursements to medical providers, for example, hasn't helped either. Unfortunately, by reducing medical reimbursement, it has forced many providers to not accept Medicaid patients.

States are trying other means of tightening up the rules. Annuities have drawn the most recent attention. These policies have been essential elements of asset transfers, under an old Health Care Financing Administration rule known as Transmittal 64. Here, as long as annuities are irrevocable, term certain, actuarially sound, and payments went to either the Medicaid beneficiary or spouse, this was a strong asset shelter. Today, states are fine-tuning this rule to add specific months and years of payments to be considered a proper transfer, and requiring level payments, eliminating the balloon payment that many advisors (and their clients) prefer.[44] It is a slow, piecemeal, case by case practice that still requires precious time, effort and money on the part of Medicaid to act as watchdog.

Medicaid today accounts for 20 percent of all state budgets and 7 percent of the Federal budget.[45] With money tight, it's fair to expect more difficulty with playing the transfer game. Medicare, in its annual "Deathwatch" report, cites insolvency projected now by the year 2026, four years earlier than last year's forecast.[46] Dollars on Capitol Hill will be watched closely for both of these programs.

But until long-term care insurance is seen as a more viable option than playing this game, the practice will flourish and may cost all of us in the long run.

Veteran's Benefits

Veterans of foreign wars may be eligible for nursing home and home health care benefits. Veterans are accepted into the subsidized VA program for health care (including long-term care) based on a priority order. Veterans with service-connected disabilities and low-income veterans are considered top priority applicants. Higher-income veterans not disabled in the service will find it increasingly difficult to qualify for any type of assistance.

On August 1, 2002, Veteran Affairs Secretary Anthiny Principi noted that the VA health system was discouraging new enrollees since they were currently experiencing problems caring for the ones already in the system. Thousands of veterans were on a waiting list for services.[47]

The Federal government addressed this problem in a roundabout way by offering veterans the chance to enroll in the new Federal LTC plan that was offered on an open-enrollment basis from July 1, 2002 through December 31, 2002. (More details on the Federal LTC plan can be found in Chapter 17, "Alternate Long-Term Care Financing Options.")

After determining the eligibility class of a client, contact the local Department of Veterans Affairs office for specific information on qualification.[48]

Summary

Medicare and Medicaid are two separate and distinct programs that can provide payment for long-term care services. But there are drawbacks to each program. In general:

Medicare – This program covers some skilled nursing care in a nursing home or at home if specific qualifications are met. Home health care is available but is subject to stringent eligibility rules. There is no coverage for true custodial care, the most common of the long-term care services needed.

Medicaid – This program pays the costs for many long-term care services for individuals at or below the poverty level. Medicaid benefits are usually not available until the individual's savings have been depleted.

Chapter Notes

1. "GAO: Time's running out on Social Security," *USA Today*, January 16, 2003, pg. 6A.

2. Allison Bell, "LTC Policies Now In Place Could Save U.S. $30 Billion," *National Underwriter*, October 14, 2002, pg. 18.

3. Allsion Bell, "Older Seniors Confused About Medicare Nursing Home Benefits," *National Underwriter*, July 23, 2001, pg. 31.

4. Stephen Moses, "Denial Is Not A River In Egypt," *LTC Bullet*, Center for Long-Term Care Financing, September, 2002.

5. Source: Center for Medicare and Medicaid Services.

6. Source: U.S. Census Bureau Report: Health Insurance Coverage 2001, released September 2002.

7. Source: A Profile of Older Americans, 2001; Administration on Aging using data from Current Population Reports "Poverty in the United States, 2001," issued September 2002.

8. "Managed Care, Elder Care and Medicare," *Health Care Innovations* (July/August, 1995), p. 20.

9. *Ibid.*

10. Source: MetLife Mature Market Institute Survey on Nursing Home and Home Care Costs, 2002.

11. General Accounting Office Report to Congressional Committees, "Skilled Nursing Facilities," December 2002.

12. Janelle Carter, "Government Wants Better Nursing Home Info," *Associated Press*, April 20, 2002.

13. Source: Centers for Medicare and Medicaid Services, Program Information, June 2002 edition.

14. "February 5 Brings Severe Medicare Cuts for Thousands of Texans," PR Newswire, January 26, 1998.

15. "Report: Medicare Coverage Authorized for Alzheimer's," *Reuters*, April 1, 2002.

16. "Special Alert: Medicare to Cover Alzheimer's Disease," *LTC Bullets*, Center for Long-Term Care Financing, March 30, 2002.

17. Donald Jay Korn, "Choice Cuts," *Financial Planning*, February 2003, pg. 49+.

18. "Senate Action On Medicare Cuts Will Stop the Hemorrhaging," *PR Newswire*, January 24, 2003.

19. "AMA: New Medicare Payment Provisions Shore Up Medicare's Foundation," *PR Newswire*, February 14, 2003.

20. "Judge: HHS Must Notify on Medicare," *Associated Press*, August 13, 2001.

21. Melissa Gannon, "Rate Increases For Medigap Insurance Slow considerably Across the Board in 2002," *HIU Magazine*, November 2002, pg. 63+.

22. Anjetta McQueen, "Report: Medicare System Lacking," *Associated Press*, August 13, 2001.

23. Source: U.S. Census Bureau.

24. Carrie Teegardin, "Public putting heavy burden on Medicaid," *Atlanta Journal-Constitution*, August 4, 2002.

25. Source: Florida Agency for Health Care Administration, "A Snapshot of Florida Medicaid".

26. Source: The Kaiser Commission on Medicaid and the Uninsured report "The Role of Medicaid in State Budgets", October 2001.

27. "Study: Medicaid cuts hurt state economies," *USA Today*, January 16, 2003.

28. Bill Hogan, "States Eye Deep Medicaid Cuts," *AARP Bulletin*, January 2003.

29. Source: "State Health Policy Brief," National Conference of State Legislatures, September 2001.

30. "Medicaid Woes Worsen," *LTC Bullets*, Center for Long-Term Care Financing, March 7, 2002.

31. "Wake Up To The LTC Crisis!" *National Underwriter*, July 29, 2002, pg. 14.

32. Source: National Association of Health Underwriters.

33. Source: National Conference of State Legislatures, "Home and Community-Based Services for the Elderly and People with Disabilities," August 2002.

34. "New Long-Term Care Office Up and Running," *AARP Bulletin*, November 2002, pg. 13.

35. Source: "Health Care Policy Report," The Bureau of National Affairs, Inc., June 3, 2002.

36. Source: National Conference of State Legislatures, "Home and Community-Based Services for the Elderly and People With Disabilities," August 2002.

37. Stephen Moses, "Denial is not a River in Egypt," *LTC Bullet*, Center for Long Term Care Financing, September 2002.

38. Source: U.S. Census Bureau, "Health Insurance Coverage Status for 2001".

39. Stephen Moses, "Denial is not a River in Egypt," *LTC Bullet*, Center for Long Term Care Financing, September 2002.

40. Liz Taylor, "Many Well-To-Do Expect a Free Ride in Old Age," *Seattle Times*, February 10, 2003.

41. Michelle Higgins, "Getting Poor on Purpose," *Wall Street Journal*, February 25, 2003, pg. D1+.

42. Laura Parker, "Medicaid Patient Dies, Who Gets The House?" *USA Today*, May 1, 2002, pg. 1A+.

43. Michelle Higgins, "Getting Poor On Purpose," *Wall Street Journal*, February 25, 2003, pg. D1+.

44. Jennifer Frazier, "The State of Medicaid-Friendly Annuities," *Senior Market Advisor*, March 2003.

45. Stephen Moses, "Long-term Care Crisis Builds," *Health Care News*, March 2003, pg. 1.

46. Janelle Carter, "Medicare Reported Closer to Insolvency," *Associated Press*, March 18, 2003.

47. "Veterans Affairs Health System To Cease Active Recruiting," *Washington Times*, August 2, 2002.

48. For further information and assistance, write or call: Veterans Benefits Department, Paralyzed Veterans of America, 801 18th Street, NW, Washington, D.C. 20006, 1-800-424-8200.

Chapter 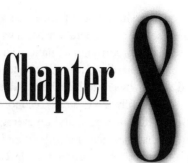 8

The Importance of Financial Planning

"I'm living so far beyond my income that we may almost be said to be living apart."

— e.e. cummings

"You can send a message around the world in one-seventh of a second, yet it may take years to move a simple idea through a quarter-inch of human skull."

— Charles F. Kettering

Sheryl and Chip Baggett were rolling along financially as they neared age 50. He's a pilot for U.S. Air, destined only a short time ago for years ahead of solid income and a building 401(k) that would ensure them $100,000/year during retirement. They have two kids in college and one in law school, with a 14-year-old still at home. Sheryl's biggest concern was picking out a color as she orchestrated the re-painting of the household. But now the airline industry is in trouble, Chip has taken a 35 percent paycut, they are up to their eyes in their children's college loans, and Chip is looking at a mandatory retirement age for pilots of 60, leaving only a few years to reverse this financial trend. What keeps Sheryl up at night these days? It's the prospect of losing their health insurance.[1]

Boomers (and others) are getting a huge dose of fiscal reality today. Long the spenders of the fruits of their labors, this generation has always thought that 'Rainy Days and Mondays" was a decent song, not a financial strategy. Now, they face an extraordinary uphill battle towards a future that suddenly looks financially desperate. The 80s and 90s now seem to have been a dream, or at best a significant aberration from the usually slow, steady economic growth that marked previous decades. But the future is near, and on average Boomers have saved only about 12 percent of what they need for retirement.[2] In the words of Harvard professor Elizabeth Warren, who studies middle class bankruptcy, "What does it mean to be 52 years old, college educated, professional, and broke – with a nice house in the suburbs and an SUV in the driveway and a 401(k) that's flat busted?"[3]

Times will, of course, change. Today's retirees' actual income sources include Social Security (44 percent), employer-funded pension plans (25 percent), personal savings (17 percent), sale of home or business (5 percent), other government programs (5 percent), support from children/family (4 percent) and employment (1 percent). Future retirees are expected to depend on these same income sources, but in differing amounts: personal savings (44 percent), employer-funded plans (21 percent), Social Security (13 percent), employment (9 percent), sale of home or business (6 percent), other government programs (less than 5 percent) and support from children/family (about 1 percent).[4] With the bulk of dependency coming from personal savings, it's no wonder fear of the future rules the day, given the deplorable savings habits of the Boomers.

Today, six in ten retirees opt to collect their Social Security benefits early (prior to normal retirement age).[5] However, this is sure to change if continued employment is necessary since earned income would offset any Social Security benefits during the early retirement stage and the financial benefits of working longer create an additional incentive to stay in the workforce. Employers can't afford to give people early retirement packages any longer, a situation that will continue to govern human resource departments in the future when older Boomers (50s and 60s) are still the dominant worker age group.

In 2003, retirees received the lowest Social Security raise in five years (1.4 percent translating to about $13 per month for the typical retiree). And part of this minimal increase would be offset by the $4.70 jump in Medicare Part B premium for 2003.[6] With Social Security the largest source of retirement dollars for the elderly, what would a long-term care burden do to this individual's (and family) finances?

Before one can consider the impact a long-term care illness will have on someone's finances, it is important to establish what type of financial picture lies in the future for the individual. Today's economic news seems to be "one darned thing after another" and financial planners have their hands full between declining incomes for seniors closing in on a long-term care need and declining savings opportunities and other monetary problems for Boomers.

Planning for the future is not only about estimating the amount of income one will need to maintain a reasonable standard of living. It's more about estimating the amount of expenses one could expect to have. Some financial advisers say your expense needs could be 40 to 60 percent of pre-retirement income depending on your needs. If a house is paid for, that means 40 percent could be a more likely figure, depending on the area of the country where you reside.[7] But long-term care expenses could change those estimates, unless some other planning is done in advance, such as the consideration of long-term care insurance.

As Boomers see their parents deal with long-term care issues, they become more definitive about protecting that part of their financial future. For Marian Ferziger, a 57-year-old New York accountant, the decision to buy her own long-term care insurance policy came after her mother-in-law applied for coverage in her 80s and was denied due to a health problem. She feels better for having bought it, not wanting to spend her assets on this type of care in the future.[8]

Women are primary targets for the long-term care aspect of financial planning. Everyone knows the longevity issue. Most women spend nearly a third of their lives financially independent. Combined with the statistics showing that 75 percent of residents in a nursing home are female, and the importance of long-term care as part of a financial planning strategy becomes obvious.[9]

Women have taken on more family financial responsibility than they have in the past. This includes sole or joint responsibility for IRAs, annuities, life insurance, and estate planning/wills, and 83 percent of women say they understand the amount of money that will be needed for a secure retirement. A 2002 Study on the Financial Experience and Behaviors Among Women also showed that eighty-four percent felt securing long-term care insurance was important, yet only 13 percent had done so.[10]

Most people realize financial planning is important but many procrastinate, thinking that there will be enough time later on to plan for the future. Yet, like Karen Parker mentioned in Chapter 1, the worse scenario is having to confront a long-term care situation without proper financial planning. With finances already in disarray or, at the least, clouded with incredible uncertainty, it is time for planners to be more proactive with their clients.

Family Discussions

Adult children should sit down and talk with their parents about their family's financial situation and decide on a plan of action for the future. If their parents haven't saved enough or planned for the possibility of long-term care, whether in a nursing home, an assisted living facility, or some other type of long-term care, this shortfall will also likely affect their children in the form of a need for financial, emotional or physical support.

Likewise, parents should willingly discuss financial matters with their children. This is especially difficult if it is a topic that has not been shared in the past. Many parents believe their finances are not their children's business and may resist their advice on financial matters even if those children are now in their 30's, 40's and 50's. Older Americans have a different view of money than today's generations, believing it to be more of a private matter and making the initiation of these important financial discussions all the more difficult.

Also critical in these "fireside chats" is what the parents would expect from their children should they become incapacitated and unable to make decisions or care for themselves. Where do they want to receive care? Who do they want to receive care from? Is it practical? Is it affordable – for parents and/or children? The financial road here runs both ways – a long-term care illness has ramification for both generations not only because of the physical need and the evident cost of long-term care, but because a number of Boomer adults today in their 40s and 50s still lean on their parents for help with the family, financial assistance and emotional support.[11] A long-term care illness can have dramatic consequences for the child even if no hands-on caregiving is required.

There are groups in America with strong family ties, making these talks more urgent than ever. The nation's fastest growing ethnic group are Hispanics, and they are "sandwiched" more than any other segments of American society. This is a product of the stalwart family bond Hispanics have, with parents often living with adult children, who in turn are assisting with taking care of their own children. This closeness is often deceiving in the case of preparedness. Because this multi-generation household is common, discussions about future planning are often avoided since there is the general philosophy that things will simply somehow work out. With thirty-one percent of Hispanics expecting to provide some financial support to elderly parents or in-laws, financial planning can't happen soon enough.[12]

But will it? There's a significant underestimation of the risk long-term care presents combined with an optimistic view of what dollars will be needed during retirement. According to a recent HIAA study, the general population perceives their risk to be about 25 percent that long-term care will be necessary in their lifetime. However, conservative estimates show there to be at least a 40 percent chance of this happening. Consumers are low in their estimates of the actual expenses involved and believe that government programs like Medicare can be relied on for constructive help.[13] These are dangerous assumptions and a recipe for future disaster if allowed to stand.

The Administration on Aging's *Profile of Older Americans: 2002* showed that in 2001 16.6 percent of the older population was poor or near-poor (less than 125 percent of poverty level). Older women had a higher poverty rate (12.4 percent) than older men (7 percent) in 2000. Older persons living alone or with nonrelatives were much more likely to be poor than were older persons living with families. The highest poverty rates were experienced by older Hispanic women who lived alone or with nonrelatives.[14] There are a number of individuals who are just getting by in their retirement years. The need for long-term medical care could destroy this already delicate balance. Two key markets for long-term care – women and Hispanics – are represented in this data.

The key to understanding the importance of long-term care financial planning is that death itself is often preceded by a lengthy disability that could cost thousands of dollars. An estate could be erased within a short period of time if proper planning has not been done.

This is where an insurance agent can play a vital role. Bridging the gap between parents and children is part of long-term care planning. The agent should be prepared to deal with a number of emotional issues as information is gathered. Some parents may not even want their children present. Others may not give the agent all of the information. There are people who still remember the "Great Depression" vividly and may not disclose the cash hidden under the mattress, or the money that is stashed away in a safety deposit box. Talking to both parents and children is the ideal situation because it often reveals most of the information that the agent needs in order to make a recommendation, and emphasizes that this is a problem every family member has a stake in solving.

How early should planning start? Obviously, as the Doan family discovered, the best time to plan is before something happens. A 1997 cartoon from *The New Yorker* showed an elementary school age boy with a briefcase talking with a girl of the same age and saying, "Do you have a minute to talk about your retirement years?"[15]

There are no communication strategies that work for all families and all situations, but the earlier planning begins the better. Parents want to control their own lives, and it's important children (and planners) keep this in mind as talks about planning progress. Parents generally do not want children to make their decisions for them, so even though children may be more motivated to make something happen, it's best to initially move at the parents' speed and see where that takes you. Their safety is an overriding concern for all involved, and it's the reason long-term care can be a vital part of the planning talks.[16]

A clear sign of the financial times today is that the majority of baby boomers no longer finance their children's weddings. Fully 70 percent of today's couples pay for their own nuptials.[17] With aging parents, children's college loans still being paid off, and retirement funds far behind the need, some traditional expenses are being passed over. It's important that long-term care insurance be recognized as a critical potential souce of funds for the future and not another insurance premium that can be ignored.

I have a friend who suffered a brain-stem stroke at age 41 and will need long-term nursing care for several years. This convinced me to add long-term care coverage to my own insurance portfolio at age 43. Timing is everything, but part of the planning process is knowing when LTC insurance rates will begin to climb for long-term care policies. Generally, by one's late 50's, new business premiums are starting to make significant jumps. Making it a part of pre-retirement estate planning is simply a must.

Data Gathering

Before any long-term care recommendations can be made, one must review the individual's assets and income that would be protected, in addition to hearing what the specific needs someone might have should a long-term care event occur.

There are two components to the data gathering process – words and numbers. Data gathering is critical to long-term care planning because the words and numbers dictate a plan of action. If the client has an attorney and/or an accountant, it is best to involve them from the beginning – along with family members – since they may play a role in carrying out part of the agent's recommendations. There are some legal and financial issues that should be carried out by most everyone.

Words

As the agent, it is important to construct a profile of your client. Asking specific questions can gauge the person's ability to comprehend and follow through on the proposals the agent makes. This will also help the agent assess whether or not this client is a candidate for long-term care insurance.

This data gathering process will help the agent identify a person's recent health history and estate planning, if any. It will also provide important contacts in the event the agent may have to call them on behalf of the client in case of an emergency and gives the agent an essential profile of the client. Figure 8.1 shows the questions that should be asked.

FIGURE 8.1

Data Gathering Questions to Ask in Long-Term Care Planning

Questions to ask:

Name: _____ Date-of-Birth _____ Age _____

Social Security Number: _____Telephone:_____

Address:_____

City _____ State _____ Zip Code _____

Occupation_____

Employer (Current or Retired From): _____

Health Benefits Provided by Employer: _____

Smoker? _____ Height & Weight_____

Current Physician_____

Have you been hospitalized in the last 5 years?_____

FIGURE 8.1 (continued)

If so, give more details, including date and current prognosis: _____

_____

Are you currently taking medication?_____

If so, please list: _____

_____

On Medicare?_____

On Medicaid?_____

Important names and phone numbers:

Attorney _____

Accountant _____

Stockbroker _____

Clergy _____

Closest relative _____

Closest friend _____

Other agent or financial planner _____

Account number and location of key documents:

Safe deposit box: _____

Bank: _____

Home: _____

Office: _____

Other: _____

Do you have:

Will? _____

Powers of Attorney   Financial: _____ Medical:_____

Special bequests: _____

Burial instructions: _____

Before proceeding in obtaining financial information, it is important to focus on several of these key data elements just collected.

1.   *Will.* This is an important issue. There are many elderly people that do not have a will. The purpose of a will is to determine how the estate is to be distributed. Financial planning may be almost worthless without this document. If a person's net worth is more than $1,000,000 (in 2003) or a couple's net worth exceeds $2,000,000 (2003), certain trusts can help avoid probate and estate taxes. The exempt estate value amounts, below which estate taxes are not required, will be increasing each year for the next several years, until a one-year repeal in year 2010. But estate taxes will revert back to 2002 levels in year 2011, making planning and periodic reviews all the more important. One should check with the family accountant or attorney for the current year information.

2.   *Financial Durable Power of Attorney.* This document allows the person appointed to sign an individual's name and to legally conduct affairs on behalf of the individual. If one or both parents are incapacitated, this document is crucial. Without it, bank accounts may not be accessed, bills may not be paid, checks may not be signed, and the entire family financial situation placed in turmoil.

While this frenzy can be avoided with a financial durable power of attorney form, it is easier said than done. Asking a parent to give someone else (especially a child) access to their hard-earned assets and a license to handle all of the financial affairs is a scary proposition to many. It's not so much a matter of trust (although it can be) as it is a matter of giving up control and the ability to make decisions for themselves. If there are concerns of this nature, powers can be designed to be triggered at a specific time such as only when the individual(s) become disabled.

Then as long as the person who is assigning the financial durable power of attorney is capable of making decisions, he or she will continue to do so. The purpose of the financial durable power of attorney is to have a contingency plan in the event of an unexpected inability to communicate. Without someone to take over the financial affairs, control is then truly lost.

Anyone age 18 or older and of sound mind generally can be designated as the holder of the power of attorney. The selection of the proper individual is an important part of the entire planning process, since much responsibility is given this person. The individual chosen should be willing to respect and honor the individual's wishes. The oldest child may not be the best choice if he lives 3,000 miles away or is not trustworthy or does not have the parent's best interests at heart. Careful consideration should be given to this issue.

3.   *Medical Durable Power of Attorney.* While the financial aspect of this legal preparation allows someone to conduct financial affairs for your client, the holder of the financial durable power of attorney cannot make medical decisions unless a medical durable power of attorney form has also been signed. This form, also called a Health Care Surrogate form, puts the appointed individual in a position one hopes never to be in – to make crucial medical decisions on behalf of another who is incapable of making decisions such as withdrawing life support systems or authorizing the donation of vital organs. Some durable power of attorney forms have both a financial and medical section.

For many hospitals, the medical durable power of attorney form carries legal authority that living wills (in many states) do not have even though both documents may contain the same requests. There are many individuals who do not wish to be kept alive in certain circumstances, for example, and these wishes would have been discussed in advance with the holder of the medical durable power of attorney.

The living will is not legally binding on a physician so in this respect it is not the same as the medical durable power of attorney. With concerns over malpractice, a doctor is not likely to carry out the patient's wishes specified in a living will. A physician could, however, carry out the directives voiced by the person given medical durable power of attorney on behalf of another.

If a person has specific medical requests, they should be discussed with the person given the authority to make medical decisions. Many people do not want to stay technically "alive" at enormous costs, especially if there is little hope of recovery. This can be avoided with the medical durable power of attorney form.

Longer life spans increasingly mean that people are likely to die of extended illnesses. Modern medicine enables a person to stay alive for extended periods of time, perhaps longer than a person would want. Machines can keep vital signs running properly even if the patient is unconscious with little hope of recovery. While it is a difficult subject to discuss, there are many who have strong convictions about these matters and will be receptive to signing a medical durable power of attorney form.

These documents are vital to the success of a long-term care financial planning program. Without them, a complete and proper job cannot be done for the client who relies on the agent's advice. Scenarios like the following, contained in a letter to the editor of the magazine *Sandwich Generation*, may develop.

A daughter has been caring for her comatose mother for nearly ten years. She has been signing her mother's Social Security checks and using the money (plus some of her own) to pay for full-time home health care (not covered by Medicare). No durable power of attorney forms, financial or medical, were signed. For some unknown reason, Social Security records indicated that her mother was deceased which would prevent any further Social Security payments. The daughter had to prove to the Social Security administration that her mother was technically "alive."

Because the daughter signed the checks, Social Security had the right to ask for an accounting of the money spent. Since the cost of home health care exceeded her mother's Social Security check, this wasn't hard to prove. However, now she has to continually provide this information to Social Security in order for the checks to keep coming in. If a financial durable power of attorney form had been signed, the checks would have been automatically deposited into her mother's bank account and she would have had the authority to write checks on her mother's account. With a medical durable power of attorney, she could also have stopped her mother's life support system some time ago.

But she didn't have these options and the documentation required by Social Security would have been substantial if the cost of care hadn't exceeded her mother's check. While there were many other expenses she could have claimed on her mother to justify the check, the monthly documentation alone would have been a considerable burden.

Fortune magazine published some questions for children to answer if they were concerned about a parent's finances. A "yes" answer to the following questions indicated that both parent and children are prepared for the financial future:[18]

"Do your parents have a will that has been reviewed within the past three years?"

"Do you know where to find all your parents' financial and legal papers and advisers?"

"Do you know the approximate annual cost of maintaining your parents' current lifestyle in retirement, and do you know if they have sufficient resources to do so?"

"Have you reviewed their assets to ensure there will be enough cash readily available to pay any estate taxes due within nine months of death?"

"Have you reviewed the tax consequences of your parents' retirement plans, including the plan balances and beneficiary designations?"

Working closely with the client and his attorney will enable the agent to recommend and follow through in getting a will drawn up and the necessary durable power of attorney forms signed. From there, the next step is the numbers.

Numbers

Figure 8.2 gives a synopsis of the financial information needed to create a financial planning analysis.

FIGURE 8.2

Data Gathering Form for Long-Term Planning

Find Your Net Worth

Assets	Amount
Checking Accounts	_____
Savings Accounts	_____
Home or other Real Estate	_____
Live Insurance Cash Value	_____
Annuities	_____
Retirement Equity	
(pension, 401(k))	_____
Stocks (market value)	_____
Bonds (market value)	_____
Mutual Funds	
(market value)	_____
Other Investments	
(collectibles)	_____
Automobile	_____
Household Appliances	
and Furnishings	_____
Loans Owed to You	_____
Other Assets	_____
Total Assets	

Liabilities	
Current Bills	_____
Auto Loans	_____
Credit Card Balances	_____
Mortgage Balance	_____
Student Loans	_____
Other Debts	_____
Total Liabilities	_____

Your Net Worth	
(Assets Minus Liabilities)	_____

Check Your Cash Flow

Income	Monthly Amount
Take Home Pay	_____
Overtime	_____
Bonuses	_____
Social Security	_____
Interest Dividends	_____
Other Income	_____
Total Cash Income	_____

Expenses	
Mortgage or Rent	_____
Credit Card Payments	_____
Alimony, Child Support	_____
Insurance (auto, home	
health, medical	
and so on)	_____
Food	_____
Utilities (heat, phone,	
electricity and so on)	_____
Child Care	_____
Personal Care (clothing,	
hair cosmetics	
and so on)	_____
Medical Bills Not	
Paid by Insurance	_____
Education Expenses	_____
Recreation	_____
Donations	_____
Savings	_____
Gifts	_____
Miscellaneous	_____
Total Expenses	_____

Income Surplus or Deficit	
(Income Minus Expenses)	_____

An asset and liability review will yield a net worth number. Married individuals with a net worth below $100,000 (not including a home or one car) may qualify for Medicaid in a relatively short period of time, thus the money spent on long-term care insurance would not be worth it as there are very few assets that need to be protected.

The $100,000 figure is merely a guideline. There may be families with a net worth of $100,000 or less that desire long-term care insurance and can afford it. There may be people with a $150,000 net worth who do not want the coverage or cannot afford it. The use of a rule-of-thumb asset guideline is dangerous in that everyone's financial situation is different. The cost of long-term care varies widely across the country, and there will be some areas of the country where the cost of LTC is relatively low and likely corresponds with the standard of living for the area. Someone with a lower net worth who lives in an area where costs are low may still be a viable candidate for long-term care insurance, while a higher net-worth person in a more expensive part of the country may not take that long to spend down.[19]

Ultimately, the agent will have to use his own judgment, based on the person's information, when recommending long-term care insurance.

The NAIC, in its model regulation for LTC insurance, suggests that consumers should be discouraged from buying a policy if the premiums account for more than 7 percent of income or if the purchaser does not have at least $35,000 in financial assets. This is only intended as a guideline, too. It has been noted that many elderly already devote a substantial share of their income to medical care and health insurance, and thus 7 percent may not be a sustainable guideline for some.[20]

A 2003 Kaiser Family Foundation Report indicated that three out of four married couples could theoretically afford long-term care insurance, using affordability criteria adopted by the American Council of Life Insurers. Yet, only one in five is adequately protected in all the other areas, including retirement savings, life, health and disability insurance. This data suggests that a great many families who can afford long-term care insurance are not yet preparing for retirement, or are not protected against life contingencies that could arise before expected retirement age, underscoring the importance of financial planning. The numbers:[21]

Age of household head	Households (000s)	Can afford LTCI	AND has adequate savings	AND has adequate life ins.	AND has health insurance	AND has disability insurance
35-44	10,323	73%	57%	30%	29%	18%
45-54	10,605	80%	52%	39%	36%	21%
55-59	3,411	72%	43%	39%	37%	25%
Total	24,340	76%	53%	35%	33%	20%

These numbers are guidelines to follow and decisions should generally be based on the client's specific needs and preferences.

As mentioned, income and expenses are equally important. Getting an idea of an individual's cash flow will give the agent information on two key factors:

1. *Income surplus.* This indicates the ability to afford the premium for long-term care insurance. Long-term care insurance is not for everyone. A large amount of discretionary income indicates both an ability to pay and a sizable income and asset base to protect.

2. *Liquidity.* The amount of cash can be important later in determining the length of time the client can self-insure before needing long-term care insurance benefits. This will help in deciding on the elimination period (i.e., the number of days before policy benefits are payable) too. For more information on this topic, see Chapter 9, "A Long-term Care Sales Presentation."

The financial analysis is critical in setting up guidelines in order to establish a financial plan. The plan should be updated annually based on current circumstances.

A new educational web site, www.PlanLTC.com is designed to help seniors and their families assess how likely an individual is to need long-term care and to explore a full range of options that can be used to pay for care. Based on the individual's need and financial situation, this site suggests generic categories of long-term care financing options for consideration. Among these options are:[22]

- self-funding

- government-financed Medicaid

- whole life insurance with LTC benefits

- deferred annuity with long-term care benefits

- long-term care insurance

- variable universal life with long-term care benefits, and

- immediate annuities.

There are ways to determine self-insurance costs for the client to compare with the long-term care insurance choice. You certainly want the client to be comfortable financially with the decision to purchase coverage. It might be worth pointing out, however, that in 2002, over $1 billion worth of annual benefits were paid to Americans who have a long-term care insurance policy. In a report by the NAIC, through the year 2000, actual cumulative incurred claims of all LTC policies ever written hit $11.1 billion.[23] Long-term care insurance can, and does, work for individuals and families.

But you also know there are reasons – other than financial – why people purchase long-term care insurance, emotional reasons that include preservation of financial independence, avoidance of dependency on children or relatives, estate conservation for heirs and avoidance of Medicaid and the resulting loss of control.

Still, there will be people who decide that Medicaid spend-down, despite federal legislation discouraging it, is the better path to pursue. They should be prepared for the potential consequences that Medicaid patients have a harder time getting into a quality nursing home because Medicaid is the lowest payer to LTC providers of any third party involved in the financing of long-term care expenses. (See Chapter 7, "Government Programs.")

Long-term care insurance can be one of several financial sources to help pay the costs of nursing home or other services. The decisions that will be made hinge on the specific information uncovered during this financial planning process. Every client is different and so, too, will be his or her needs. Ask the questions, take down the information and their wishes, and help your clients plan accordingly.

The client will probably ask many questions during this process. Be prepared to answer as many as possible and elicit the assistance of other key players (e.g., an accountant or attorney) and family members.

Reverse Mortgages

A reverse mortgage allows people to borrow on the equity in their home, creating a stream of monthly payments or a line of credit. For those who rely only on Social Security, this could be a critical flow of income. People like Helen Grady, for example. A 76-year-old Pennsylvania widow, living on her $1,008/month Social Security payment with rising property taxes, a leaky roof, a contaminated well and a broken dishwasher. She was in real danger of losing the house and having it sold off to pay taxes, leaving her without shelter. A reverse mortgage let her stay in her house, and generated a monthly payment stream that let her make the necessary repairs and pay her taxes.[24]

You must be age 62 or older to receive income payments. The "loan" is paid when the property is sold after the owner's death, with the heirs splitting the remaining equity.

Some data suggests that there are a significant number of homeowners over age 70 whose low income stream may make them viable candidates for this option. There are even some insurance carriers reinsuring the risk that the homeowner lives too long, much like an annuity calculation.

Seniors should be careful about this option, however. There are substantial costs that are associated with reverse mortgages that are often rolled into the loan, so it is easy to ignore them. These include initial mortgage insurance premiums, origination fees, and other costs normally associated with a mortgage.[25]

There are also numerous reverse mortgage scams that have surfaced over the last few years. The National Center for Home Equity Conversion warns homeowners about reverse mortgage "specialists" who offer them monthly income payments for a fee and then refer them to a reverse mortgage lender when homeowners can go directly to reverse mortgage lenders themselves without the necessity of paying a fee.

The National Reverse Mortgage Lenders Association reported for the fiscal year ending September 30, 2002, that lenders closed a record 13,049 reverse mortgages, a remarkable 63 percent increase over the previous record of 7,982 in 1999. Los Angeles, Denver, New York, Detroit, San Francisco, Chicago, Seattle, Santa Ana, Richmond and Newark were the top 10 areas where seniors sought these loans.[26]

Summary

If an agent has done a thorough job of gathering data, he will be prepared for the variety of questions and emotional issues that will surface. Despite the enormous challenges of today's tumultuous economic climate, this data gathering will make it easier to prepare a financial plan and, if appropriate, a long-term care insurance solution. Failure to understand what long-term care is, how it is financed, and the resulting impact on lifetime savings, exposes clients to potential financial ruin, and planners to lawsuits for breach of fiduciary obligation.[27] Yes, long-term care planning is that important.

Chapter Notes

1. Betsy Morris, "Is Your Retirement at Risk?" *Fortune,* March 17, 2003, p. 58.
2. Stephen A. Moses, "Wake Up, Little Susie, Wake Up," *LTC Bullet,* Center for Long-Term Care Financing, June 22, 2002.
3. Betsy Morris, "Is Your Retirement at Risk?" *Fortune,* March 17, 2003, p. 60.
4. Source: Employee Benefit Research Institute, "Paying for Retirement," *2002 Retirement Confidence Survey,* with American Savings Education Council and Mathew Greenwald & Associates.
5. Dan Moreau, "Payday: Sooner or Later?," *AARP Bulletin* (November, 2002), p. 26.
6. Martin Crutsinger, "Lowest Social Security Raise Since '98," *Associated Press,* October 18, 2002.
7. Fred Brock, "How Much Will You Need to Retire?" *New York Times,* March 17, 2002, p. BU8.
8. Eileen Alt Powell, "Boomers consider costs of future skilled-care needs," *Daytona Beach News-Journal,* July 7, 2002, p. 3E.
9. Merry Mosbacher, "Why Insurance Is Attractive To Women," *National Underwriter,* Life & Health/Financial Services Edition, January 13, 2003, p. 11.
10. Marcella De Simone, "Survey Highlights Planning Gap Between Knowing and Doing of Baby Boom Women," *National Underwriter,* Life & Health/Financial Services Edition, November 4, 2002, p. 28.
11. Sandra Timmermann, EdD, "Financial Gerontology," *Journal of Financial Service Professionals* (September, 2001), p. 36.
12. Chuck Jones, "Heavily Burdened," *Advisor Today* (March, 2003), p. 28.
13. Scott Perry, "Raising America's LTC IQ," *Best's Review* (November, 2002), p. 75.
14. Source: "A Profile of Older Americans: 2002," Administration on Aging and U.S. Census Bureau.

15. Cartoon appeared in *The New Yorker*, double issue of April 28 and May 5, 1997.

16. Sandra Timmermann, EdD, "Financial Gerontology," *Journal of Financial Service Professionals* (September, 2001), p. 38.

17. Amy Baldwin, "Boomers no longer expected to pay for kids' weddings," *Daytona Beach News-Journal.*

18. Susan E. Kuhn, "Dealing with your Parents' Finances," *Fortune*, September 30, 1996, p. 275.

19. Marilee Driscoll, "Setting Asset Level Guidelines for LTC Can Be Dangerously Simple," *National Underwriter*, Life & Health/Financial Services Edition, January 20, 2003, p. 8.

20. Source: Kaiser Family Foundation Report, "Long-Term Care Insurance: Who Should Buy It and Why Should They Buy?" (March, 2003).

21. Source: 1998 Survey of Consumer Finances, using ACLI premiums and thresholds, from Kaiser Family Foundation (March, 2003).

22. "New PlanLTC.com Website Helps Seniors Assess Potential Need for Long-Term Care," *PR Newswire*, February 12, 2002.

23. "Consumers Benefit," *Advisor Today* (March, 2003), p. 30.

24. Janelle Carter, "Reverse mortgages catching on with cash-poor seniors," *Daytona Beach News-Journal*, January 12, 2003, p. 1F.

25. Source: NAHU Long-Term Care Working Group, Reverse Mortgage Project, 2003.

26. Janelle Carter, "Reverse mortgages catching on with cash-poor seniors," *Daytona Beach News-Journal*, January 13, 2003, p. 1F.

27. Harley Gordon, "Planners Have a Fiduciary Obligation to Recommend LTC Insurance," *National Underwriter*, Life & Health/Financial Services Edition, August 6, 2001, p. 17.

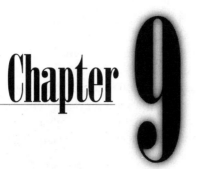

Chapter 9

A Long-Term Care Sales Presentation

"Wisdom doesn't come automatically with old age. Nothing does – except wrinkles. It's true, some wines improve with age. But only if the grapes were good in the first place."

— Abigail Van Buren

Obtaining financial data from a client is only the beginning of the sales process. As noted in Chapter 8, "The Importance of Financial Planning," data gathering gives you enough information to tailor a solution to the client's long-term care needs. That solution must be arrived at from the client's own individual numbers. The second interview is when you present the answer to funding this critical health care financing need.

The market is extensive, as detailed in Chapter 2, "Today's Changing Demographics." There are more than 40 million Americans ages 50-64, and 35 million people ages 65 and older.[1] The government, in the form of the Health Insurance Portability and Accountability Act of 1996 (HIPAA), has sent the message that it is not assuming any more long-term care risk. That leaves it up to individuals to take personal responsibility for the financing of this potential health care risk.

The long-term care market has been in a relative holding pattern for the last few years. The number of insurers has not grown and the number of policies sold actually declined for a couple of years. For a time, people waited to see if the Clinton health plan (proposed in 1993-94) would provide significant long-term care benefits. It did not, and never saw the Congressional light of day anyway. Then, along came HIPAA, and tax clarification came, both favorable and controversial. But it only boosted sales briefly, with a fire sale in the last quarter of 1996 as agents rushed to "grandfather" in tax-qualified plans. Since then, progress has been slow.

The passage of HIPAA did give consumers some direction in addressing their long-term care needs. But there is more to a market than seeing an opportunity. To be truly successful at assisting people with their long-term care needs, you need to believe unequivocally in the product's value.

My first long-term care client was my mother. Approaching your own parents and relatives for the purpose of selling long-term care insurance is an excellent way to enter this market. Writing that policy on her several years ago opened up this market for me and gave her peace of mind about the issue. She did not want her children burdened with either the cost or responsibility of taking care of her should the need arise. With long-term care insurance, she has relieved herself of this concern. I learned from the experience and was able to "practice" solving these needs with my own mother. What more natural market is there than your own family?

To successfully present a product, you must firmly believe in the product yourself. With insurance, that usually means purchasing coverage on yourself. This also applies to long-term care insurance. Depending on your age, selling long-term care insurance to a family member is just as effective.

However, selling to family members may not be that easy. Long-term care is a very emotional subject and, like your clients, family members might be "guarded" on issues involving long-term care insurance. Many parents are not enthusiastic about sharing financial information with their children, nor do they want to discuss nursing homes, moving into a child's home, or anything related to long-term care.

However, never forget that the long-term care insurance sale is about family. As has been previously pointed out in this book, the need for long-term care will impact more family members than just the one who needs the care. This is true with yours as much as anyone else's family. Solving one need also helps take care of potential problems for others. You are just as likely a candidate for caregiving as for needing the care.

Approaching parents on this subject is good practice to perfect your sales presentation. This will help you prepare for any objections that might arise from recommending long-term care insurance as an alternative financial solution to a potentially devastating situation. Parents can also be excellent centers of influence.

There are three essential types of prospects for long-term care insurance. These are: people over age 65, people under age 65, and employers and their employees. Each of these units likely has a different motivation for considering long-term care insurance as a solution to a need. Once you understand what these key beliefs are for each group, you should be successful at implementing long-term care insurance, when appropriate, as a financing vehicle for long-term care expenses.

The Benefits of Long-Term Care Insurance

In September 2002, the Health Insurance Association of America (HIAA) published a report regarding the benefits of long-term care insurance to consumers. A summary of their findings, is as follows:[2]

Benefits to Policyholders:

- Having long-term care insurance allows disabled elders to remain in their homes and delay or avoid using institutional services.

- Disabled elders with private long-term care insurance receive an average of 14 more hours of personal care per week than similarly disabled non-privately insured elders.

- Having a long-term care insurance policy reduces by 66 percent a person's chances of having to spend his or her assets to pay for nursing home care to the point of impoverishment and Medicaid eligibility.

- Long-term care insurance reduces the out-of-pocket expenses for disabled elders. The average reduction of out-of-pocket nursing home costs is between $60,000 and $75,000 and can total more than $100,000 for assisted living costs.

- Buying long-term care insurance makes purchasers feel more secure about their future and better about the way they plan to secure that future.

Benefits to Family Caregivers:

- Family caregivers suffer less stress if the disabled elder they are caring for has private long-term care insurance.

- Working age family caregivers double their chances of remaining in the workforce if the disabled elder they are caring for has private long-term care insurance. These caregivers also experience significantly fewer work disruptions and social stresses.

As you work in any of the three identified market segments for long-term care, keep in mind these insurance benefits as this is information you will want to share with a prospect, either in obtaining the appointment or in making the presentation. Yours is a difficult job in many respects – you have to motivate healthy people to consider a possible unhealthy future. But the benefits of insurance for the right prospect can often carry the day. The disabled person with long-term care insurance will have eased at least one burden of an injury or illness – the financial one. This can help the person focus on physical recovery without the economic worry that can slow down, or often derail, a recovery.

Networking

A considerable amount of publicity in the last few years concerning long-term care insurance has heightened consumer interest in this product. From *Consumer Reports* to *USA Today* to *Money* magazine, people of all ages have read something, somewhere, about long-term care insurance.

With this public awareness, you have an opportunity to start building a base of potential prospects. It is easier to approach individuals about a subject that is in the news on a daily basis.

There are four areas in which to prospect: (1) parents, relatives, and their referrals; (2) existing clients; (3) professionals and organizations that are involved in long-term care situations; and (4) businesses and their employees.

1. *Parents* – This is the beginning of a long list of prospects. In addition to parents, your aunts, uncles, grandparents, in-laws, and other family members are a great source of prospects for long-term care insurance. Referrals from family members will provide daily activity and an opportunity for making long-term care presentations and recommendations for a long time in a generally warm market atmosphere.

2. *Existing clients* – If you already have existing clients, this is another excellent place to start. An agent with a large number of disability income clients can begin identifying the ones age 50 and over. The need for disability income coverage will begin to taper off in one's 50s and the need for long-term care protection will ultimately replace it. If a client already understands disability income, it is an easy transition to long-term care. (See Chapter 10, "Long-term Care versus Disability Income Product Design.") If you do not sell much disability income coverage, look at your client list over age 50. These are all potential long-term care prospects. Chapter 8 gave you some guidance on the income and asset requirements for a good prospect. If you have this information, review it against your guidelines to pre-qualify the prospect.

3. *Professionals and organizations* – These prospects easily recognize the need for long-term care insurance and may be receptive to the idea themselves. With continual association with the elderly in some aspect or another, these prospects should be able to provide a long list of additional potential prospects. This group includes:

    Health care providers. What better group to talk to about long-term care insurance than home health care workers, nursing home employees, private duty nurses, durable equipment salespersons, hospital workers, and physicians? As the population continues to age, the need for long-term care will increase. The medical field – providers and health care services organizations – is rapidly expanding each year into long-term care services. The fastest growing occupations in the job market over the past decade are consistently in the long-term care field. This prospect list alone can be extensive.

    Attorneys. Specializing in elder care law, these attorneys deal with clients who are concerned with protecting themselves and their wealth. Making these attorneys aware of your services in the long-term care insurance area could result in qualified prospects for you. When contacting these professionals, prepare a long-term care sales presentation as you would for a client. This will help the attorney in understanding the need for long-term care insurance and how it can benefit his clients (and his own family – don't forget that he is a prospect, too). It will also make it easier for the attorney to refer clients to you for long-term care insurance.

CPAs. The same approach used for attorneys would also apply to CPAs. Knowledge of long-term care insurance will assist CPAs in their financial discussions with clients. Clarification by Congress of the tax consequences of the long-term care product has helped give CPAs more confidence in this financing solution. The American Institute of Certified Public Accountants has recently created a "senior-specialist" CPA sub-specialty, so if you can, look to this group of CPAs first.

Bankers. These individuals do a considerable amount of trust work with older people and can be an excellent source for prospects. For example, a person who has established a living trust indicates a willingness to do some financial planning and may be agreeable to a presentation on long-term care insurance. Banks tend to do well with seminars. Bank customers are often more comfortable coming to a bank-sponsored event, and many of them have questions about this subject, so long-term care insurance as a topic would likely be a good draw.

Churches and synagogues. Your own religious affiliation can provide you with another source of prospective clients. While a minister, priest, or rabbi deals with family long-term care issues, these organizations also focus on older, senior members of the congregation and provide activities designed exclusively for them. Contacts here can further add to your list of prospects.

Rotary Clubs, Kiwanis, etc. These types of group meetings are always looking for speakers, especially those with a timely topic. What could be more relevant than long-term care needs? Senior groups would seem to be a natural audience, but often you are better accessing seniors through one of the other outlets noted above. Look for investment clubs, especially female-oriented ones. The recent stock market slide has forced people to reevaluate their needs and investment choices, and asset protection is a critical subject. Long-term care insurance is a great asset protection tool.

4. *Businesses and their Employees* – Without question, a number of people in their 40s and early 50s are discovering through firsthand experience the emotional and economic impact of a parent or relative requiring long-term care services. They have become caregivers and their work absences have likely contributed to some type of deficit at work – in revenue or work load. Due to these personal experiences, they want to preserve their independence and protect their assets – two solid reasons to consider long-term care coverage. With these "younger" prospects showing an interest, insurers have begun to develop and market employer-based long-term care coverage. Employers, especially those with 50 to 75 employees or more, are sensitive to employee benefit programs. With respect to how an employee would seek medical assistance and the restrictions put on health insurance, employers are softening the blow by offering additional coverage options. One of these options is long-term care. If you have employer-clients already, you should contact them about this valuable employee benefit. The premium savings generated by buying younger can be substantial over the long haul, due to lower initial premiums, and a lesser impact of potential future rate increases. Property & Casualty agents should include long-term care proposals for the principals of any commercial account each year they return to implement that year's renewal coverage. You have taught them how to protect their business assets and now is the time to focus on protecting their personal assets as well. For more on employer-sponsored long-term care, see Chapter 19, Employer-Sponsored Long-term Care Insurance."

The Approach

Now that you have a list of contacts, the question is what is the best way to approach them on the concept of long-term care insurance? The best approach will vary with your own strengths and experience.

Telephone Calls

For individuals with whom you have some relationship, either personally or professionally, the phone is often the best way to try and secure an appointment.

At this point, you should not attempt to sell a concept or product over the phone, but to secure an appointment to discuss a few estate planning ideas that can save money. It may be that your contact has no need for your services but this is not easily discerned over the phone. You should at least discuss the idea briefly with the prospect. Remember, unlike life insurance, long-term care does not protect against the inevitable. Some people will die peacefully in their sleep and never need a day of long-term care services. Resistance to a discussion about the possibilities of long-term care is a trait this product shares with disability income. Healthy people need some prompting to discuss a potential unhealthy future. Be sensitive to this early objection and advise that you only want a few minutes of the individual's time to discuss some pre-retirement estate planning concepts. You can discuss long-term care insurance in detail at the interview and fact-find. The telephone call is only meant to secure a prospect. Use some of the HIAA LTC insurance benefits listed earlier to help solidify the reason for an appointment.

Letters

Mass mailings are a numbers game. The more mailings you send, the more responses you are likely to get. There are lists available that can be purchased and, depending on your criteria, they can identify ages, income, or net worth of people in your community. The list might initially be limited to the more likely qualified buyers of long-term care insurance. These are individuals ages 65-74, who have more than $40,000 in annual income, $100,000 to $600,000 of liquid assets, and live in single-family homes, retirement communities, or senior high-rises.[3] Your letter should be brief and to the point. Depending on your approach in soliciting business, there are several options available. A letter can indicate that you will be calling them to set up an appointment or it can invite the reader to attend a free seminar on long-term care. Letters #1 and #2 in Figures 9.1 and 9.2 are samples for such approaches. In Figure 9.3 Letter #3 is a sample letter for a professional or an organization. This letter suggests working as a team to meet the long-term care needs of their members or clients. After all, that's what you plan to do. If this was a campaign slogan, you could call it "It's Their Numbers, Stupid." A letter should also state the intent to follow-up whether it is with a phone call or a postage-paid return envelope. It is up to you to decide which action to take. The most common is a phone call as a follow-up to a letter.

FIGURE 9.1   **Letter #1**

June 1, 2003

Mr. And Mrs. Alfred Bridge
1050 Tara Boulevard
Atlanta, GA. 30328

Dear Mr. And Mrs. Bridge:

It's a tragedy!

Perhaps you've read about it happening to someone in your town; a person whose lifetime savings is spent on health care that's not fully covered by Medicare. The costs associated with health care and aging are increasing and the alternatives to financing these necessary services are few.

If your desires are to:

1.   Maintain your independence;

2.   Retain your dignity;

3.   Avoid depending on your children;

4.   Eliminate the financial concerns of a long life span; and

5.   Provide an inheritance for children and grandchildren,

you will be interested in hearing a few ideas that can let you accomplish these important wishes and goals.

I will be in your area the week of _____ and plan on calling you in advance to see if we can schedule some time to discuss these important ideas to help you avoid future financial concerns.

I look forward to meeting you.

Sincerely,

FIGURE 9.2

Letter #2

June 1, 2003

Mr. And Mrs. Alfred Bridge
1050 Tara Boulevard
Atlanta, GA. 30328

Dear Mr. And Mrs. Bridge:

Lately, you may have noticed an increasing number of news stories on the subject of long-term care. Perhaps you, like many people, are both confused and concerned about this important issue.

The need for long-term care is unpredictable, but the risk is higher than you think. According to the author of *J.K. Lassers's Choosing the Right Long-Term Care Insurance*, 60 percent of Americans age 50 and above need to look into a private source of funding a future long-term care need.

I am personally sponsoring a free seminar on the facts concerning the issue of long-term care. In this 45 minute session, I will provide you with data and information that can help you sort out your own concerns about this subject.

The seminar, entitled *Everything You Need To Know About Long-term Care* will be held at the Embassy Suites in Dunwoody at the following times: 10:00 A.M., 2:00 P.M. and 7:00 P.M. Light refreshments will be provided. There is no charge to attend.

I look forward to seeing you there.

Sincerely,

___ YES I'd like to attend your seminar at: ___ 10:00 AM ___ 2:00 PM ___ 7:00 PM

___ NO, I cannot attend, but please send me more information about long-term care.

FIGURE 9.3 **Letter #3**

June 1, 2003

Ms. Michelle Truman
205 State Street, Suite 214
Springfield, MA 01106

Dear Ms. Truman:

A loved one in need of long-term care services is an emotional event that we all would like to avoid. Yet, in increasing numbers, many of us are facing the necessity of arranging for care for loved ones suffering from a chronic health condition.

As a professional servicing the mature individual, you hold a unique position. You will often be sought for advice and direction on this issue of long-term care. As such, my firm may be able to assist you.

The improvement in long-term care policies over the last few years has made this product a viable option for many mature individuals with assets to protect. This product is becoming the program of choice for those planning ahead for their financial future. Long-term care insurance can let individuals maintain independence, avoid depending on their children, retain their dignity, and provide an inheritance for their loved ones.

A recent report on the benefits of long-term care insurance found that having a long-term care insurance policy reduces by 66 percent a person's chances of having to spend his or her assets to pay for long-term care to the point of impoverishment and Medicaid eligibility.

From one professional to another, I am enclosing my card. I would like to schedule a convenient time to stop by and discuss how we can work jointly on behalf of your clients.

I will call you next week to identify an appropriate date and time to get together. I look forward to meeting you.

Sincerely,

Note that the letters are all less than a page and simple and on point. People are more likely to read something that will only take a few seconds to absorb.

Sending a letter is one way to secure an appointment but it can be an expensive process depending on the number and frequency of your mailings. Generally, a letter should always be followed up by a phone call. This will help to increase the number of appointments you will have to schedule. A general rule to follow when mailing several letters at the same time is to mail only the amount that you are able to follow-up on a timely basis by telephone. For example, mailing 25 letters a week is usually sufficient when following up by telephone the following week to schedule appointments. Keeping the letters within a zip code makes organizational and logistical sense in making the follow-up practical and reasonable for you.

Addressing different audiences – seniors, 40-50 year olds, the professional – requires a variation in the letters sent. These groups may all have different motivations with regard to long-term care, and you should be sensitive and knowledgeable about these differences. This will help you convey enthusiasm for your prospect's circumstances over the phone, an energy vital in obtaining an appointment.

Insurance companies may assist you with a targeted direct mail program. Simple mailing pieces alerting the individual as to the long-term care concern can be successful, depending on the piece, the quality of the mailing list, and your follow-up. There are also highly qualified direct mail companies. Look for ones that have consistently done mailings to people over age 50. They will understand what design layout and message is likely to meet with success. This is a potentially effective way to generate qualified prospects.

Earlier in this book, it was noted that Boomers are increasingly remodeling their homes in anticipation of a long-term care event for a parent, relative, or themselves. That means they have thought about long-term care, but probably have done little to investigate the financing end of the issue. Targeting a list of home re-modelers could result in a high return rate simply because this potential health situation is on these individuals' minds.

Seminars

Seminars are a very effective tool in communicating the need for long-term care insurance. A number of insurance professionals using this mass marketing approach have been very effective. Many seniors have plenty of time to attend seminars and many come just for something to do. The larger the audience, the greater the likelihood of finding a few good candidates for long-term care insurance.

When sponsoring a seminar, light refreshments such as coffee, tea, soft drinks, and water accompanied with a couple of snacks should be made available. Mid-morning and mid-afternoon seminars are usually the best time for seniors. Boomers and professionals are more likely to attend evening sessions. It is a good idea to follow up with a phone call to those who did not respond to your invitation. The ideal size of an audience is 25 to 30 people. Don't try to pack in any more than that. It's a comfortable-sized audience and attendees are likely to be lees intimidated about asking questions. Location should be convenient with plenty of parking available. Check the senior centers because they may have space available at no charge.

Keep your session on an informative and educational level. The purpose of holding a seminar is to advise how long-term care insurance can be a solution to a potential financial problem, not to sell your product. Long-term care can be a very complicated subject and using visuals such as cartoons will keep the presentation reasonably light. The entire seminar should not be more than an hour and audience participation by way of questions should be encouraged. You can do an effective job within that time frame. If the seminar runs more than an hour, it should be only because people are still asking questions. They are probably there because they have a specific issue to raise and are trying to secure an answer; this should be encouraged in every respect, without letting any one audience member dominate the talking. Remember, it's important to keep the audience's attention by telling them everything *they* want to know about long-term care and not everything *you* know about long-term care. Keep it light and simple.

In concluding a seminar, be sure to have your appointment book handy. Either yourself or an assistant (or two) should be at the back of the room to set up an appointment for people who are interested in further discussing their own situation with regard to long-term care. This is vital, as people who are truly interested can probably make the appointment right there. While you can follow up all the attendees by phone, you will have more success with the more interested prospects who are willing to commit right then to a time to talk to you.

One way of having the attendee stop in the back to talk to you or an assistant is to hand out an evaluation form as shown in Figure 9.4 and ask them to complete and turn it in. This form will not only provide you with feedback on your presentation and with important information on a prospect that could possibly result in a sale, but it also ensures the chance to see if the individual would like to schedule a time to go over their own individual situation.

FIGURE 9.4   **Sample Evaluation Form**

Please indicate your rating of this seminar:

	Excellent	Good	Fair	Poor
Subject Matter				
Presentation				
Material				
Location				
Time				

Additional comments and suggestions: _____
_____
_____

Your name: _____ Spouse's name _____
Date-of-birth: _____ Date of birth: _____

Address: _____
City _____ State_____ Zip Code_____

Home Phone: _____

Please check one:

____   I would like to review my long-term care insurance options. I would like to sign up for an appointment tonight or contact me for an appointment (best time to call is _____).

FIGURE 9.4 (continued)

___ I already have a policy with _____. Please sign me up for an appointment tonight or contact me (best time to call is _____)to receive a free analysis of this program to ensure that it is up to date with my needs.

___ Please send me more information about your long-term care insurance program.

When the seminar evaluation form has been turned in, distribute a prepared packet of information that should include the *Shoppers Guide to Long-term Care Insurance* (available from the National Association of Insurance Commissioners, your state insurance department, or many insurance companies), one or two articles about long-term care insurance, and a copy of the outline of your presentation with key topics highlighted. The *Shoppers Guide* is an excellent summary of long-term care insurance and can be used in conjunction with the contract you are marketing to show your prospect how your policy works. It is an excellent third-party piece.[4]

The seminar approach is an excellent tool for making a sales presentation to many people at the same time. Individual attendees are relaxed and don't feel pressured in this environment. If you give a strong, informative presentation, appointments will be made, probably that evening. Specific details can be addressed during a follow-up appointment. In the follow-up, people will ask even more questions about the subject, especially if they have read the material you sent home with them after the seminar. Encourage these attendees to discuss the subject with friends, family, and their accountants or attorneys, and encourage these people to also come to the follow-up interview. You want everyone on the same page and getting the same information from you, rather than having it filtered through a third party. Long-term care will affect family members, and these individuals can often help the immediate prospect to make up their mind about the coverage.

Meeting with the children of your senior prospects and clients will also automatically help you tap into the next generation of prospects for your product. You are giving them an out on full-time caregiving responsibilities for their parents and you can now help them set up (on an earlier, perhaps more cost-effective basis) their own asset protection plan.[5]

This is one potentially successful way to enter the long-term care insurance market.

Video

Another possible pre-approach to potential prospects is with a video. Contact your local community-access cable channel and try to arrange a show on long-term care. Some of these stations have a need for better local programming. A long-term care show can involve members of the community, such as a director of admissions of a local nursing home or a home health care nurse. These people can speak to the access to long-term care, the cost of care, and the problems of qualifying for medical assistance. Many of these channels already have a local community talk show that you may able to link into to bring yourself and your community guests (along with one of your own policyholders or, if possible, claimants).

PBS recently sponsored a highly-watched show on long-term care, so there is an audience for it, and television and community-based cable stations may remember "And Thou Shalt Honor," which ran in 2002. PBS is already planning a follow-up to that well-received and highly successful program.

If you are able to appear on local cable channel show, ask for a video copy. You can then bring these to interviews with potential clients, or send them out to highly qualified prospects. Mailing a video may seem like a costly expense, but it does separate you from your peers. People are used to receiving videos today for almost anything, whether to view a potential retirement community or to get a tutorial on the new dishwasher they just bought. A long-term care video can speak volumes within a short period, and not just in the agent's voice. Agents utilizing such a video can add tremendous, legitimate credibility to the idea that long-term care planning should be discussed.

Advertising

Finally, there are numerous outlets to advertise yourself as a pre-retirement estate planning consultant, long-term care insurance salesperson, or whatever the appropriate title should be. In addition to placing advertisements, you can accomplish the same objective at a much reduced cost by using the media in other ways.

Most communities have a local newspaper. It is usually of the weekly variety and is geared toward homeowners with news that is relevant just to their local area. These publications are always looking for material. In the Daytona Beach area, for example, there is a publication called *Seniors Today.* Granted, Florida has a large, established senior audience for this type of publication, but America is growing older *everywhere.* Many older citizens are opting to stay within their own community when they retire, rather than relocate, so this type of newspaper is becoming more prevalent. If you volunteer to write an article about long-term care insurance for this type of publication, you have a better than even chance of getting it published, once your credentials for writing the story are verified. In this article, you can discuss generally the need for long-term care. If there is a local story you are aware of that illustrates the importance of planning for this potential problem, then you increase the immediacy of the problem for your audience.

Writing an article is a good way to generate calls from interested people who read the article and have further questions. That's also what direct mail solicitation is intended to do. You are simply utilizing another media outlet to generate your prospects on a far lower cost basis than either advertising or direct mail.

There are also plenty of radio talk shows on the AM dial today. You know the ones in your area. Contact the station manager (or the host) to see if you can come on as a guest to talk about long-term care issues. These guest chats often generate a lot of phone-ins. Consumers have questions about long-term care and often don't know where to go to get answers. An "appearance" on the radio further boosts your credentials, especially if you can turn that into a once-a-week, or twice-a-month segment. The talk show host wants the call-ins, and you might even find local assisted living facilities, retirement communities, or home health agencies to advertise during that segment of the show. These advertisers will help ensure that you have a regular gig, and increase your prospecting chances with only an outlay of your time.

Straight advertising can also be effective. Today, insurers require you to use only some camera-ready copy of a state-approved advertising piece. In many states, regulators require that only the material they approve is allowed to be used in the prospect of, and sale of, long-term care insurance. If you are using your company's name, then it is a must to check with your carrier's compliance department before you submit anything to a media outlet for publication.

Today, even article reprints should come directly from the home office of your insurer. Typically, the insurer seeks permission to reprint a set level of copies of an article for distribution to its field force. These are often good third party pieces that can help establish the credibility of financing long-term care expenses through insurance.

The message here is follow the insurer's guidelines and don't run afoul of your state insurance department. Using set advertising pieces prepared and sanctioned by your insurer is your best bet if you utilize this method of reaching a prospect base.

Working With Your Prospects

The long-term care insurance market is now nearly four decades old. Needs have evolved over time, and it is safe to say that long-term care is no longer "ahead of the consumer curve" and more people experience a long-term care event through need or caregiving every day.

During this time, different prospect pools have emerged. The over-age-65 individual has long been the primary source of business in this market. The under-age-65 and employer markets are now emerging as individuals are attempting to square away their pre-retirement planning early, while employers deal with lost productivity due primarily to the loss of an employee to caregiving duties rather than just disability.

Each market has their own set of priorities in addressing this coverage. They have different motivations for buying and it is important to keep those in perspective as you carry on your daily long-term care insurance work.

Buyers' priorities have also changed over time. Ten years ago, 30 percent of long-term care buyers worried most about depending on others, while 24 percent were more concerned about protecting assets. These reasons have swapped places in the last decade. Today, 30 percent of U.S. long-term care buyers named protecting their assets as the most important reason to buy long-term care coverage, while only 19 percent worried about having to depend on others as their primary reason for the insurance purchase.[6]

While involving family members, note that older parents and their adult children have different ideas about where the parents would like to live if they become unable to care for themselves. Older parents would prefer not to move in with their kids, even though their adult children thought that they would. In addition, from a financial standpoint, this recent survey found that 32 percent of parents believe they will need financial assistance from their children, while only 44 percent of adult children expect to help their parents financially.[7]

Stay up on trends like this so that you have in your mind how parents and their children might view long-term care differently. Do not assume that this is how they are going to think – every situation is different, but know that the generation gap probably exists for this product, too.

Senior Prospects:

Seniors often view the insurance industry and related services in a negative light, including long-term care, due to personal (and not necessarily heart-warming) experiences with other insurance agents, Medicare, doctors, nursing homes, and other topics related to their health. This negative perception initially arose out of the Medicare supplement scandal involving seniors who purchased and carried several extra (and worthless) Medicare supplement policies, and evolved through the bad taste left by the Medicare+Choice managed care practice, where many seniors were abandoned by their HMO program. Although the insurance industry is trying to rebuild its reputation in a positive way, there is still a mistrust that exists among seniors.

To be successful in working with mature individuals, a bond of trust must be established. This can be accomplished by building credibility with the potential client. A seminar on long-term care, for example, may firmly establish you as an expert in the area of long-term care insurance. A referral from a family member, relative or friend can also assist in building their trust in you as an agent.

Once you have gained that trust, you can maintain your credibility by asking questions and listening to their answers. Their answers will tell you a lot about their situation, both emotionally and financially. Completing the financial analysis covered in Chapter 8, "The Importance of Financial Planning," assures the senior client that you are working to find a solution for them and not just trying to make a sale. Tell them at the outset what you hope to accomplish and then review these key points to reinforce your recommendation.

As an agent, you will need to educate your client on Medicare, Medicaid, and other statistical data with respect to long-term care services and cost. This background information is of great interest to the client because it directly affects them. During your presentation frequently ask your client whether he agrees or disagrees with what you are saying. This approach allows you to keep the client involved in the process and at the same time allows you to continue with your sales presentation.

At times, you will be a counselor more than an agent. Many seniors have spent time trying to learn about long-term care and they have many questions, a large majority of them basic. Take the time to let them ask and for you to answer them to the senior's satisfaction. You need to build a consumer's confidence about this subject so that they see not only their own financial protection needs on paper, but have emotionally accepted that they are doing the right thing. If the prospect is given time and space to deal with the issues involved, and you remain available and stay in touch, the sale will ultimately be made.[8] Patience is a virtue that will be rewarded. People who are buying long-term care insurance are keeping it (persistency on this business is abnormally higher than on other lines of health insurance). This is a direct result of letting the consumer feel comfortable enough with the idea that the older one gets, the more one potentially needs to use the policy benefits.

For seniors today, you are insuring an independent lifestyle for them in the future.[9] Seniors are very concerned about becoming dependent late in life and want to do something to allow them control their own destiny should health deteriorate or a catastrophic event occur. Long-term care insurance is that lifestyle choice, creating a myriad of options at the point of disability in terms of what services can be rendered and where these treatments can be delivered.

Seniors tend to pick an advisor who is knowledgeable, but who does not make them feel foolish by talking about technical details they do not understand.[10] Their questions during a sales interview tend to be basic ones, and you should not stray too far into the realm of complexity from which there is no retreat. Make sure the client understands what they are buying, but keep it as simple and easy to digest as possible. Leave the insurance acronyms and jargon at the office.

For those who feel they do not want to invest the proper time into making the suitable sale to a senior prospect, remember that these are the most motivated individuals as they are closing in on a potential need for the coverage, and that they also control the majority of wealth in this country. Translation: they have assets to protect and thus are the most important potential users of the product.

There is also a certain amount of self-preservation that agents should incorporate into their daily practices. Some courts have found that consumers are well within their rights to sue an insurance agent who fails to mention long-term care insurance as part of a financial planning program and as a result there is no coverage when a disability occurs. The agent had access to and the ability to write long-term care insurance, but never brought it up. Unquestionably, the agent's Error & Omissions coverage is going to be tested. This should not come as a surprise to those who have worked in the health insurance industry. A disability to an individual has generated the same type of backlash — why didn't my insurance agent tell me about disability income coverage? Long-term care represents the same issue. Hopefully, those of you reading this book do not need that kind of motivation to begin talking about long-term care insurance. But the risk of a litigious situation will always be there if you don't.

Under Age 65 Prospects:

Younger buyers sometimes have difficulty relating to the need for long-term care insurance. However, many of these younger income-earners can relate to the need to preserve quality of care later in life and they have the desire to protect a nest egg they are fighting an uphill battle to build. When long-term care is incorporated into the retirement planning process, it helps motivate the under-age-65 prospect to buy. More and more workers are thinking that long-term care insurance is part of a retirement plan and not just for after retirement.[11]

While seniors represent a more motivated group of prospects, you can utilize the McDonald's theory of marketing to expand your potential audience base. McDonald's runs markedly different television ads during Saturday morning cartoon shows than they do during adult-oriented prime time.[12] So, too, should you remember that this age category will have a different perspective on long-term care insurance. When in Rome ...

Younger buyers (ages 40-64) can already see the financial handwriting on the wall as far as their employers go. Many businesses have switched over to cash balance pension plans, leaving some older workers a little short of what they thought their pension fund was going to contain. Analysts have been saying for years that economic necessity – that gap between the cost of promises made and the companies' ability to keep that promise – leaves corporate management no choice but to reformulate, rethink, and in some cases, renege on post-employment benefits for workers. Benefits are going to continue to be cut in the future, in some way or another. The share of American workers with company pension plans has progressively slipped in each decade, from nearly 40 percent at the beginning of 1980 to about 20 percent today.[13]

Young people understand the fragility of their retirement plan *without* a disability event. It is not a major mental leap to see the importance of asset protection that is better done early when it is most cost-effective. A recent U.S. Chamber of Commerce survey found that 56 percent of all workers are concerned about the future need for long-term care coverage.[14] If you approach these individuals and stay on message about incorporating this protection vehicle into their retirement plans, this will be a successful market segment for you.

It is important to overcome the belief that this is insurance only for the elderly. It's not! An agent describes a situation where a 25-year-old was on his way home from his engineering job driving his motorcycle, when a truck pulled out in front of him. The resulting head injury not only disabled him, but caused his 23-year-old spouse to lose her job as she had to help him with all of his bodily functions over the succeeding three-year period. The spouse's view? She said, "I guess you couldn't have enough insurance for something like this."[15] According to the 2000 Medical Expenditure Panel Survey Findings 12, published by the Agency for Healthcare Research and Quality (a division of the Department of Health and Human Services), nearly 50 percent of Americans receiving long-term care are under age 65.[16]

Buying long-term care insurance can be especially motivating from a health perspective for people in their 40s and 50s. These are the decades when chronic degenerative diseases like Parkinson's Disease (actor Michael J. Fox) and multiple sclerosis (featured as a plot point on the hit TV series *The West Wing*) begin to strike more frequently.[17] These are classic examples of medical conditions that will require long-term care services.

Younger prospects (under age 65) need to hear this medical news. They understand financial downturns. Medical problems are harder to relate to, but no less important. Long-term care coverage is for them to make a part of their pre-retirement estate planning portfolio.

Business/Employee Prospects:

As noted in the "Under Age 65" prospect base above, employers are cutting back on defined benefit pension programs, and employees have been seeing 401(k) plan balances tumble with the new century market slide. Much of the employer pullback can be attributed to the December 1990 Financial Accounting Statement No. 106, issued by the Financial Accounting Standards Board. This ruling required most private companies to significantly alter the way they account for retiree health benefits. Unfunded retiree health liabilities (those that lay out in the great wide future based on current employer promises) were required to be recorded on their financial statements, creating a large liability and an instant desire to limit them in an effort to improve the paper bottom line.[18]

So, employers know costs. They are not interested in adding more to their profit & loss sheet. That being said, what has their attention today is the increasing amount of missed work taken by employees. It is not necessarily because employees are sick; more often, it is because they have caregiving responsibilities. It's déjà vu for the employer, as child care nightmares from the 1980s and 90s come flooding back in, when the baby boom echo created a large number of working parents who simply had to leave or miss work entirely when a child was sick.

Lost productivity and an easy way to solve it will get an employers attention as you explain that long-term care programs can include not only employees on payroll deduction, but spouses, parents, in-laws, grandparents, and grandparents-in-law. The employer does not just care about insuring the employee for long-term care, but more importantly, insuring the people that may make caregiving demands on the worker if something happens.

Employees will be told the same essential motivating information you would tell any under-age-65 prospect. They know they must take charge of their own retirement program in today's corporate atmosphere, and that includes long-term care. In addition, they need to understand their loss of control if something happens to a loved one, and they are pressed into caregiving service. This will cost them dearly in terms of finances as well as the physical and emotional commitment that are the centerpiece of caregiving responsibilities.

According to the American Council on Life Insurance, the lost income tax revenue because of family caregivers leaving the workforce breaks down like this:[19]

Situation	Year 2000	Year 2030
Employee took early retirement	$ 700,000,000	$2,600,000,000
Employee left workforce for caregiving	$1,500,000,000	$5,400,000,000
Totals	$2,200,000,000	$8,000,000,000

Lost income tax revenue simply means lost income to the employee, in far greater numbers. So, an employee must deal with two issues: their own health and financing issues, and their loved ones, since it can also impact them.

The Basic Sales Presentation

Establishing the need and providing a solution by identifying the alternatives are basic steps used in a long-term care sales presentation no matter which type of prospect you are facing. It does not matter whether it is in a one-on-one interview or in a seminar environment.

Establishing The Need

This initial phase of the presentation can be handled in two parts. First, a fact finder must be completed to gather important financial details. This will assist you in making a sound recommendation. Much of this phase is accomplished by the financial data that is gathered as discussed in Chapter 8, "The Importance of Financial Planning." By identifying your client's assets, including a spouse's assets, and their cash flow situation, the need for long-term care insurance is established.

During the fact-finding phase, you might want to gauge their long-term care IQ. Ask them if they have any specific concerns about a long-term care policy, any benefits that they know about that they wish to include, and if they have any knowledge of the underwriting process to qualify them for this insurance.[20] This way, you can include the benefits they have expressed an interest in, and prepare answers to the questions they already have.

Prospects should already have priorities set for their retirement years. To further establish the need for long-term care insurance, certain questions need to be asked. Do they plan to see their families as often as they can? Do they want to travel? Do they have the finances to accomplish these goals? Reinforce the fact that they have worked hard to build up their assets to make their retirement a pleasurable one and then ask what they think the need for long-term care will mean to them financially.

At this point, you are into the second part of establishing the need – indicating the likelihood of needing long-term care insurance. Simple statistics are best: For every 1,000 people, according to the Insurance Information Institute, 5 will face a house fire, 70 will have an auto accident, while, according to the Agency for Health Care Planning & Research, 400 will require long-term care. We all have a tendency to overdo statistics, and these few numbers say it all about mandated coverage versus insurance we need to think about on our own.

As noted earlier, most people believe the need for long-term care happens to someone else. My 87-year-old mother-in-law looks at her neighbors as elderly and infirm, but does not see herself in that way. "They're elderly," she'll proclaim, with the implication that she is not. That is the type of thinking, though, that also believes long-term care will happen to someone else. The statistics cited above may help convince the prospect that the risk is too high to gamble, and that the chance one takes is not only with their life but with family members, too.

Since the likelihood of a nursing home stay has already been factored into your client's financial analysis, now you must identify the potential cost to your client. It is the cost factor that can now be brought to the forefront and discussed in relation to your client's financial situation.

To illustrate the costs involved, you must be aware of the average cost of a quality nursing home in your area. The national average cost for a nursing home today, according to the MetLife Mature Market Institute is $61,320 a year.

Using this national average cost of $61,320 a year, a five-year nursing home stay (should your client be one of the 21 percent who stays in a nursing home for five years or longer) would cost over $300,000. Now, ask your client if he has this much money "tucked away for a rainy day" when the need for long-term care arises.

Most people do not have an extra $30,000, let alone $300,000, nor do they realize the potential devastating impact that long-term care can have on their finances. What about assisted living facility costs? These are $25,908 annually, on average, according to Life Care, Inc. That's still $130,000 to account for over a 5-year period, and the average assisted living facility stay is likely to be longer than a nursing home stay data because the patient entered the residence in better health. It is still a major financial hurdle to leap.

Using local nursing home and assisted living facility rates (plus home health care costs at an average of $18 per hour, four hour minimum charges typically apply), and the occurrence statistics, you can "bring home" these calculations to relevant status for your client. And, while the likelihood of a long-term care need is greater for someone age 65 or older, there are many younger people that need and receive long-term care services. An auto accident, a boating mishap, or a skiing incident can leave anyone with a long-term care need. A spinal cord injury, for example, necessitates physical dependency on someone else for the rest of the victim's life. It can and does happen and, as such, you can make long-term care relevant for people of almost all ages.

Identifying the Alternatives

How is long-term care paid for today? An exploration of who pays the cost today can set the stage for dispelling the myths that Medicare and Medicare supplements pay for long-term care.

The majority of funds come from either an individual's own finances or from Medicaid. A large percentage of older adults still has blind faith in Medicare, but the numbers belie that belief.

The following is a breakdown of the responsible parties that paid long-term care costs in 2000.[21]

Families	25%
Medicaid	43%
Medicare	14%
Private Insurance	10%
Other (V.A., Church, Charity, etc.)	8%

Sixty-eight percent of all long-term nursing care costs are paid by the individual needing care or by Medicaid, because the individual has little or no income or assets. This remains the largest unfunded liability in the country.

In Chapter 7, Government Programs, a detailed study breaks down what Medicare will cover. The result is an overall fourteen percent contribution to the total costs of long-term care. This certainly dismisses the notion that Medicare pays much of the long-term care costs, and what is reimbursed has more to do with home health care than nursing home costs.

Reviewing various financial options to paying for long-term care:

1. *Medicare* – Medicare is clearly designed to cover acute medical expenses such as doctor's visits, hospital stays, and surgery. This government program does not reimburse for personal care or custodial services, which are the primary reasons long-term care is administered.

2. *Medicare Supplement* – This policy is important to seniors because it covers many of the acute medical expenses that Medicare does not pay for, including deductibles and coinsurance. There is virtually no coverage for custodial or personal care and additional benefits are not substituted in the ten mandated Medicare supplement plans available.

3. *Savings* – How much will be enough? A financial analysis of your client's liquid assets compounded with nursing home, assisted living facility, and home health care costs, will indicate how long his savings will last. People do not want their entire life savings spent on health care. What if they eventually recover? What happens if their savings are nearly depleted? This alternative can help determine the elimination period (the number of days before benefits are paid). As statistics indicate, savings can help fund a short-term long-term care need, but savings are not likely to last in the event long-term care is needed on a continual basis.

    Our general savings rate as a nation has been plummeting since the early 1970s. This does not bode well for general retirement living let alone paying for long-term care services. Baby boomers' emphasis on investments is in full reverse with the recent market slide and children's college costs are sure to cut into any respectable saving gain over the next few years.

4. *Family members* – Children and other members of the family are often placed in the position of caregiver because of a lack of any other alternative. Today, this option has become more difficult with two income earners, single parents, long distances between parents and children, and delayed parenting which places potential caregivers in the position of raising young children.

    This option can be an emotional burden for all parties involved. Many parents do not want to move in with their children and, should that be the only option, resentment between the caregiver and caretaker and of the entire situation will affect all concerned.

    This option may not be financially feasible for the children either. If a parent has very little money and the only choice is to try and care for this person, the added expense of another dependent may be overwhelming to the family budget.

While this alternative is often utilized instead of Medicaid qualification, it is one that both parent and child usually would like to avoid.

5.   *Borrow/charity* – Borrowing money, unless it is from a relative or
     friend, is unlikely because an elderly person or disabled individual is
     not considered a good risk to loan money. However, some banks will
     consider reverse mortgages (see Chapter 8, "The Importance of
     Financial Planning").

     With the many volunteers assisting senior-based groups, char-
     ity might be a possibility. Many churches and synagogues have pro-
     grams for those in need of long-term care. As long as the care need-
     ed is custodial, or preferably, homemaker-type services, these organ-
     izations can furnish help. If nursing assistance is necessary, however,
     it is unlikely these charitable groups can be of assistance.

6.   *Medicaid* – This is often the last resort. When personal funds are
     exhausted and family members are not able to provide care, applica-
     tion for Medicaid is the only other option. (For a full discussion of
     Medicaid, see Chapter 7, "Government Programs.") If state guide-
     lines are met, Medicaid will pay for nursing home and now, in some
     jurisdictions, assisted living facilities, and home health care. The
     drawback of this program is that the person needing care must find
     and go to a facility or home health care agency that accepts Medicaid
     payments. Because Medicaid reimburses at a low rate, many facilities
     and agencies do not accept this form of payment.

     Nursing homes accepting Medicaid patients are generally
     packed three or four to a room because of the low reimbursement
     rates. Some of these facilities would not be selected if the individual
     had a choice. With Medicaid, for the expenses to be covered, you take
     what you can get.

     For those individuals who transferred assets in order to qualify
     for Medicaid, this money was simply a loan from the government.
     State governments have legally promised to look for the money spent
     on long-term care services after the patient and the patient's spouse
     have passed away. A large percentage of all long-term care services
     needed in a skilled nursing facility are paid by Medicaid because of

the transfer of assets "loophole." However, if states are successful at changing the penalty period beginning date from the date of transfer to date of Medicaid application, this may slow down this practice.

Transferring the Risk

The alternatives described above are less than perfect and it makes sense to look into private long-term care insurance. The sole purpose of insurance is to pay for significant financial events that otherwise cannot be easily handled. Long-term care fits this definition nicely. The nature of long-term care from the onset will likely require medical services on a long-term basis. High cost for long-term care medical assistance will eventually deplete someone's personal finances.

This product also gives consumers choice, a flexibility they (and their family members) will appreciate when a claim occurs. Maintaining control over your long-term care treatment should be a high priority, and long-term care insurance can make that happen, rather than create a dependence situation with a government program.

With long-term care insurance, the insured pays an allotted premium today for the insurer's promise to take care of the larger, ongoing bills later. The younger the individual, the lower the premium cost. People in their late 40s and 50s should seriously consider this product, given that they have taken care of other financial priorities, because the price is lower. Waiting until someone is 65 or 70 will have a significant impact on the premium rate for a long-term care policy, and the total outlay for this coverage.

Long-term care insurance is the best solution for those that can comfortably afford the premium. People with few assets to protect and very little income after expenses are not usually good candidates for this type of coverage. These individuals will probably qualify for Medicaid in a short period of time after the need for long-term care begins.

For people in the middle to upper class in assets and income, long-term care insurance presents a wonderful opportunity to plan in advance. By not planning for future long-term care expenses, the entire family will be at a disadvantage when the need for long-term care arises. This is what happened to the Doan family, described in Chapter 1.

Long-term care insurance policies can cover both nursing home and home health care in the same plan. In addition, most policies now cover care provided in a variety of assisted living facilities. Depending upon how accurate the daily benefit selection was, out-of-pocket expenses will often be small once the claim commences.

Long-term care insurance provides an excellent alternative to financing the long-term care need.

It might also be helpful to point out the tax advantages of an insurance answer to this funding problem. Tax-qualified long-term care insurance policies hold out the possibility for a deduction of the premium paid (more likely for a business than an individual who must itemize to obtain it), and the benefits are received income tax-free. If one self-insures the risk, there is a strong possibility that, depending on income, not all of these costs will be personally deductible, especially if these numbers exceed income, a probable scenario during retirement years. If one relies on Medicaid and transfers assets, the family who eventually sells these assets faces potentially high capital gains taxes, and a possible bill from the state for Medicaid costs.[22]

That's it! You have just been through a basic sales presentation. The concept of long-term care insurance is simple; the financial analysis portion is more complex. Once the financial details are filled in – liquidity, income, and assets, the remainder of the presentation should proceed smoothly.

Objections

Naturally, there will be some objections. This is a normal reaction when buying most items. Most of the objections come down to cost – and buyer's remorse. Here's how to answer some of the objections.

"I'd like to think it over."

This objection generally masks a larger concern. Ask the client why he wants to think it over. At this point, the real objection should surface – most often the concern is the cost of coverage.

The cost issue comes down to two scenarios. Outline each one (as shown below) and ask the client which one he would feel more comfortable with.

Scenario #1 – The client pays $150 per month for $100 a day of long-term care coverage in any type of facility or at home.

Scenario #2 – The client pays $3,000 per month for long-term care services when needed.

If the insured pays a premium of $150 a month for 25 years before using the policy, total premiums paid (without any rate increases) would be $45,000. If the cost for long-term care services remains at $3,000 per month (which is unlikely in today's economy), it would take 15 months to recoup the total premiums paid of $45,000. Twenty-five years of premium repaid in 15 months!

Then ask the client which expense is more likely to alter his retirement lifestyle, $150 a month or $3,000 a month. The $150 a month is a known expense, while the $3,000 a month could be needed next week, next month, or next year.

Ask your client again if there is a reason to wait since the $150 per month premium will increase based on an age change.

Another chart that can be utilized illustrates the number of nursing home days that it takes to equal the premium paid. The chart below shows the number of days, based on the daily benefit amount, required to recover the premiums paid. The daily benefit amount is assumed to have an inflation feature added that increases the amount by five percent each year. The calculation is based on $100 per day benefit, with no elimination period and a lifetime benefit period with the inflation feature.

Age at Issue	Annual Premium	5	10	15	20	25	30
				Years Premium Paid			
				Days to Recover Premiums Paid*			
50	$1,410.00	58	91	107	112	109	103
55	$1,785.00	73	115	135	141	138	160
60	$2,030.00	84	131	154	161	157	148
65	$2,840.00	116	183	215	225	220	207

* Calculated as total premiums paid divided by the nursing home daily benefit payable that year.

Cost will always be a problematic issue. Long-term care insurance is not inexpensive. However, there is a growing tendency for agents to stray toward the lowest priced product on the market. As has been true in the past with other health insurance-related coverage, this can be dangerous.

There have already been examples of carriers that have had to raise their rates dramatically due to adverse early claims experience. For example, an older policyholder who has held coverage for four years suddenly receives a 75 percent premium increase, and simply cannot afford it. What does he do now? Drop the coverage as he inches ever closer to actually using it? Or try to pay the premium even if it causes him a financial hardship?

Chances are the agent is long gone and the policy holder is stuck. He could shop around for a lower rate, but what about health? People have to qualify to acquire coverage. Depending on his age and health since he bought the policy, this may no longer be possible.

It is an unconscionable situation, but there are a number of policyholders holding potentially under-priced policies that may create serious difficulties in the future. If the agent has done the proper data gathering job and identified the income and asset situation of the client and the present cash flow, what the client can afford will be identified. Obtain several quotes and look to the policies priced closely together and tailor the benefits around affordability. This will help avoid the cost objective, but more importantly help to prevent a future problem for the client trying to financially withstand a large rate increase.

Many states have passed suitability requirements requiring consumers be given a disclosure form stating the insurer's renewal rate history. This can help distinguish those carriers that are more likely to raise rates in the future. While the NAIC is working on cracking down on under-priced carriers, the agent can be proactive by doing proper due diligence prior to a sales presentation.

"I'd like to talk with my children first."

This response can come up often and can be avoided by involving the children in the presentation and discussion. There may be a considerable distance between the parent's and children's residences so this is not always practical.

Ask your clients what their children would think about long-term care insurance. Would they rather take care of their parents if the need for long-term care arises or would they rather purchase long-term care insurance that promises to pay the bills for future long-term care services?

When interviewing prospective clients, I ask them if they would like their children to receive copies of all the materials. If so, I mail proposal information along with a letter of explanation. Children rarely balk at their parents' attempt to protect assets that will eventually be passed along. In some cases, the children have offered to pay the premium if the parents object to the coverage, understanding the consequences even better than their parents.

The kids honestly do not want to be caregivers if it can be avoided. It is not that they do not love their family, but work and child-caring demands, along with financial pressures, make informal caregiving a tough choice today. Those that bravely assure their parent that they will take care of them and there is no need to spend the money on insurance typically do not understand what the caregiving process involves. An agent told me that she always asks a child who makes this assertion if he or she comprehends the tasks involved, such as bathing or changing a diaper. Getting the child (and parent) to face the reality of what the caregiving responsibility means can help you make the sale and turn this work over to those most qualified to deliver the services, courtesy of the insurance policy.

Involving your client's family in the solicitation and presentation of long-term care insurance usually strengthens your overall position. You have nothing to hide – long-term care insurance is an alternative to financing future long-term care services. The more up-front you are in demonstrating a willingness to work with family members, the greater is the likelihood of making a sale.

"I'd like to talk with my attorney (or physician or CPA)."

As with family members, you should ask the client early on who he would like involved in the discussions. If not included originally, ask your client why, at this time, he needs a professional's advice. Would an attorney, CPA, or doctor sign a statement advising a client *not* to purchase long-term care insurance?

Advise that the physician's input will be important later on when the need for long-term care arises. Otherwise, this objection is another smoke screen for the concern about the cost of the plan. If this is the case, you can respond with the same explanation concerning costs used earlier (see the objection entitled "I'd like to think it over."), or refer to the section, "To Buy or Not To Buy – That Is The Question!" presented later in this chapter.

"I would like to shop around a little more."

This objection can be avoided by doing the shopping yourself. To satisfy your client, you should have at least three quotes from companies offering long-term care insurance. For a complete listing of long-term care companies, please refer to Appendix A, "Companies Selling Long-term Care Insurance." In addition, several industry publications including *Life Insurance Selling* and *Advisor Today* have issues devoted each year to reviewing long-term care insurance companies and their products.

In the financial analysis phase, ask your client if there are any insurance companies or policies he is interested in. If possible, obtain quotes from the companies he has identified. This gives you the opportunity to shop for your client. If only one quote is presented, this does not offer him the opportunity to compare quotes and, thus, the objection is valid.

"I'm not going to a nursing home under any circumstances."

This objection occurs if you dwell only on the nursing home aspect of long-term care. However, since the majority of claims are home health care oriented, it makes more sense to place a greater emphasis on this aspect of long-term care services. The product you are recommending should have benefits payable in a number of settings. It is vital that this be stressed when reviewing the policy benefits as part of the proposal process.

Very few people voluntarily enter a nursing home. A nursing home confinement is generally the alternative if no other means of providing long-term care services is feasible. The client needs to know that if a nursing home is the only alternative for treatment, the insurance policy will provide reimbursement.

"I'd like to wait since I'm in good health now and don't need the coverage."

This is another excuse used to delay having to make a buying decision. Delaying the purchase of a long-term care policy will not only drive the cost higher, but ultimately will not save money. It also runs the risk of your client incurring a health problem which may hinder his chances in the future of purchasing long-term care insurance.

Use this monetary example of the cost of waiting:

Coverage purchased: $130/day, 0 day elimination period, lifetime benefit period, simple inflation of 5%
Cost: At age 45: annual premium is $1,182.35   At age 65: $3,463.59
By age 85:   40 years of payments will equal $47,294.00
              20 years of payments will equal $69,271.80

So if this person needs care by age 80, by waiting 20 years, it has cost the individual over $20,000, let alone left a potential underwriting exposure that may prevent the person from qualifying for coverage at age 65.

Many consumers do not yet realize that there is an underwriting component to long-term care insurance An application must be completed and detailed medical questions must be answered to pass the eligibility test for coverage. The longer the wait, the more expensive the policy will ultimately be. But, perhaps more important, the ability to obtain the coverage may be gone by the time the individual wants to buy it. So often, people who procrastinate this decision incur a medical problem which reawakens their interest. Unfortunately, this condition could prevent the policy from being issued at a standard or preferred rate, or even at all.

Although your client is not planning on getting sick, he is probably paying for some type of medical insurance. He is not planning on getting in a car accident, yet he is paying for automobile insurance. He does not think his house will catch on fire, but he is paying for homeowner's insurance.

Insurance is always a gamble. Clients should not take the chance and wait because the need for long-term care services is unpredictable and could cost them the opportunity to transfer a significant potential liability to a third party. If the premium is affordable now, there is no reason to wait.

"The government is going to take care of long-term care."

This objection came up during the months of debate over President Clinton's national health care plan. Even that program, as wide in scope as it was, failed to do much in the way of long-term care. Nursing home coverage was not covered. Home health care was covered for a short time, but the qualification to receive it was more stringent than most private insurer's policies. Even the Clinton administration realized that the cost of long-term care was too high to be rolled into a federal health care program.

Considering the heated debates over the solvency of the Medicare and Medicaid programs, private long-term care insurance still emerges as one of the stronger viable ways to finance this risk.

Part of the concept of pre-retirement estate planning is to identify how health care costs will be handled. The Medicare program, a Medicare Supplement, and a private long-term care insurance policy will often be enough to protect against the significant unknown of health care expenses as one ages. Should something unfortunate befall the government programs, the individual has not placed all his bets on those public sources of paying these health costs later in life.

"I have plenty of assets to pay for my care."

That may be true. Do not assume, though, that because a person is wealthy they will have no interest in protecting their assets. These people did not get to be wealthy by accepting risks they can easily and more cost-effectively transfer.

An agent relates a story that illustrates this point. A woman worth $30 million opted to purchase long-term care insurance even though she might have enough money to actually purchase a facility. But she was worried about the day her heirs, ever aware of the inheritance windfall they might be close to receiving, would be making medical decisions for her. Long-term care insurance gave her the peace of mind that the highest quality care would be available to her and the nest egg would likely not be affected.[23]

To Buy or Not to Buy – That Is the Question!

As a final means of closing the sale, you can illustrate the difference between someone who buys long-term care insurance and someone who chooses to self-insure the risk.

At age 70 the premium for long-term care insurance is significantly higher and the key to understanding the coverage for some is to see how the numbers work.

Both candidates, age 70, own their own home and one car. They have a comfortable retirement income of $2,250 per month and $120,000 in other liquid assets. The $120,000, invested in various vehicles, earns an average of six percent per year. They would like to pass along as much of that $120,000 to their heirs as they can. Both are interested in buying the following coverage:

- $100 per day in long-term care coverage

- 20 day elimination period (number of days before policy benefits begin)

- unlimited benefit period (policy pays for as long as LTC services are needed)

- inflation option (which increases the daily benefit of $100 by five percent each year)

The premium cost for this plan is $3,800 annually. One individual pays the premium despite the high cost, using money from his brokerage account. The other individual decides against purchasing the coverage, citing high costs. He assumes that the $120,000 will be more than sufficient to cover the costs of long-term care.

Both individuals live another ten years before the need for long-term care arises. When the need does arise, both individuals' medical conditions require skilled nursing care and personal care assistance. The individual with long-term care insurance chooses home health care, which averages about $140 a day. The inflation option benefit in his policy increased benefits to $145 a day, ensuring him there will be enough in the policy to pay the increase. The person who elected to self-insure chooses to enter a nursing home for $125 a day because it is less expensive than home health care. See Figure 9.5.

FIGURE 9.5	
Insured vs. Self-Insured	
INSURED	**SELF-INSURED**
$120,000 in various investments earning 6 percent	$120,000 in various investments earning 6 percent
Needs long-term care at age 80	Needs long-term care at age 80
Spent $41,534 in total premium payments	Elected not to buy long-term care insurance
Age 80, liquid assets have Accumulated to $157,589	By age 80, liquid assets have accumulated to $214,901
Care at home: $140/day	Nursing home costs: $125/day

FIGURE 9.5 (continued)

Insured vs. Self-Insured

INSURED	SELF-INSURED
Costs:	Costs:
1st year: 20 day elimination period insured pays $2,800 ($140 x 20)	1st year: Nursing is $45,625
	2nd year: Nursing home costs $49,275 (assume 8 percent nursing home inflation)
2nd yr +: insured pays –0- as policy (daily benefit is sufficient to pay full costs. Unlimited benefit period and inflation rider should continue to assume full costs	3rd year: Nursing home costs $53,217
	4th year: Nursing home costs $57,474
Liquid asset balance left after 4 years of long-term care: $195,796 and growing, earmarked for children's inheritance.	Liquid asset balance left after 4 years in a nursing home: $34,302. This individual will qualify for Medicaid in the 5th year. $120,000 original nest egg for children's inheritance is gone.

Demonstrating how a third party (such as an insurance company) can assume the financial risk of long-term care better than an individual is a powerful argument. The costs of long-term care can quickly erode even a presumably safe nest egg. Most people are not in a financial position to pay for long-term care on their own for a long period of time and will be eligible for Medicaid sooner than the fifth year as in this example.

Moreover, the insured *elected* to receive the care at home because his long-term care policy covered it. The individual who was self-insured had little choice but to enter a nursing home in order to stretch his dollars as far as possible.

This financial scenario should help in closing cases where there is an objection to a high premium. The premium must be affordable. In the example above, both individuals had the means to pay for the coverage. When working with clients with different financial situations, you can alter benefits such as the daily benefit, elimination period, benefit period, or inflation feature to fit within a person's budget.

The Waiver Statement

For any number of reasons, people will turn down long-term care insurance as a financing alternative. If this is the case, it is important to have the prospect sign a waiver form, a copy of which you and the prospect will keep.

The waiver form itself is not legally binding, but it can be a powerful closing tool or used to discourage a potential lawsuit later on down the road. As a closing tool, this form will give the prospect a second chance to reconsider purchasing the coverage. Once he has read the form, he may question the reason why the form needs to be signed.

You can point out that it is necessary to clarify the result of the sales interview for both parties and, because the insurance was not purchased, a signature attesting to this fact will go in the prospect's file. Offer to follow-up at a later date (usually three to six months) to further discuss long-term care insurance as a financing alternative. The individual may sign the form or may reconsider and ask for an explanation one more time. Sales have been made when this form has been presented. A sample form appears in Figure 9.6.

In any event, secure a signature! Insurance agents have been sued over the lack of a certain coverage within a person's portfolio. Don't take that chance!

FIGURE 9.6

Acknowledgment of Responsibility

I understand the risk of needing long-term care insurance as explained to me by
_____. I understand that neither Medicare nor Medicare Supplement policies will satisfy that need.

I choose to decline the insurance protection shown to me at this time and, in so doing, acknowledge that I am assuming responsibility for arranging funding of any long-term care services that I may need in the future.

_____	_____
Name	Date
_____	_____
Signature	Agent's Signature

The agent might also consider having a form signed stating that coverage accepted is less than the amount recommended. This waiver of liability form would indicate that the individual had the opportunity to purchase one amount and elected another. Claims have occurred where the reimbursement received was less than what the insured expected. The insured's memory may not be as good as the agent's file records. This form will help to clarify the position taken by the insured at the time the application was made. A sample form appears in Figure 9.7.

FIGURE 9.7

Waiver of Liability

By my signature below I acknowledge that I have elected to obtain long-term care insurance that provides less coverage than that recommended by _____ who has offered this coverage as protection for my assets.

The plan recommended would have paid a daily benefit of _____ with an elimination period of _____ and a maximum benefit period of _____.

Instead, I have selected a daily benefit of _____ with an elimination period of _____ and a maximum benefit period of _____.

_____	_____
Name	Date
_____	_____
Signature	Agent's Signature

Both your client and you should each sign this form and keep a copy. This can clear up any confusion in the future.

Other Considerations

Impaired Risks

Initially, underwriters of long-term care coverage adopted an "accept or decline" approach and people that had health problems were automatically declined because of high risk.

Today, several insurers have classified health risks and created rate classifications that allow insurance companies to insure people with health conditions by adding a table rating for the coverage. While the cost for the health-impaired individual is higher, insuring the extra risk means that there are no restrictions on the coverage when a claim occurs. The benefits, elimination period, and benefit period are unaffected.

Some companies may choose to insure a risk by decreasing the daily benefit amount, increasing the elimination period, reducing the benefit period, or offering a facility-only policy. The more serious the condition, the greater the likelihood that these approaches may be taken rather than offering no coverage

This openness to writing impaired risks has resulted in long-term care coverage issued for people who have osteoporosis, arthritic conditions, cancer, pulmonary problems, history of heart problems, diabetes, high cholesterol, or current high blood pressure that is controlled by medication. One company even has a lengthy book of underwriting guidelines and classes, listing a number of conditions and their respective rate classes. There may even be an offer to review the modified coverage at a later date, or the extra premium may be only a temporary charge removed after a specified time if there are no changes in the insured's health.

Substandard cases are sometimes easier to close because the applicant is perfectly aware of his medical condition that requires the modifications in the coverage. Impaired risks have a higher probability of needing long-term care in the future than healthier individuals and, as such, usually desire the coverage more than the healthy person.

For more information on underwriting, see Chapter 17, "Underwriting and Claims Experience."

Why Long-Term Care Insurance Works

In March 2003, the American Council of Life Insurers released a report illustrating the reasons people are buying long-term care insurance. These may be helpful as you construct your own sales presentation to help motivate people to buy this coverage.[24]

- Women baby boomers are buying long-term care insurance as a result of their experiences as a caregiver.

- Almost half of Americans 45 and older have discussed their possible need for long-term care with their children.

- At least 22 states are offering long-term care insurance to their own employees.

- More than one-third of large firms are offering LTC coverage as an employee benefit.

- Life insurers have paid out more than $11 billion in long-term care benefits.

Long-term care insurance remains a viable financial alternative to funding this potential risk. People are buying coverage in greater numbers as evidenced by the increase in private insurance money picking up the long-term care insurance tab (now 10%). Gary and Jene Comfort decided to purchase long-term care insurance recently. They started to recognize that if one of them needed long-term care, their assets would take a substantial hit.[25] There are millions of people like the Comforts out there, seeing the need on their own.

So – start prospecting! The basic long-term care sales presentation works because it is simple and uses the prospect's own numbers. You cannot do a proper financial analysis and recommendation without the individual's financial picture. Your presentation is based on selling a program that is a financing alternative for long-term care costs. The presence of insurance coverage gives people more of a choice about their long-term care when it is needed. It is a control issue, one that is very important to stress as many fear losing independence more than going to a nursing home. Remember this, and your sales presentations will be very successful.

Chapter Notes

1. John M. Connelly, "Profile the LTC Insurance Buyer," *National Underwriter*, October 28, 2002, p. 30.

2. Source: HIAA, Mark A. Cohen, "Benefits of Long-Term Care Insurance," Research findings published September 2002.

3. Wilma G. Anderson, "Direct Mail: The Key to the Long-Term Care Gold Mine," *HIU Magazine*, November 2001, p. 33.

4. "Selling LTCI," *Advisor Today*, November 2002, p. 46.

5. Tom Doherty, "LTC Can Tap the Next Generation," *Advisor Today*, March 2001, p. 24.

6. Allison Bell, "LTC Buyers' Priorities Are Changing," *National Underwriter*, December 11, 2000, p. 3.

7. Marcella De Simone, "Adult Children, Aging Parents Have Different Views on LTC: Study," *National Underwriter*, October 7, 2002, p. 41.

8. Nancy P. Morith, "The Counseling Approach to Long-Term Care Insurance Sales," *Life Insurance Selling*, December 2002, p. 56.

9. Cheryl McNamara and Mary Madigan, "Insuring An Independent Lifestyle," *Best's Review*, April 2002, p. 82.

10. Trevor Thomas, "Advisor: Seniors Can Be A Tough Sell, But Well Worth It," *May 6, 2002*, p. 49.

11. Source: American Council on Life Insurance, as reprinted in *Best's Review*, August 2001, p. 95.

12. Jesse R. Slome, "Want To Sell LTC To Younger Buyers? Take A Tip From McDonald's," *National Underwriter*, January 21, 2002, p. 11.

13. Janice Revell, "Bye-Bye Pension," *Fortune*, March 17, 2003, p. 65.

14. Kelley M. Blassingame, "Tips for buying long-term care insurance," *Employee Benefit News*, February 2003, p. 48.

15. Phyllis Shelton, "What My Survey Revealed About LTC Market Trends Today," *National Underwriter*, October 28, 2002, p. 37.

16. Kevin P. McCarthy, "Expecting the Unexpected," *Best's Review*, August 2001, p. 93.

17. Wilma G. Anderson, "Long-Term Care Insurance Isn't Just For Seniors," *HIU Magazine*, July/August 2002, p. 77.

18. "New EBRI Research: Retiree Health Benefits Likely To Keep Shrinking, New Report Finds," *PR Newswire*, August 15, 2001.

19. Source: American Council of Life Insurers, 2001.

20. Ben Lipson, "Ways to Help Consumers Evaluate LTC Insurance," *National Underwriter*, August 19, 2002, p. 8.

21. Source: General Accounting Office, 2001 Testimony before Senate Finance Committee.

22. James G. Blasé, "The Tax-Efficient Approach To Long-Term Care Insurance," *Life Insurance Selling*, March 2003, p. 35.

23. Debra C. Newman, "Overcoming LTC Insurance Objections," *Advisor Today*, October 2002, p. 60.

24. "Long-Term Care Insurance: Consumer, Business Awareness Translating Into Action," *PR Newswire*, March 26, 2003.

25. Michelle Singletary, "Do your homework for LTC Insurance," *Tallahassee Democrat*, December 24, 2002, p. 1E.

Chapter 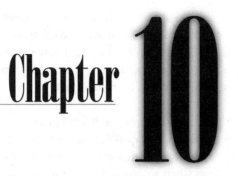 10

Long-Term Care vs.
Disability Income Product Design

"The secret to life is to replace one worry with another."

— Charles Schulz

E arly long-term care policies were narrow in scope and easy to explain. If an insured entered a nursing home, the policy paid a specified daily benefit, usually in cash, directly to the individual, in indemnity fashion. When home health care policies became available, the arrangement was the same – the daily cash benefit was paid directly to the insured.

The early policies were popular with agents who specialized in the Medicare supplement market. The products were targeted at seniors and could usually be handled in one sales interview. Insureds could easily see what they were buying.

Today's long-term care products take a more comprehensive approach toward the reimbursement of long-term care expenses. There are several reasons for this approach:

1. The NAIC adopted a model program that prompted a more comprehensive policy form. The program has allowed the NAIC to refine contract language while expanding the range of benefit options.

2.   Insurance companies, while struggling to get a handle on the proper design of the policy form, turned to the actual providers of long-term care services for input. Feedback resulted in the expansion of benefit choices and a variety of settings in which long-term care services could be administered and be reimbursed.

The feedback from the providers was also helpful to companies when modifying contract language in the areas of qualification for benefits and types of covered services. For the first time, insurance companies in the marketplace began developing a comfort level when an actual claim occurred – how services were rendered and who was administering the care. It also helps them keep up with the latest developments in long-term care delivery services, including the advent of assisted living facilities a few short years ago. In effect, policies today are far more practical and accurate in providing benefits for most long-term care situations. This evolution might never have happened had the industry not tapped into the growing medical field for its knowledge of long-term care.

Good News for the Disability Income Specialist

Agents that are apprehensive about the long-term care market and lack an understanding of its products can take solace in the knowledge that today's long-term care product is very similar to a disability income policy. While product development has moved long-term care policies beyond the scope of traditional Medicare supplement plans, the long-term care policy of today closely resembles a disability income policy.

We shouldn't be surprised. As explained in Chapter 7, "Government Programs," the Medicare program is not a disability-based plan. Therefore, the largest gap in Medicare is treatment of chronic conditions with long-term care services. If long-term care policies are to be truly effective, they must be disability-oriented in their coverage.

When I first explored the long-term care market in the late 1980's, I did so in search of a program for my mother. She had read an article about long-term care insurance and called me to find out if it was in her insurance portfolio. Upon hearing that it was not, she instructed me to search out this coverage.

I contacted several companies I knew that were marketing long-term care insurance and requested quotations. The questions asked by the marketing representative concerned elimination periods and benefit periods. It wasn't until the question, "Do you understand that if your mother is disabled, there are several ways to qualify for benefits?" that I realized: (1) I obviously knew very little about this coverage, and (2) it was going to be easier to learn than I thought.

I read all the information including the specimen policies sent. The long-term care product was indeed a disability-based product with a design similar to the disability income policies I'd been marketing. Now, I was on familiar ground.

More importantly, it was a product I could market to my existing clients. My disability income clientele was aging and starting to focus on retirement. For many of them, it was only 10 or 15 years away and preparing financially for retirement had taken on an immediacy previously missing from our discussions. A long-term care policy would be central to their retirement planning because a disability could severely hamper their lifestyle at retirement just as easily as it could threaten income flow during their working years.

The more I thought about it, part of the traditional definition of "own occupation" in a disability income contract was similar to the disability definition in a long-term care contract. The last line of the "own occupation" definition of disability read:

> "If you are not working, your duties will be considered to be that of a retired person."

What did this mean? The first part of the definition addressed eligibility for benefits if a person was unable to work at his own occupation – the job held at time of claim. What did not working have to do with it?

I called a claims administrator for the answer. Because the disability policy was a guaranteed renewable and non-cancellable policy, the company could not cancel the policy for any reason other than for non-payment of premium. It was anticipated that there would be individuals who might retire from work, but continue to pay the premiums for their coverage. Even though no occupation was involved, the insured was still eligible for benefits if he suffered a disabling injury or illness.

This meant that another measurement had to be established to determine the insured's inability to perform duties – the essential key to qualifying for benefits. If not working, the insured was assumed to have retired, hence the policy language stating that supposition.

What are the duties of a retired person? Golf? Tennis? Gardening? Actually, the disability claims department uses an activities of daily living measurement – bathing, dressing, eating, mobility, for example – for ordinary activities performed every day. If these were modified in any way, the insurance company at least had a way to measure the disability and any subsequent recovery. Activities of daily living, as you will see, are the primary disability definition in a long-term care product.

Understand that this was all conjecture on the part of the claims administrator. This particular insurance company had no claims that were filed utilizing this language but it was a perfect transition to understanding a long-term care policy.

Two basic concepts resulted from this research:

> *Disability income* policies protect the insured during his working years.

> *Long-term care* policies protect the insured primarily during his retirement years.

To explain it simply, disability income benefits could be paid to retired people. Certainly, long-term care services are reimbursed to a number of people under the age of 65.

I don't want you to have the impression that long-term care and disability income are mutually exclusive. Someone could qualify for both coverages (if they owned both) during a disability. DI replaces income, while long-term care is intended to pay for services rendered – two different needs. That both are potentially payable during a disability tells you there is a strong connection between the two programs.

Both disability and long-term care policies should be purchased early on – disability income for people in their 20's and 30's and long-term care for people in their 40's and 50's. Disability income is protection in the event of a disability while working and long-term care is primarily protection against a disability after retirement (when the need for long-term care is the greatest).

If an agent sells disability income coverage, he can easily move into the long-term care market. I made some minor alterations in my basic disability income sales presentation and created a basic long-term care story to share with existing clients and prospects.

Other Parallels

The basics of my disability (and now long-term care) sales presentation are:

1.   Explain the need.

2.   Introduce statistics.

3.   Identify financing alternatives.

4.   Present the product as a better financial alternative.

In reviewing each of these key areas, you will see how a minor change in wording or emphasis placed on a particular benefit can transform a discussion on disability income into one about long-term care.

Explain the Need

During a sales presentation for disability income, prospects are asked what is their greatest asset. Their reply will vary (spouse, car, home, children – not necessarily in that order) and eventually they are steered towards understanding that income is their central asset. Loss of income would be a serious financial setback for them and their family.

Disability insurance is intended to protect the insured's ability to work and earn an income. There are tables available that indicate the potential earnings a worker will make over the course of a career. It is the potential income and assets derived from income that disability insurance is designed to protect.

Long-term care is intended to protect income and assets, too, except it is designed to protect income and assets already built up. The lifestyle of the person who is retired is dependent upon money accumulated during that person's working years and any investment income. This can be reduced drastically should the need for long-term care arise. Recovery is not certain at this point in life. If anything, a return to normal health will take longer.

Introduce Statistics

For disability income, the statistics on the chances of a disability occurring are currently based on the 1985 update of the Commissioner's Disability Table (CDT). A measurement of the chances of being disabled for 90 days or longer, noted at benchmark ages (25, 30, 35, 40, 45, 50, 55, and 60) is introduced during the sales presentation to give the client some idea of the frequency and chances of becoming disabled. Other statistics include the rate of recovery based on the length of the disability and the chances of a disability versus premature death for any given age. In addition to a discussion about the risk to income and assets should a disability occur, the chances of a disability occurring can be clarified by using these statistics.

Long-term care has a growing amount of historical data and statistics similar to disability income. The data is primarily concentrated in the nursing home arena, simply because that is easier to measure. Home health data is harder to come by, because it can be used so sporadically. You could use data cited earlier where 600 out of 1,000 Americans will need long-term care in some form at some point in their lifetime.

Or you could use data aimed specifically at women, the gender that should consider long-term care for several reasons. Generally, they are likely to outlive their husbands. The average age of widowhood is 56.[1] This means no at-home spouse is likely to be around to provide informal care in the initial stages of need. You can add to this information by noting that women are twice as likely to remain unmarried after age 65, and three times more likely to be alone after age 75, ages where the possible need for long-term care begins to accelerate.[2] Women also are less likely to have substantial assets and income to fall back on. A recent Census Bureau survey pointed out that women were less likely to reach the higher salary brackets during their working years. Almost 16 percent of men age 15 and older who worked full-time in 2001 earned at least $75,000 a year, compared with only 6 percent of women.[3] A greater need and less money to meet that need should help you sell to this important market segment.

More and more studies and statistics will emerge in the future, but these numbers give the prospect some idea of the need for long-term care insurance.

Identify Financing Alternatives

Prospects are aware of the impact a disability will have on their income, especially during their working years. They know how much they make and how much they spend. They understand that a disability can completely eliminate that income.

With long-term care, the agent must quantify the income need. It is important to know the average daily nursing home rate for your state and surrounding counties where you work. On average, the annual cost for a nursing home stay is over $60,000 nationwide. A five-year nursing home stay would cost $300,000 – a major financial setback. Using local data is important and it is up to you to provide this information, since costs will vary based on location. In Miami, Florida, for example, the average cost for a nursing home stay will be close to or above the average $60,000 per year costs. A nursing home in a rural setting would average a lower rate. See Appendix B for a complete listing of the state agencies on aging where you can obtain more information about your local costs.

For disability there are several financing alternatives – savings, borrowing, relatives and friends, unearned income, Social Security, other disability income coverage, a working spouse's income or selling one's assets. The financing alternatives for long-term care are the same except Medicare replaces Social Security and selling one's assets is replaced by Medicaid. Other long-term care coverages available are Medicare supplements.

Some of these financing alternatives may provide sources for replacing income during a disability. In all likelihood, the gap between what is needed and the money coming in will be substantial.

Present the Product as a Better Financial Alternative

Generally, setting aside an allotted premium for a disability income or long-term care policy is better than any of the alternatives to fund the income need should a disability occur. A disability can occur any time, any place, anywhere. It is often unexpected and there are few ways to properly prepare for the financial need occurring during the recuperation period. Transferring the risk of funding the income need during disability makes sense for many people, whether it is to replace a salary to pay basic living expenses or to provide money to pay providers of long-term care services.

With a few modifications, your disability income sales presentation has become a long-term care story. The audience may have changed somewhat, but the story is still essentially the same. But, the parallels between disability income and long-term care don't end there.

Product Similarities

The plan design of a long-term care policy utilizes language comparable to a disability income policy. The key plan parameters are:

Disability Income	Long-term Care
Monthly Income	Daily Benefit
Elimination Period	Elimination Period
Benefit Period	Benefit Period

Indemnity versus Reimbursement Plans

Disability income products are indemnity-type plans. An individual purchases a monthly benefit based on income, and should a disability occur that is covered under the DI plan, this monthly benefit will be paid in full during a total disability. In a total disability situation, the actual current income is not important, the company has agreed to indemnify the insured with the monthly benefit purchased.

Long-term care can be paid on this basis, too. Many agents feel that indemnity contracts are more consumer- friendly and easy to explain since they function similar to a DI policy. Once the insured qualifies for benefits, the daily benefit amount is paid without regard to the cost of care.[4]

This has changed, however, as most LTC insurers today offer a reimbursement-type policy for long-term care coverage. With this plan type, the cost of care actually matters, and policies reimburse the cost up to the amount of the daily benefit. As a result, this policy may take longer to pay out all of its benefits than an indemnity product that pays the amount regardless of the actual expense incurred for long-term care services. For this reason, it is also less expensive than an indemnity plan.

Still, a number of agents like indemnity plans, even though they are scarce today. With an indemnity-type plan, the insured and his family are not required to submit a record of expenses (or arrange for the provider to be paid directly). The benefits can be used to cover other out-of-pocket expenses should the daily benefit amount exceed the cost of care.[5]

Monthly Income vs. Daily Benefit

Monthly income versus a daily benefit is a primary difference between plan designs. For long-term care you will have to do a little more homework so that you can make a daily benefit recommendation. The information is available and should be updated on an annual basis. Look for newspaper articles about the costs of nursing home and home health care in your area and state. Contact your state Ombudsman or Department of Health and Human Services or Area Agency on Aging for specific data for your area. Long-term care is a popular subject and this information is an excellent source for making daily benefit recommendations.

Elimination Period

The disability income salesperson will recognize this plan parameter. This, in effect, is the policy deductible – the number of days that the policyowner must self-insure before benefits are payable.

With individual disability policies, we have witnessed the demise of the shorter elimination periods. The plans with 14-day, 30-day, and 60-day elimination periods have been shelved for the professional and executive disability risk. Gray and blue-collar applicants will likely find 30-day and 60-day elimination periods still available. For the rest of the working world, the starting point of elimination period discussions is a 90-day elimination period.

For long-term care, first day eligibility with a zero-day elimination period is available. This means as soon as the insured qualifies for benefits, reimbursements begin, providing immediate coverage. So far, the premium for a zero-day elimination period is not substantially higher than other elimination periods available in a long-term care policy. For example, when presented with a choice of several elimination periods, my mother selected the zero day option since the premium difference between a zero-day elimination period and a 30-day elimination period was minimal. I cautioned her that claims experience could subject her to future rate increases, but that didn't deter her. Since she purchased the policy she has had thirteen rate renewals and is still paying the original premium quoted.

In addition to the zero-day elimination period, long-term care elimination periods are also available for 15-, 20-, 30-, 60-, 90-, 100-, 120-, 150-, 180-, and 365-day periods. Some states place limitations on the longest elimination periods. A 20-day elimination period is a common choice because Medicare's skilled nursing coverage ceases full payment of the approved amount beginning on the twenty-first day. The primary selection, however, has been a 30-day elimination period, less expensive than zero, but more cost-effective than waiting a longer period of time and using assets to pay for care during this self-insured period. Whether these short options will expire over time, in the face of deteriorating claims experience, is still not known at this time.

The longer one can wait before benefits begin, the lower the premium cost. How long one can wait depends on the retirement cash flow and the availability of liquid assets to pay the premium. In Chapter 8, "The Importance of Financial Planning," there is a detailed discussion on how to arrive at these numbers.

Carriers are also adding, if states will approve them, 2, 3, and 4-year elimination periods. The reason for their existence is that a lot of early purchasers of long-term care insurance selected 2, 3, and 4-year benefit periods. Now there is concern that this is insufficient to meet the need. By adding an elimination period that ends at the same time as the prior policy's benefit period, you can stack coverage to expand the benefits.

Long-term care elimination periods may need to be satisfied only once in a policyholder's lifetime, meaning that if one qualifies for benefits by satisfying the elimination period, and then recovers, there is no longer an elimination period to satisfy to obtain benefits, making it a first-day plan from that point forward. This is more liberal than disability income, although chances of recovery following qualification for long-term care benefits are not as optimistic as with a disability income definition that may emphasize a return to work in its benefit approach.

Benefit Periods

Benefit periods are familiar ground for the disability income agent. A benefit period determines the maximum length of time that benefits will be payable. For disability income, the choices generally range from 12 months to age 67, coinciding with Social Security's latest retirement age at the moment. Benefit periods for two and five years and "to age 65" are also available.

For long-term care, the lifetime benefit period (often called "unlimited") is available – for now. Combining a zero-day elimination period with an unlimited benefit period offers a more complete financing alternative to fund the income need during long-term care than any other alternative. The lifetime (or unlimited) benefit period is likely to be phased out over the next couple of years as insurers replace their current portfolios.

Also available are two-, three-, four-, five-, six-, and ten-year benefit periods and there may be more options to come. The longer the benefit period, the greater the premium. With different benefit periods available, the agent will be able to reduce the premium and stay within a prospect's budget. Medicaid requires a five-year grace period when transferring assets irrevocably from a trust before becoming eligible to apply for reimbursement under this federal/state government program, as long as the transfer was not for the purpose of qualifying for Medicaid benefits, so there may be a reason to elect this length of time.

A five- or six-year benefit period could save premium dollars and provide ample coverage for the risk involved. There can be a significant premium difference between an unlimited benefit period and a five- or six-year benefit period, and while lifetime coverage provides more peace of mind, the historic length of claims is generally short (most under 5 years). This could be because the definition to qualify for coverage is tougher with the ADL requirement, and people are more disabled with less longevity by the time they begin to access coverage.

As one can see, the similarities of long-term care and disability income should help the agent with marketing long-term care insurance.

Product Definitions

Renewability

For years, the disability income industry touted its non-cancelable renewal provision as a benchmark of quality coverage. Non-cancellability meant that the insurer not only could not cancel the contract (except for non-payment of premium), but rates could not be increased until age 65. This was a strong unilateral policy provision with the insured holding most of the cards.

Recently, poor claims experience has caused most disability income carriers to steer away from this type of renewable provision. It's not the cancellable aspect of the renewal that has been the headache, but the inability to adjust the rates on a particular block of business. Because of this, the non-cancellable feature has become expendable.

Instead, for some of their disability products, insurers are substituting a guaranteed renewable provision which retains the non-cancellability feature, but allows the insurer to raise rates in the future on a class basis. The class basis is often a specific policy form (insurers cannot isolate individual bad risks) that incurs the rate increase. These increases are not an automatic adjustment. Due to the extensive requirements in obtaining approval of premium changes from the state insurance departments, rate increases are made only when absolutely necessary.

The NAIC established the guaranteed renewable provision as the minimum standard for long-term care policies, meaning that virtually all long-term care plans have conformed to this requirement even in states that have not adopted the NAIC model. Insurers have yet to emerge with a non-cancellable provision for this coverage, although some carriers have provided short-term rate guarantees (up to 20 years). However, given the lack of credible experience for the long-term care product to date, combined with the inability of insurers to raise rates on existing business in the non-can DI market when claims experience headed south, there is little chance the renewal provision will advance beyond the reasonable guaranteed renewable language.

Definition of Disability

The definition of disability is considered the core of disability income and long-term care contracts. It determines how an insured qualifies for benefits, which is certainly an important matter to discuss with a prospect. There are distinct parallels between the two products in this area.

"Own Occupation" vs. Activities of Daily Living. Earlier in this chapter, it was mentioned that the "own occupation" definition of disability based qualification on the ability of the insured to perform the duties of a retired person – the ability to perform activities of daily living.

The disability income definition is considered met if the insured cannot perform the typical duties of his own occupation. Each occupation may have a different set of key tasks upon which eligibility for benefits will be considered. The long-term care definition is based on the inability of the insured to perform such activities as bathing, dressing, eating, toileting and transferring positions. While Chapter 12, "Phase Two: Provider-Aided Design," will look at these activities of daily living in more detail, know that the primary method under both policies of qualifying an individual for benefits is based on the ability to perform tasks – work duties for disability income and essential activities for long-term care.

Presumptive Total Disability vs. Cognitive Impairment. In a disability income policy, another way of qualifying for benefits is a catastrophic-type event that automatically makes the insured eligible to receive benefits. These catastrophes are the irrecoverable loss of sight, speech, or hearing, or the use of two limbs. Should one of these types of disabilities befall the insured, no other qualifications need to be met and benefits are often paid from date of loss, thus the elimination period no longer needs to be satisfied.

The long-term care equivalent is called cognitive impairment. Part of the NAIC model policy's objective was to ensure that benefits would not be denied for organic mental disorders like Alzheimer's disease. A diagnosed cognitive impairment – any kind of organic brain disorder – is another way to qualify for benefits under the long-term care policy. No other qualifications need to be met with a cognitive impairment diagnosis.

Under A Doctor's Care vs. Medical Necessity. Most disability income policies require the insured to be under a doctor's care to be eligible to receive benefits. This condition could be waived if future treatment would have no impact on an individual's recovery.

For a long-term care policy (until HIPAA), a "medical necessity" (under a doctor's care) resulting from an illness or injury is another possibility for benefit eligibility. The insured could qualify for benefits if a physician directed that long-term care services were needed to help further an individual's recovery. Under the 1996 HIPAA legislation, "medical necessity" was not made a part of tax-qualified plans. Some insurers are still marketing policies with "medical necessity" contained in the policy definitions despite its absence in the HIPAA legislation. (See Chapter 13 on "Tax-Qualified Plans" for more information.)

The definitions for disability income and long-term care are very similar and the experienced disability income salesperson can easily transfer the disability income concept to long-term care insurance.

Residual Disability

It took disability income carriers several decades to add the residual disability benefit to disability income policies. Under a total disability definition (as described above), there was little provision for benefits should the insured actually return to his own profession. In the early 1970's, claims experience indicated that the majority of claimants did go back to their own jobs – without much in the way of benefits.

The development of the residual benefit established an intermediate definition of disability for the insured. If the insured's time, duties and income were partially reduced as a result of an attempt to return to work, a portion of the total monthly disability benefit based on the actual earnings loss incurred was payable. This allowed the insured to return to work without being penalized. Studies have shown that the earlier the insured returned to work the shorter the duration of the claim.

Currently, for benefits to be paid in a long-term care policy, the insured must require full assistance in an activity such as dressing or toileting to qualify under this definition. HIPAA regulations also defined "standby assistance" as qualifying for long-term care services. Here, there is supervision of an activity of daily living without a hands-on requirement. Unlike many residual disability cases, this may not signify recovery, but deterioration of ability. The person's ability to perform the task may ultimately require full hands-on assistance. This similarity to residual disability where a type of partial assistance is required is a regular feature in insurers' tax-qualified long-term care insurance plans.

Critical Illness Disability Plans

A new product beginning to take hold in this country is typically called *Critical Illness*. Under these policies, if the insured suffers a specific major illness or injury, a lump-sum benefit is payable. This differs from the usual disability income policy that provides a weekly or monthly income stream if one qualifies under the definition of disability in the contract, without regard to the specifics of the ailment.

This product is not geared to every disability situation. But the idea of lump-sum payments rather than monthly benefits mirrors a product situation in long-term care. Indemnity-based long-term care pays benefits on a daily basis, as this text has described. However, there are alternatives that pay either for long-term care services or a death benefit if the individual passes away, a linked-benefit policy with both long-term care and life insurance present. These policies usually have similar long-term care benefits to their indemnity counterpart, however, with the added lump-sum death benefit feature. This often functions as a safety net for people whose disability becomes fatal rather than a lengthy claim. Read more about this alternative product design in Chapter 15.

Chapter Notes

1. Wilma G. Anderson, "Marketing LTCI to Women Is Powerful," *National Underwriter*, Life & Health/Financial Services Edition, April 22, 2002, p. 8.
2. Carroll Busher, "Agents: Sell LTC Policies to Women," *National Underwriter*, Life & Health/Financial Services Edition, April 30, 2001, p. 11.
3. "Census Report: Women's pay lags," *USA Today*, March 25, 2003, p. 15A.
4. Marc. G. Sigel and Howard S. Wacks, "An Age-Old Remedy," *Financial Planning* (January, 2003), p. 54.
5. Sheri Strange, "Baby Boomers Are a Missed Market for Long-Term Care Insurance," *HIU Magazine* (November, 2001), p. 18.

Chapter 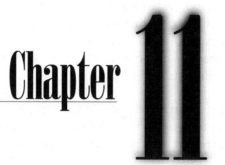 11

Phase One: Early Bad Press

"A child of five would understand this. Send someone to fetch a child of five.."

– Groucho Marx

"I believe in equality for everyone, except reporters and photographers.."

– Mahatma Gandhi

A person seeking automobile and homeowners insurance, which is generally required by a third party, looks toward an insurance company for these coverages. Products such as long-term care insurance, however, are sales driven. The need for this type of product is not always apparent despite the avalanche of publicity that has been accorded long-term care.

The need for long-term care must be identified and alternative solutions presented using the basic sales presentation described in Chapter 9, "A Long-Term Care Sales Presentation."

If the media views a product in a negative way, as was originally the case with long-term care insurance, this often will surface during a sales presentation. Bad press can represent an obstacle in establishing long-term care insurance as a viable financial alternative.

Long-term care insurance has been both praised and reviled by the mainstream press. This product has received more media coverage in its youthful stages than more traditional plans that have been around decades longer. Of course, media outlets are far more plentiful today then they were when long-term care was first introduced in the mid-1960s.

That it is a plan many seniors are interested in may explain some of the widespread media interest. Past episodes with Medicare Supplements have conditioned the raising of the red flag when plans surface that may again bring together insurance agents and the elderly.

But there's more to the story than what has generally been printed in consumer publications. Timing has been a predominant issue in the media reviews of long-term care insurance. Change has happened so rapidly to this insurance coverage in its brief lifespan that by the time the media records a trend, a newer one has already begun. This can create, at best, some confusion in the minds of both agents and clients.

This chapter will trace the history of long-term care as a product, from its modest early beginnings and questionable policy forms, to a more liberal approach of underwriting and payment of benefits, to the Federal government's influence on policy design with the Health Insurance Portability and Accountability Act of 1996 (HIPAA). The rapid developmental changes in long-term care insurance have made it difficult for the media (and consumer and insurance agent, for that matter) to keep pace.

The Birth of Long-Term Care

There are two key points to remember:

1. Long-term care coverage was created virtually without data.

2. Long-term care coverage is one of a handful of products developed during the information age.

When a product is introduced, there is an expectation of profit by the insurance company. Affordability and profitability are two considerations with product development. Insurance company actuaries rely on data and experience for the predictability of usage. Without the data and experience, claims frequency is a guessing game that most insurers (and reinsurers) don't want to play.

In the beginning, actuaries had very little information available – only a few tables showing the admissions and duration of stays in nursing homes – to rely on for the development of a long-term care insurance product. The first long-term care policy nearly 40 years ago (by the CNA Companies) covered nursing home care on a supplemental basis only. Home health care was a fledgling industry, with only a few agencies and arrangements with private duty nurses to provide care. Home health care was not incorporated as a benefit in a long-term care policy for nearly two decades after the first policy was written.

Pricing a policy without historical data and experience in order to predict future usage is an actuarial nightmare. Assumptions, generally made with a high degree of certainty, gave way to a pure stab in the dark. Moreover, there was no way to predict who the average buyer of long-term care insurance would be since the product was not in existence. Insurers pioneering long-term care were placed in the difficult position of developing and pricing a policy based on pure assumptions. To avoid high claims experience, the companies implemented "gatekeepers." These safety nets were:

- a requirement of a three-day hospital stay prior to becoming eligible for benefits;

- requiring that skilled nursing care be administered prior to becoming eligible for policy reimbursement for intermediate or custodial care; and

- high premiums.

Most long-term care services are custodial in nature and quite often a three-day hospital stay is not necessary prior to long-term care being administered. The purpose of this requirement was to eliminate all but the most severe claims from being paid under the early long-term care policies.

When long-term care insurance was introduced in the late 1960's and early 1970's, the only other program available to pay anything for long-term care services was Medicare. As a result, much of the language used in policies by the insurance companies was identical to Medicare. For nearly forty years, coverage under Medicare, except for a few improvements, has remained the same.

Insurers have handled their products differently. Long-term care insurance was developed during the information age, a time in our history where data availability had become greater and more easily accessible. As more reliable data became available, insurance companies were able to fine-tune their long-term care products. As a result, eight or nine generations of the long-term care product have evolved. Many insurance products developed 100 years ago have not seen nearly that many changes.

The three-day hospitalization requirement mirrored Medicare's language. The skilled care requirement reduced claims from individuals who only needed assistance with activities of daily living. The conservative premiums were priced high based on the data available at the time and assuming the worst in terms of claims experience. It was reasoned that it would be easier to lower premiums later, rather than underestimate the potential for high claims experience and run the risk of financial jeopardy for the entire company.

The goal was to effectively reduce the number of potential claims. With the three-day hospital stay and skilled care requirements under private policies, the insured could count on assistance from Medicare for the first few days of nursing home treatment. The high premiums diminished the product's attractiveness even further. Long-term care products early on were clearly not as helpful or as affordable as insurance was intended to be.

It is difficult to place the entire blame on the insurance companies. The development of long-term care policies was an answer to a growing need – certainly a prediction that has come true. Without substantial and reliable data however, it is nearly impossible to feel comfortable with either price or policy language. The early long-term care policies were available for an extended period of time because it takes several years for this type of insurance to accumulate reliable claims experience and allow contract adjustments to be made.

Nursing home costs varied widely geographically, making it difficult to predict the benefit amount that would consistently be elected. As mentioned earlier, home care costs were virtually unknown, as the current medical technological advances permitting most health care to be administered in the home were still several years away.

Mortality (death) and morbidity (disability) rate tables have been around for decades and patterns used in developing a life or disability product could easily be discerned. So, one can feel some empathy for the long-term care trailblazers – it wasn't an easy job. They knew the insurance need existed – how to fill it required experimentation in product design and pricing. These early insurers and their policyholders became the long-term care market's guinea pigs.

The media backlash for long-term care products took some time to emerge. Nursing home plans enjoyed relative obscurity for twenty years until Medicare's diagnostic-related groups (DRGs) brought the skilled nursing facility to national prominence. (See Chapter 2, "Today's Changing Demographics.") By then, up-to-date nursing home data was available, home health care was beginning to emerge as a major growth industry, and there was a rapidly increasing community focus on the need for long-term care. Product sales began to accelerate, often by selling a Medicare supplement and pointing out the scarcity of nursing home coverage under both Medicare and Medicare supplements. The country's population was beginning to age and the time for this product had come.

Battered

Early policies didn't change as quickly as the demand for them did. During the early 1980's a number of claim denials and the obvious similarity in safety nets between private insurance and Medicare became more apparent and attracted a hailstorm of criticism. These opinions were echoed in the following headlines:

Chicago Tribune, Section One, September 21, 1988:

"Study finds big holes in home care coverage"

Greensboro North Carolina News and Record, page A-15, September 23, 1988:

"This insurance doesn't pay"

U.S. News and World Report, page 62, August 13, 1990:

"Many long-term care policies are too restrictive to offer much genuine protection"

Harsh criticism or an accurate appraisal? These headlines did not surprise many buyers of earlier generations of long-term care coverage. These buyers had experienced the safety nets when filing claims against their policies. They were naturally upset when measuring the dollars paid for the product versus the lack of dollars the plan paid for long-term care services.

There were two other factors that made the media (and insurance regulators) suspicious of early long-term care policies. First, the age range of the individuals eligible for the earlier policies was generally limited to those 60 years and older. This meant that the policies were being sold to the age group with the highest probability of utilizing policy benefits. Marketing an insurance product to its primary users makes it impossible to properly distribute the risk. The principle of insurance is based on the *law of large numbers*. Many people pay for a product and only a few actually use the benefits. Healthy people subsidize the unhealthy, but because everyone is at some risk, there are many buyers who gladly purchase the plan and hope never to use it.

With long-term care insurance, the odds that most seniors will use the policy benefits are good, making the pricing of the plan even more difficult. When in doubt, insurance companies price high.

Secondly, abuses in the Medicare supplement market were beginning to emerge and the public was genuinely outraged. Senior citizens who had paid a lot of money bought seven or eight Medicare supplement policies when one policy would have been sufficient. Seniors demonstrated a lack of understanding about the coverage and insurance agents apparently were hesitant in filling in the gaps necessary for their clients to make an informed buying decision. The complexity of the Medicare supplements made it difficult for both the insured and the agent to sort through the different policy benefits. The federal mandate of ten specific Medicare supplement policies over a decade ago has lessened this lack of understanding and has made selling supplement policies more manageable.

At the time these problems were identified, it was easy to compare the abuses in the Medicare supplement market with another product aimed directly at the senior market – long-term care insurance. When the gatekeepers reared their heads on these contracts, the media was ready to pounce.

Correction

Long-term care products and sales presentations to the public began evolving more rapidly from the mid-1980's forward. Insurers hurried to improve their products based on more substantial data. While these new, improved products in no way resemble the early products, several factors (aside from negative media) have contributed to the positive product changes in the late 1980s – early 1990s.

NAIC

The National Association of Insurance Commissioners (NAIC) is composed of state insurance commissioners across the country. Insurance is not federally regulated as a result of the McCarran-Ferguson Act passed in the 1940's by the House and Senate. Instead, each state regulates the insurance industry in its own state. State insurance commissioners attempt to bring consistency to this jurisdiction by meeting regularly and adopting model laws for each state to add to its own specific statutory law. Despite this apparent semblance of order, not every state sees fit to adopt the model laws as is; still other states don't adopt any of these laws, and opt to do their own thing instead.

Medicare supplements eventually had to be sorted out by a federal law mandating standard plans. This had to be embarrassing to the NAIC and further gave impetus to those in Washington who would love to see the McCarran-Ferguson Act repealed and the federal government regulating the insurance industry. The NAIC was determined not to lose control of the new product line for seniors – long-term care insurance.

The late 1980's saw the NAIC's creation of standardized language for long-term care insurance. One of the first corrections to the existing policy language was the removal of both the three-day hospital stay requirement and the necessity of skilled care administered before any benefits for intermediate or custodial care were allowed. This effectively eliminated two gatekeepers that stood in the way of benefit eligibility.

The purpose of the model policy is to give the states statutory language for long-term care policies. Once the states adopt policy language, insurers filing policies with that state must use contract language that conforms to the state's statutory language. Companies that do not comply are rejected by the state.

A model policy is intended to cover essential aspects of a policy. This gives the states and insurers leverage to add other provisions to expand coverage. This type of flexibility, along with the reluctance of some states to use the model policy language, results in a number of policy variations for insurers that marketed long-term care insurance, adding to administrative costs that is part of the premium pricing equation.

The NAIC has continued to work with and update its original long-term care model policy. For example, a requirement that home health care benefits be offered as part of, or as an optional benefit to, a long-term care plan has given these policies a wider scope of coverage beyond the early nursing home only plans. Age banding to determine rates was eliminated: rates can only be increased on a class basis, not on a predetermined basis. The NAIC's Long-Term Care Task Force also required insurers to offer compounded inflation coverage and non-forfeiture benefit provisions in the early 1990s. Their recent activity has been directed at controlling premium rate increases and ensuring that long-term care insurance be sold appropriately to a qualified consumer.

The model policy immediately improved policy benefits under a long-term care policy and steered insurers towards offering plans with more flexibility.

Increased Competition

With an interest in long-term care insurance and the emergence of more thorough data on the usage of long-term care services, more and more insurance companies have introduced new products in the last part of the 1980s and the early 1990s. Insurance companies offering long-term care coverage peaked at nearly 150 insurers, but have since dropped back somewhat, with ten insurers accounting for the sales of the majority of coverage.[1] For a complete, current listing of long-term care companies, please refer to Appendix A.

Early on, when more companies entered the long-term care market, competition forced insurers to stay abreast of long-term care industry trends, resulting in rapid product improvement. While insurers have been tempted to follow the same liberalization steps taken by disability insurers during the 1980's (which resulted in a claims disaster), some caution prevailed due primarily to the "newness" of the benefits and a decided lack of claims experience. It was clear that some insurers entering the market had no idea how to design, price, market, and underwrite this product. Some of those carriers have since withdrawn their contracts, preferring to focus instead on programs they are familiar with and understand. This may explain the drop in the number of insurers in the long-term care marketplace from its early 1990s high, even though the market for this product is clearly growing in numbers for now and the foreseeable future.

Another reason for the diminishing number of insurers in the long-term care market is the regulation of the product by state insurance departments. Certainly, this has to be the most regulated product the industry has ever introduced. Much of that is due to the Medicare supplement debacle that the NAIC does not want to see repeated.

Marketing of long-term care insurance has now been going on long enough to begin accumulating thorough and valid experience, which should lead to better predictability of claims and assurance of accuracy in the pricing of long-term care policies.

Expanding the Age Range

Insurers began to incorporate a *law of large numbers* philosophy when they branched out to offer long-term care insurance to younger people. While consideration of this product may not be a priority for younger people, those ages 40-45 and older should give serious consideration to this coverage. It's important in the overall design of a pre-retirement plan which people should consider well before they reach retirement age.

The initial success in the sale of long-term care insurance was due to the efforts of those agents specializing in Medicare supplement sales. But it soon became apparent that as policies changed and acquired more complexity as a disability-based product, long-term care insurance was a different type of sale and involved more detailed financial planning. A long-term care sale often requires 2-3 interviews, while Medicare supplements are usually sold on the first appointment. The agents working in the long-term care insurance market today are more traditional and focused on financial planning for all age groups. With long-term care insurance expanded to younger age prospects, it is a product many agents propose routinely now as part of an overall financial plan.

The younger buyer (age 40+) likely will not use the policy for several years, but it's easier to qualify for the coverage and the premium is much lower if purchased early on. Since the NAIC banned automatic age band increases (where premiums typically increased every five years), any rate increases filed by an insurer for a class of policies will be exercised on lower premiums if the policy is purchased at an early age.

The younger buyers help spread the risk from the older age buyers who are more likely to use the benefits. The effectiveness of spreading the risk steers long-term care insurance into a "comfort zone" for insurers and allows insurers to continue offering better policy benefits.

The long-term care insurance market is unprecedented in insurance history. While it usually takes years for a product to reach a second generation of language revision, long-term care has seen multiple revisions over a period of nearly four decades. These swift changes make it difficult for insurance agents, let alone consumers, to absorb these alterations to the product and to explain them to the insured or prospect.

While these changes have been generally positive for the consumer, it is more complicated for the insurance agent, as a full examination of both product and price is necessary to properly compare and evaluate long-term care insurance policies. While some policies are in their ninth generation, there are others that have not seen current changes. Chapter 12, "Phase Two: Provider-Aided Design," reviews the basics of current plans, giving the agent a basis upon which to compare other programs.

Gotcha!

Although long-term care products improved, initial media reaction did not. The June, 1991 issue of *Consumer Reports* placed long-term care insurance on the front page with the tag line "Gotcha!" By this time, however, product changes had created a better product design. While this assessment of long-term care policies was considered unfair given the improvements made, the assessment of a lack of knowledge on the part of the agent concerning long-term care was more likely accurate. Change had come so fast that few agents (and obviously the media) could comprehend it well enough to explain it to a prospective buyer.

Insurers and states moved quickly to rectify this "gap" in education. Educational programs for agents were implemented by insurance companies, while states began introducing continuing education requirements for an agent in order to retain his license. Some states had pre-licensing requirements specifically for long-term care.

As agent knowledge progressed and coverages improved, even *Consumer Reports* begrudgingly acknowledged long-term care insurance as a viable financing alternative – for some. The September 1995 issue of *Consumer Reports* stated "…another way to pay for a nursing home stay is with a long-term care policy – a relatively new form of insurance coverage."[2] Even though the article was cautionary in its praise, this was a long way from "Gotcha!".

However, not all consumer magazines were endorsing long-term care insurance. In the December, 1995 edition of *Smart Money* (a *Wall Street Journal* publication) an article stated, "The numbers certainly suggest you can do without this insurance…" and went on to state, "If you are among the unlucky seniors who do need a nursing home, chances are that it will cost you no more than $57,600."[3] The implication at the time was that most people have $57,600 in liquid assets that can be spent on long-term care services. And this was a consumer financial publication? Maybe the unlucky senior who took this advice can send his bill to the magazine.

Despite the aforementioned articles, by the mid-90s long-term care insurance had made a remarkable rebound from a rocky start. The products were better even as prices began descending. The early "fat" that had been factored into the policies to cover any and all actuarial guesswork was being trimmed. Naturally, the negative media focus generally missed these trends. Consumers and financial planners were starting to view long-term care insurance as a viable financing alternative to long-term care needs.

Consumer magazines today are still hit and miss as far as accurate long-term care information goes. The typical article today is similar to one appearing on *Money* magazine's web site in August 2002, where the writer gives some decent information, but also spends every third paragraph, tossing the reader an out from considering coverage if they wish to take it. These outs, that can usually be found in a lot of high-profile consumer publications, include "the richer you are, the less you need a policy" (and using hazy definitions of "rich"), "make sure premium does not exceed 5 percent of your income" (the United Seniors Health Cooperative recommends 7 percent), and "although it's a smart move for many people, for others it may be a waste of money."[4] Consumers reading these comments who are hoping to see that they won't have to buy this coverage may include themselves in the category of "don't need it" as a wish fulfillment without qualifying it further.

More helpful media articles are ones such as this posted on the *Kiplinger* web site in September 2002. This article begins "How would you pay for long-term care if you needed it? When baby boomers were asked this in a study, only 5 percent said they would rely on long-term care insurance. Most said they expected life, health or disability insurance or government programs to cover the costs. If that's what you're counting on, think again."[5]

Ideally, this is how media coverage should be. Take away the wishful thinking, give some overview information, and send the consumer on a quest to see if they are truly a viable candidate for long-term care insurance or not.

Tax Clarification

By the mid-1990s, there was one remaining issue that needed clarification. The taxation of long-term care insurance was still not defined in the tax code. This made some buyers hesitant, and some professionals like CPAs and attorneys reluctant to totally endorse the product. Employers, who had initiated the progress towards group long-term care insurance in the late 1980s, generally backed off further expansion of this line into their overall employee benefits picture.

Enter HIPAA. The Health Insurance Portability and Accountability Act of 1996 was primarily about health insurance. However, one section of this legislation included – at last – long overdue tax regulation of long-term care insurance. Federal legislators had been trying in earnest to accomplish this for over a decade. The new tax clarification treats long-term care insurance similar to health insurance. Benefits are not taxable, employer premiums are deductible without any compensation attributable to the employee, and, in a surprise move, limited premium deductibility is also extended to individuals who itemize medical expenses on their tax returns.

This tax favorability came with a price. In defining long-term care insurance for the purposes of tax clarification, HIPAA eliminated one way to qualify for benefits under these policies and limited another. (For a full explanation of tax-qualified plans, see Chapter 13.) Insurers, agents and state regulators were stunned by these developments. The product evolution that currently had insurers marketing fair and competitive products was about to take another turn – backward.

Insurers had to re-file policies to conform to the new federal language. State regulators had to revamp statutory law to accommodate the new federal law. Sales of existing long-term care insurance went sky-high during the latter part of 1996 as agents rushed clients to decisions on the basis that pre-HIPAA policies were better than what would follow. Insurers, agents and consumers were unsure as to whether HIPAA represented tax progress or a serious step back in product development, or both.

In keeping with the practice of staying behind the current LTC trend, the media initially missed this HIPAA paradox. The October 1997 issue of *Smart Money*, in a special report about taking care of aging parents, noted that long-term care insurance was "an increasingly popular alternative." These were not "the same suspect products" the magazine had criticized in the previously cited December 1995 issue. "Back then the sales pitches were sleazy, the policies inconsistent and the payoffs uncertain." But, thanks to HIPAA, which "forced long-term care insurers to conform to national standards, including covering cognitive impairments like Alzheimer's and incorporating inflation protection, much has changed."[6]

The article goes on to discuss the lowering of premium rates by as much as 30 percent. These two issues of this consumer publication illustrate an inability to keep up with the changing trends in long-term care insurance. The December 1995 article reported a 1980's trend that was long gone. The October 1997 article illustrated the early 1990's progress in long-term care plans. It was anyone's guess when *Smart Money* would discuss the true difficulties presented consumers by the enactment of HIPAA, as it came down to choosing between tax-qualified and non-qualified plans.

Far from being the final word on long-term care insurance, HIPAA created a state of confusion in the insurance industry. Both pre- and post-HIPAA long-term care insurance is currently being sold, and both agent and consumer must thoroughly understand the consequences of each before making a decision.

The mainstream press added to the confusion. Much of the coverage of HIPAA's effect on long-term care has been devoted toward the tax angle. A number of publications have praised the tax-deductibility of the policy premiums for individuals. This has placed the agent at a slight disadvantage since the expectation of premium deductibility has to be initially tempered during the establishment of the need for the coverage. Only those individuals who itemize on their tax return can claim the deduction. According to some Treasury Department estimates, less than 5 percent of the taxpaying public itemized medical expenses since they must first exceed 7.5 percent of adjusted gross income.

So, for many, the news delivered by the insurance agent that the premium may not be deductible is a setback, if the prospect read consumer articles noting the tax-deductibility of the premium.

While one can argue over whether the new policies are as good as the previous generation (see Chapter 13), the post-HIPAA plans are still highly competitive and offer far more coverage than the early policies did. The industry has not returned to the "dark ages" of the mid-1980s. Coverage is still much broader than early product generations, and better data continued to place pricing on new policies into more of a comfort zone than the early days. Insurers and agents may have to overcome product objections in their efforts to sell plans that conform to achieve favored tax status.

The October 1997 issue of *Consumer Reports* further added to these difficulties by ranking long-term care coverage again. The magazine's first eight top-ranked plans did not meet the specifications of the HIPAA legislation and its favored tax status. In a sidebar article, the magazine pointed out that benefits paid out by its recommended non-HIPAA qualified plans might be taxable, and that the Treasury Department has been silent on the issue.[7] Readers, of course, may not take notice of this disclaimer, leaving the agent to explain the difference.

This particular issue (and subsequent ones as well) of *Consumer Reports* warns readers to be leery of insurance agent presentations of long-term care insurance. In this way, the magazine information is both valid and helpful. Agent education is a critical issue and those individuals selling long-term care insurance may or may not be well informed on the subject.

The industry seems able to absorb bad press and keep on ticking. Agents should strive to learn the product and its issues thoroughly as many consumers still depend on them for guidance in this area. Consumers themselves try to stay informed, but the hit-and-miss coverage of subjects like long-term care insurance make it difficult to be properly educated on the subject. It doesn't help to have *Money/CNN* run an article like the aforementioned one on August 26, 2002, giving consumers a number of reasons (some valid, some not) to ignore insurance as a funding solution for this problem. Then, on August 27, 2002, *Money/CNN* turns around and publishes a positive article about LTC insurance, in their "Armchair Millionaire" column, with a lead-in saying "Consider that the cost of a long-term care policy can be downright cheap compared to the cost of long-term care", and ending with "For protecting your assets and offering peace of mind, there may be no better deal than long-term care insurance."[8] Good days, bad days.

The next two chapters describe many of the features found in today's long-term care policies and their purpose. Understanding these provisions can assist agents interested in doing proper planning for their clients.

Chapter Notes

1. Jeanne Sahadi, "Playing the odds on long-term care," *Money/CNN*, August 26, 2002.

2. "Who Pays for Nursing Homes?," *Consumer Reports* (September, 1995), p. 591.

3. "Shelter from the Storm?," *Smart Money* (December, 1995), p. 130.

4. Jeanne Sahadi, "Playing the odds on long-term care," *Money/CNN*, August 26, 2002.

5. Cameron Huddleston, "Why You Need Long-Term Care Insurance," *Kiplinger.com*, September 26, 2002.

6. "Changing Places," *Smart Money* (October, 1997), p. 134.

7. "Ratings and Recommendations: Long-Term-Care Insurance," *Consumer Reports* (October, 1997), p. 49.

8. Lewis Schiff, "The long-term care debate," *Money/CNN*, August 27, 2002.

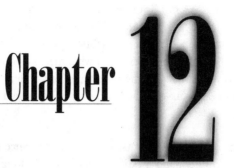

Chapter 12

Phase Two: Provider-Aided Design

"An expert is one who knows more and more about less and less."

– Nicholas Murray Butler

In the early to mid-1990s, long-term care products went through the same evaluation process that disability income policies underwent fifteen years earlier. In the late 1970s through the early 1980s, companies selling disability income policies were rewriting policy provisions, adding new features, and evaluating contract language. This created a wide disparity in the products offered. Insurance agents and consumers found that a comparison of various policy forms required a review of a dozen or more provisions to ensure a thorough and accurate analysis. Premiums fluctuated depending on the benefits and definitions included in any given policy.

Until passage of the Health Insurance Portability and Accountability Act of 1996 (HIPAA), long-term care products were experiencing the same evaluation process. There were a wide variety of definitions and policy provisions that had (and still have) a significant effect on the amount of the premium. How disability is defined, what long-term care services are reimbursable and where these services can be rendered made for a diversity of products. Sorting through the policy language is still important for an in-depth understanding of the product that is offered. It will also ensure a reliable explanation of the information when recommending long-term care insurance to a prospect.

The enactment of HIPAA has (for now) changed the product rules. By defining long-term care insurance in this federal legislation, the end-result has been to standardize long-term care policies' disability definitions to qualify them under the tax code. (For a thorough review of what makes a policy tax-qualified, see Chapter 13.) However, many of the product enhancements achieved in the 1990s are still sold in both tax-qualified and non-tax qualified polices that are sold today.

The involvement of the National Association of Insurance Commissioners (NAIC), and its development and modification of a model long-term care policy, accelerated product changes and impacted on the rate at which a number of individual states imposed specific requirements on policy design. Mandated policy provisions, varying by state, add another layer of complexity to the analysis of the product. While nowhere near the number of mandates health insurance faces, these requirements still presented a challenge to long-term care insurers during the late 1980s and early 1990s. The result was an increasing variety of products at an agent's disposal, making it difficult to keep a reasonable learning pace, and adding to confusion among potential buyers who found it difficult to both compare policies and to judge the value of a given policy provision.

For those selling (and buying) long-term care insurance, it is imperative to take the time to carefully review the coverage that is offered in a policy – specific limitations, policy exclusions, definitions of disability, and premiums. The number of insurers that have been in the long-term care market has dropped over the last several years. Merger and acquisition activity had, and continues to have, an impact on competition and product development. A number of companies entered the long-term care market with little health or disability insurance experience, and early slow sales disappointed many. Industry consolidation has forced a number of carriers to rethink product strategy, resulting in a number of marginal long-term care companies exiting the market, which is not necessarily a bad thing.

According to industry figures, about 3.8 million long-term care insurance policies were sold between 1987 and 1994, at an annual growth rate of 25 percent. But in 1993 and 1994, growth rates slowed to 16.6 and 12.3 percent, respectively,[1] while sales rebounded in 1995, with a 13.4 percent growth rate, bringing the total of in-force policies to 4.35 million.[2] Growth rates remained steady with a 14 percent increase in 1996 (which included the marvelous HIPAA grandfathering fourth quarter), before backing off. In 1997, an 11.7 percent increase was achieved (to 5.5 million policies). By year-end 2001, repercussions from HIPAA had worn off somewhat and 8.3 million policies were on the books.[3]

While the post-HIPAA sales downturn (after 1996) was predictable, the sales "slump" in 1993-95 ironically occurred during a period of rapid product change that thoroughly enhanced the quality of coverage that was available. Insurers, smarting from exposure in the consumer press about selling policies that did not pay, turned to outside help to enhance their product offerings. Seeing that early policy models reflected a lack of understanding of the nature of a long-term care claim, carriers asked the providers of long-term care services and treatments for input into the design and definition of events that triggered claims payments.

So, during the time the Clinton Health Plan was undergoing a national debate, with health and long-term care a potential government-provided program, insurance companies were examining in detail the types of care and settings currently utilized in the long-term care industry. This resulted in diversifying the products available to an even greater degree, at some risk. While experienced insurers enhanced their products and adjusted their premiums accordingly, inexperienced insurers began offering broader policy benefits and reduced prices without regard to potentially high future claims experience. This has proven costly as the financial results on these changes were starting to emerge by 2002, and future claims liability for some insurers appears to be far higher than the premiums that have been charged (More on this in Chapter 14). Like disability income coverage, a block of written long-term care business takes several years before results of any profit or loss are realized.

Working with providers changed portions of the long-term care policy in the latter 1980s and early 1990s, and an educational gap grew in the insurance industry. It was important for producers (and consumers) to absorb and understand these new enhancements, as knowledge of the key policy provisions (and their variations) helps the insurance agent, financial planner, and consumer comprehend the benefits and potential claims liability.

A significant lesson from the disability insurance industry was looming for the long-term care market. While it is important to avoid the truly restrictive products, it is equally critical to stay away from the very liberal plans where poor claims experience can translate into substantial rate increases and possible insurer insolvency.

The consumer counts on the insurance agent for guidance. When the federal government introduced its long-term care insurance plan to its employees, there were no insurance agents who were compensated to review the suitability of this product, identify assets and income to protect, and recommend a solution. As a result, while many responded by purchasing coverage, they overwhelmingly elected one of three pre-packaged plans, rather than trying to match product design to their specific need.

Despite the significant amount of press long-term care insurance receives, it is still a product that must be sold by identifying a need and matching the right product to the client's specific situation. Consumers who are interested in long-term care insurance are a diverse lot, ranging in age from late-40s to mid-80s, with their incomes, assets, health conditions, and ability to pay premiums varying widely. Finding the best policies for consumers means finding the best match between their needs and specific policy provisions.[4]

The Policy Design Basics

The key design parameters of a long-term care insurance policy are daily benefits, elimination periods, benefit periods (or maximum amounts), and inflation protection. Recommendation of these policy elements is based on the agent's own research combined with the financial analysis completed on each prospect.

Daily Benefits

The cost of care in a nursing home is generally the criterion used to initially choose the benefit amount, even though a nursing home stay is a low-frequency event in the long-term care claims world. The price for this type of institutionalized care is generally higher than for most all other forms of long-term care services and settings, due to the potential need and likely prevalence of skilled nursing providers at hand. This means the daily benefit amount, set at nursing home cost levels, should be adequate for other forms of long-term care services.

Information should be available in written form on the average cost and specific costs of nursing homes in a given area. A visit to several nursing homes is also important in eliminating those that fall below recommendable standards. It is one thing to have an average cost. But daily benefit recommendations should be done on the basis of the average cost of *acceptable* facilities.

In some policies, the daily benefit amount selected is used to determine the coverage payable for other long-term care services such as home health care. Often a percentage of the daily benefit amount can be chosen to dictate the amount paid for home health care and adult day care, two reimbursements that are usually less than the cost of staying in a nursing home.

For example, if your client has chosen a $100 a day benefit based on local nursing home costs, the policy may pay 50 percent of this amount (or $50 a day) for home health care services and 25 percent ($25 a day) for adult day care that is needed. These percentages can vary, allowing flexibility in selection. Home health care can be 50, 75, 100 or even 150 percent of the daily benefit amount selected for nursing home confinement.

Many policies offer level daily benefit amounts without regard to the service needed. For example, if an individual chooses a daily benefit of $100, the coverage, whether it is for a nursing home stay, home health care, adult day care, or other covered services, would be $100 a day. Other plans allow a selection of individual daily benefit levels for primary services.

Indemnity versus Reimbursement

The daily benefit amount can be paid two different ways:

1.   Pay the full daily benefit (or appropriate percentage) selected regardless of the actual charges for long-term care services provided, or

2.   Pay the actual charge incurred for long-term care services provided up to the daily benefit amount selected.

There is a difference and the policy language should be reviewed to determine how the daily benefit is paid. The first option pays the insured the specified amount elected under the policy for long-term care services provided regardless of the actual cost (higher or lower) of the services rendered. For example, if an insured receives home health care at a cost of $60 a day, the selected daily benefit amount of $75 is paid to the insured regardless of the actual cost. This is an "indemnity" type payment, similar to disability income coverage. As you will see in Chapter 13, this type of payment could have tax consequences for the insured. It is also slightly higher in premium than the second option for paying benefits.

The second option pays either the daily benefit amount elected or actual cost if it is lower than the daily benefit. Using the same example, if the selected daily benefit amount is $75 and the actual cost for home health care is $59, the policy will pay $59 as the actual cost is lower than $75. If the actual cost is higher than the daily benefit amount, the policy will pay $75, the maximum daily benefit amount selected. This is called a "reimbursement" type policy, and is by far the most common type of payment plan offered for sale in the long-term care market.

Inflation Protection

Daily amounts should also be indexed annually to offset the effects of inflation. Health care costs, including those dedicated to long-term care treatment, rise each year, often at a pace faster than the Consumer Price Index. You have a choice of electing an inflation option to help the daily benefit increase each year to potentially keep pace with the regular upsurge in long-term care costs. Usually the percentage available for increase is 5 percent, and it can be selected on either a simple or compounding multiple basis. This is a critical choice, especially for those buyers of coverage who are under age 65.

This is usually an optional benefit for the policy and will be discussed in Chapter 16, "Optional Benefits."

Zero Day Elimination Periods

The zero day elimination period (see Chapter 10, "Long-term Care versus Disability Income Product Design") is still available in the long-term care insurance market. When balanced against a policy that offers reasonable benefits, the zero day elimination period has so far withstood the test of time. A zero day elimination period allows benefit payments to begin immediately and many insurers have not yet experienced the anticipated adverse claims.

A word of caution to anyone considering the zero day elimination period – a few insurers have begun to eliminate this choice among elimination periods due to claims losses. If it is sold in combination with a remarkably easy qualification for benefits provision, the results will undoubtedly be high claims and equally high rate increases. The downside is for those policyholders who are now in their late 60's or early 70's (when the likelihood of long-term care increases). If they have had the policy for some time but not yet made a claim, they will soon be facing a rate increase which may render the policy unaffordable. What kind of service does the agent and the industry provide when a policyholder has to drop the plan or significantly modify the coverage at a time when the product is most needed?

The health insurance market continues to face this problem and inevitably will bring us back to the brink of a national health insurance program run by the government. The disability insurance industry expanded benefits and reduced prices in the early 1980's and paid for it with losses every year from 1986 to 2000. The result was a conservative marketing, underwriting, and claims atmosphere that suffocated sales, from which the disability income market is only just emerging.

So use caution when recommending the zero day elimination period. The long-term care market stands on the edge of feast or famine at present, and the agent and consumer must find the right balance between fair coverage and a reasonable premium. A 30-day elimination period can work just as well, save some premium dollars, and eliminate some of the frequent, small claims that can erode the insurer's loss ratio and justify future rate increases.

Benefit Periods

There are two types of benefit periods that are available today. The first type is the traditional benefit period where policy benefits can be paid within a specified number of months, or years. Typically, 12 months, 2, 3, 4, 5 and 6 years are examples of benefit periods. Policies can also be sold with an unlimited benefit period – as long as the insured needs covered long-term care services, benefits will be paid. This is a popular benefit period despite its higher cost in comparison to the potential payout with shorter benefit periods.

Historically, the choices in benefit periods began with a six-month maximum introduced in CNA's first long-term care policy in 1965. Today, many states require a minimum of 12 to 24 months for payout of benefits.

The second type of benefit period available is not measured in days, months, or years, but rather in dollars. This is called a "pool of money concept" and is becoming popular among insurers, agents, and consumers. Rather than specify a period of time, benefits for long-term care services are paid from a single lifetime dollar maximum. Benefits are payable for as long as the maximum amount lasts, regardless of the time period.

The lifetime maximum amount is calculated using the daily benefit selected multiplied by a specific number of days elected by the person buying the coverage. The specified days may be 1,000, 2,000, 3,000 or 365, 730, 1,095, 1,460, etc. The following are examples of the lifetime maximum:

$100/day x 2,000 days = $200,000

$100/day x 1,460 days = $146,000

It can be compared to purchasing a lump sum amount except the benefits will be disbursed over an unspecified period of time instead of all at once.

Pool of money plans typically pay expenses as they are incurred in an amount up to the daily benefit level (see #2 in the daily benefit explanation above). Thus, expenses that are consistently below the daily benefit amount likely mean a longer payout period than the number of days (the original benefit period) used to calculate the lifetime maximum.

At least one insurer has introduced a pure "face amount" approach to covering long-term care. Here, the consumer can elect both the daily benefit amount and the total face amount, without the need for a calculation. For example, the policy could have a $150/daily benefit amount and a $450,000 total face amount, both options selected at time of application. The thinking was that if a pure face amount was used, perhaps more life insurance-oriented agents would be comfortable in a plan design that bears some similarity to life insurance.

Renewability

Once the agent has recommended the basic policy selections to the insured, careful review of the various policy provisions is necessary. The first discussion should be about renewability.

This policy provision is usually found on the face page of the policy itself. As noted previously, the minimum renewal provision called for by the NAIC is guaranteed renewability. This means that the policy cannot be arbitrarily canceled (except for non-payment of premiums) nor can any policy provisions be altered in any way except for the betterment of provisions. However, insurers do possess the right to impose a rate increase on a specific class of long-term care business.

The term "class" consists of a specific policy or policy series. State insurance departments will allow reasonable and justifiable rate increases on a policy form because it affects all purchasers of this product.

Nearly all comprehensive long-term care policies have this type of renewal provision. This makes it easy to compare this product feature. There are no true non-cancelable renewable policies for long-term care. Given the recent troubles of the non-cancelable renewable provision in disability income policies, it is not likely to be a policy feature offered in the near future. However, some insurers are offering a premium rate guarantee for a specific number of years (anywhere from three to 20 years). Combined with the guaranteed renewable provision, this gives the consumer a period of time when the policy has, in effect, a non-cancelable provision. Recent reinsurance and claims problems may ultimately result in these types of guarantees being eliminated from future policy filings. (See more on this subject in Chapter 14.)

Be wary of policies *not* written on a guaranteed renewable basis. Policies that pay for a specified service rather than taking a more comprehensive approach may offer renewability on a conditional basis. This type of renewal, while keeping premium costs low, also gives the insurance companies the opportunity to refuse to renew the policy based on poor claims experience. Policies that provide benefits for nursing home coverage only or for home health care could contain this type of provision. These plans are not considered long-term care insurance in most states, and thus may not be advertised as such.

Definitions of Disability

This product feature dictates how a prospect qualifies for benefits. The definitions of disability, as in a disability income policy, are the key measurements of a long-term care policy.

Until the passage of HIPAA, long-term care policies utilized a "triple-trigger" means of qualifying for policy benefits. This approach gave the insured three possible ways of qualifying for benefits.

The insured's ability to function independently is the framework for benefit eligibility. The three definitions for benefit eligibility are:

1. Inability to perform a certain number of activities of daily living (ADLs).

2. Suffering from a cognitive impairment, such as Alzheimer's or Parkinson's disease.

3. A medical necessity, as prescribed by a physician, for long-term care services.

This triple-trigger feature allows the insured to qualify for benefits by meeting the requirements under any one of these definitions. The primary definition is the inability to perform a certain number of routine activities of daily living (ADLs).

The most common activities of daily living are bathing, dressing, eating, toileting, transferring (mobility or transporting), continence, or taking medicine.

Insurers generally list and define these qualifying activities of daily living in their policies. A HIPAA-sanctioned tax-qualified plan must take into account at least five of these six ADLs: Eating, toileting, bathing, dressing, and continence. (See Chapter 13.) Other policies that are considered non-tax-qualified may have other ADL definitions.

To qualify under the primary definition, the inability to perform a certain number of ADLs, usually a minimum of two must be evident. Thus, this definition was usually written as "the inability of the insured to perform two or more activities of daily living." Some insurers have required the loss of three (which you don't see anymore), while a few insurers required the loss of only one ADL to activate a claim, a dangerously easy qualification as previously mentioned.

The requirement that an insured lose three or more ADLs was strict and under-competitive, while the loss of only one activity made it too easy to qualify for benefits. Insurers marketing the latter were, in effect, competing by policy liberalization, and were making the same mistake the disability insurance industry did in policy liberalization. The ease of qualification would inevitably lead to higher than expected claims experience and necessitate the application for an increase in policy rates. This is a great definition of disability to use during a sales interview (just like "own occ" was for disability income), but the client could be subject to a heavy rate increase later that could leave him in a vulnerable position if premium affordability becomes an issue.

The loss of two ADLs is liberal enough if bathing and dressing are among those activities listed. According to UNUM Provident, a long-term care and disability income insurer, in over 85 percent of long-term care cases, bathing and dressing are the first ADLs requiring assistance. Think about it. Getting in and out of the bathtub can be dangerous because of a slippery surface. A fall can immobilize an already frail person or compound problems for someone who already has health problems. Likewise, dressing requires being somewhat limber when bending down to tie shoelaces or simply buttoning a shirt. Arthritis can significantly hamper someone's ability to get dressed. The loss of these two ADLs first triggers benefit payments quicker than the other activities.

One of the quirks of aging is that the ability to perform activities of daily living is generally lost in the reverse order in which they were learned. The last activity a parent lets a child do independently is bathing. The chances of an accident are too numerous to mention. Dressing, such as buttoning a shirt or tying shoelaces, also requires a parent's help for some time. Yet these same two activities, last learned, are the first activities lost for the elderly.

The importance of how the inability to perform activities of daily living is defined has prompted much speculation. Initially, most companies preferred to take a "black and white approach" to claims adjudication. An insured was either independent, needing no assistance, or dependent, requiring assistance. The problem was that a number of people received long-term care assistance because of an activity which they could still occasionally perform themselves. A person could put on clothes without assistance but needed help tying shoelaces. This is not independence – this person cannot leave the house without shoes (although someone could buy shoes without laces). But is it truly dependence because other articles of clothing can be negotiated?

There is an interim level of care between dependence and independence which most insurers were slow to recognize. However, when some insurers enlisted long-term care providers to help them understand the nature of a long-term care claim, it became evident that there was a "partial" gap through which a number of claims were falling. Partial assistance with certain activities of daily living was more commonplace than believed and, as such, should somehow be recognized in a long-term care insurance policy.

Similarly, it took disability income insurers many years to acknowledge the importance of residual disability. Residual disability pays a portion of the total monthly disability benefit upon the insured's return to work and is based on the percentage of loss of earnings incurred as a result. Partial assistance, the middle ground between independence and dependence, was introduced into a few long-term care policies prior to the enactment of HIPAA. The federal law identified this claim trend as "standby assistance," a term insurers had to define in the new "tax-qualified" policies. (See Chapter 13 for more details on "standby assistance.") Its appearance in HIPAA indicated the importance of including this type of care in long-term care policies.

The second definition in qualifying an insured for claim benefits is usually an alternative to the primary definition. One of the most severe disabilities affecting the elderly is Alzheimer's disease, an organic brain disorder. As millions of Americans battle this difficult disease, the condition poses a difficulty for insurers using the "ability to perform ADLs" test. Under the primary definition of disability, it is necessary for the insured to suffer a continuing inability to perform two or more ADLs. Alzheimer's patients may enjoy days they function normally, and are thus disqualified from satisfying the continued loss of an ADL requirement.

In addition, as part of the NAIC Model Act, it was mandated that insurers cover Alzheimer's disease, Parkinson's disease, and other organic brain disorders that occur after the policy has been purchased. To do this, a second definition of disability, "cognitive impairment," was developed, where the insured automatically becomes eligible for benefits. Policy language for this definition may read:

> "Cognitive impairment means the deterioration in, or loss of, the insured's intellectual capacity and may include exhibition of: (1) abusive or assaultive behavior; or (2) poor judgment; or (3) bizarre hygiene or habits, which requires continual supervision to protect the insured or others. Cognitive impairment is measured by clinical evidence and standardized tests and is based on the insured's impairment as indicated by loss in the following areas: (1) his/her short or long term memory; or (2) his/her recognition of who or where he/she is, or time of day, month or year; or (3) his/her deductive or abstract reasoning."

There was no universal definition of cognitive impairment recognized by insurers so terminology differed from policy to policy. Language was standardized after HIPAA.

Nearly 4 million Americans have Alzheimer's disease and it is believed that without a cure or method of prevention, that number will grow to 14 million by the middle of the 21st century. Approximately 10 percent of people age 65 years or older are affected by the disease, rising to nearly half of those over age 85. The U.S. spends more than $100 billion a year on Alzheimer's disease, a largely unfunded expense forcing Americans to have to pick up the tab.[5]

This explains the government's insistence in including a special qualifying definition to recognize conditions like Alzheimer's disease. The onset can often be long after the policy is purchased, and a means of benefit qualification was needed to be sure long-term care expenses needed to treat the disease were covered. While the majority of Alzheimer's patients are treated informally at home, many of these individuals end up in some type of long-term care facility because family caregivers find it difficult to care for loved ones with this condition.

While virtually all plans used the first two definitions to qualify an insured for benefits in the late 1980s, a growing number of insureds needing long-term care were not meeting these definitional requirements for policy payment. If, according to a doctor, the insured needs long-term care services, but does not meet either of the first two definitions, what happens? Providers assisting insurers with product design pointed out that this situation was more common than believed. Providers helped develop a third definition under which insureds could qualify for long-term care benefits. This gave the newest long-term care plans in the early 1990s three methods of benefit eligibility.

For those policies with the triple-trigger definitions, this third method of qualifying is called medical necessity. This definition allows eligibility for benefits to be established if the need for long-term care services is substantiated by a physician, usually the insured's own physician. It is, in essence, a fall back provision if the need for long-term care services is warranted, but neither the first nor second method of qualifying for benefits can be achieved.

Under "medical necessity," if an illness or injury occurred and it necessitated the use of long-term care services, verified by a physician, benefits were payable. Some insurers required that the medical condition precipitating the need for long-term care be the same as the original injury or illness. Other insurers required the physician to certify the need for the care. Continuous verification of the long-term care need from the physician was necessary for benefits to continue under the medical necessity definition.

The HIPAA legislation effectively disposed of this third method of benefits qualification. Tax-qualified plans are defined by two benefit triggers – loss of two of six ADLs and cognitive impairment. This was a substantial setback to provider-aided advances in long-term care policy design. (See Chapter 13 for a more in-depth discussion of this change.)

These definitions were a fair and flexible approach in qualifying for benefits and seemed to satisfy most insurers and insureds. These "triple-trigger" policies were certainly far more generous in qualifying for benefits than earlier policies. The HIPAA legislation has now rendered these plans outside the definition of "tax-qualified" plans. But these policies are still available, although they come with "warning labels" as to possible adverse taxation. At this point, the future of the "medical necessity" trigger lies in doubt.

Long-Term Care Benefits

Chapter 5 identified the types of long-term care services offered today. Now let's see how the following benefits are treated in long-term care policies:

skilled nursing care   intermediate care
custodial care   ·   home health care
home care   adult day care
respite care   hospice care

Most comprehensive policies cover these services in some fashion. Look for reference to them and their definitions in every policy.

Skilled care – Requires the service of trained medical personnel with the authorization of a physician. Skilled care can be administered in a skilled or intermediate nursing facility, a hospital, at home, or in an assisted living facility. These various settings can be found in comprehensive long-term care policies. Actual reimbursement can vary based on where the services are rendered.

Intermediate care – Requires the skill of trained medical personnel on a less frequent basis than skilled care and with the authorization of a physician. Intermediate care is generally administered to patients who need medical care or therapy to resume their ADLs. In a skilled or intermediate care nursing facility, the nursing home daily rate would likely be paid. Home health care, adult day care centers, and assisted living facilities would also receive reimbursement, possibly at a different payment level.

Custodial care – Primarily assisting with ADLs, this level of care does not have to be authorized by a physician or require trained medical personnel. Most often custodial care is received at home and delivered by qualified home health aides. If care is received in a custodial care facility, the nursing home rate would likely apply. Reimbursement at a different level for care received in an assisted living facility is also possible.

Home health care – Medically necessary skilled or intermediate care with the authorization of a physician and performed by trained medical personnel. Benefits could be paid as a percentage of the nursing home daily benefit, at the same level, or a larger reimbursement depending on the design of the product. Many policies pay home health and home care benefits on a weekly or monthly basis rather than a daily amount like nursing home or assisted living care. Facilities typically charge by the day, so this translates well to the daily benefit amount in a policy. But home health care visits are all over the map, with an increasing tendency of home health care agencies to stack visits on given days. If benefits are paid daily for home health care, it could leave the insured short on those multiple-visit days. A weekly or monthly calculation means the claimant is working from a larger sum of money from which to pay for the visits, thus ensuring a closer approximation of policy benefits to expenses incurred.

Home care – This is custodial care – assistance with ADLs and household chores. Benefits could be paid as a percentage of the nursing home daily benefit amount, at the same level, or a greater amount. This care is usually delivered by a home health care aide or possibly a licensed practical nurse. As noted above, claims benefits are often calculated on a weekly or monthly basis to help ensure fewer if any out-of-pocket costs to the insured.

Adult day care – This long-term care service is considered custodial care or intermediate care provided in a licensed adult day care facility. Caregivers who work during the day will find this a convenient alternative. The policy may have a specific rate for adult day care reimbursement or could pay from the pool of money at rates up to the daily benefit level.

Respite care – This benefit provides temporary relief for those in a caregiving role by hiring temporary help to care for a dependent adult. Depending on the policy language, more than one temporary helper can be hired at the same time. This help is reimbursed up to the limits of the policy. Typically, the policy pays for a specified period, such as "up to 21 days" for temporary help. The substitute can most often be obtained from a local home health care agency.

Hospice care – Many long-term care policies provide some benefit for hospice care, a program primarily designed for pain and symptom control for terminally ill patients. Benefits could be paid as a percentage of the nursing home daily benefit, at the same level, or a larger reimbursement level depending on the complexity of the product design. In addition, an amount may be paid for bereavement counseling for other family members. Medicare also provides some assistance for bereavement, and policies paying daily benefits on a tax-qualified plan (see Chapter 13) will involve coordination with Medicare.

These are the most common services and reimbursement structures in long-term care today. It is vitally important to be as accurate as possible in choosing the daily benefit amount because virtually all benefit services and reimbursements are based on this selection. It is important to do your homework in the areas of long-term care you plan to market so that the proper recommendations are made. (See Chapter 4, "The Financial Strain of Aging," for more details on identifying local area long-term care costs.)

Alternate Plans of Care

The focus of early long-term care policies was on reimbursing the costs of qualified nursing home stays. Later, home health care was added as a coverage feature. But long-term care services today are delivered in a variety of settings, and long-term care insurance policies have responded accordingly.

Because of the number of potential facility settings, most long-term care policies today contain a provision that allows claim payments for long-term care services delivered outside the scope of the usual policy definitions. Most insurers recognize that the long-term care industry is still evolving and advances in medical science will create services and even facilities that may not be specifically described in the policy. Still, the insurer may want to cover these services for a variety of reasons.

For example, a long-term care insurance claim involved a woman who was in a skilled nursing facility recovering from a stroke. Once the need for on-hand skilled care abated, there was the opportunity to return the patient to her home, with only some outpatient therapy treatments to be done. The problem? Her house was not wheelchair accessible. A contractor reviewed the situation, and estimated about $30,000 for wheelchair ramps, an elevator, grab bars in the shower, and a lowering of electric sockets, among other changes. The insurer was paying a daily benefit amount while the individual was in the facility. Claims expenses would be limited once she returned home, and her likelihood of a better future rested with a day-to-day existence in comfortable surroundings. For all those reasons, the insurer negotiated with the contractor, reducing the bill somewhat, and paid for the home improvements under the "Alternate Plan of Care" definition in the policy.

The illustrates the idea that basing reimbursement on the benefit triggers, as providers suggested, rather than more narrowly defining the types of services and facilities for which payment is eligible, leads to easier claims adjudication and the recognition that claims will vary considerably depending on the individual and circumstances.

Those familiar with disability income claims know that every case is different even if two people suffer a similar ailment. People adjust differently to adverse medical circumstances, and what works for one may not necessarily work for another. Long-term care insurers have been contracting case managers to assist in fully evaluating each claim, making recommendations based on the most effective treatment at the most reasonable cost, taking into account the wishes of the family, and the circumstances which would either speed recovery or make one more comfortable. Not all of this can be defined in the policy language, so carriers include "alternate plans of care" to cover other, non-contract options.

Under this option, a number of assisted living facilities like adult congregate living facilities (ACLFs) are recognized by the insurer as a setting for receiving long-term care services. Whether it is a "home for the aged" or the most expensive nursing home in the area, alternate plans of care can encompass the entire range of services. Growing at a phenomenal rate, the variety of long-term care services and facilities is expanding far beyond the capacity of an insurance policy to include the latest service or type of facility. The terminology for the policy option, alternate plans of care (and with one carrier, the catchier phrase "Emerging Trends"), alleviates the burden to keep up with the trends on paper. Insurers are always looking for ways to improve coverage, and careful monitoring of long-term care trends is constant.

Insurers have also begun recognizing that many people receive care from a family member or friend. As a result, benefits like *caregiver training* have been incorporated into the basic plan design. This feature pays a set amount (a multiple of the daily benefit) to provide training lessons for the informal caregiver. Since circumstances often dictate that family or friends adopt the caregiver role, this benefit can be especially helpful. Some insurers will even pay these individuals under the policy to provide care once they are trained and certified.

Other Policy Provisions

Waiver of Premium

This policy feature is designed to eliminate the burden of premium payments by the insured during the time of claim. Unlike disability insurance, under long-term care insurance there are an assortment of definitions as to what conditions trigger a waiver of the premium once a person is disabled. Depending on the insurance company, policies can begin waiving premiums once the elimination period has been satisfied. Other insurers do not waive premiums until the insured has been collecting benefits under the policy for a specific period of days, generally consecutive. Still other carriers will waive premiums after a specified period of days regardless of the elimination period.[6]

Some policies waive premium for only a stay in a nursing home, others for any type of care received. There are policies with split waivers – one for home care and the other for facility care.

Thus it is important to read this policy feature carefully as there are many definitions of waiver of premium. Most insurers include it in the policy, but some have it available as an option. It is vital that this option be elected, as it makes no sense for an individual to be receiving policy benefits and simultaneously paying premiums indefinitely.

Restoration of Benefits

When an insured selects a benefit period other than "unlimited" or "lifetime" periods, this policy provision will restore claim days already used. If the insured has a claim, then recovers, and is claim-free for a set period (usually 6 months), the claim period can be fully restored back to its original level or amount. For example, an individual with a three-year benefit period has a claim for a year, then eventually recovers and goes treatment-free for six months. The three-year benefit period would then be restored in full for the individual.

This provision works for the "pool of money" benefit, also. For example, assume an individual had a $146,000 policy benefit, had a claim, used $57,000 of it, and then recovered for a six month period of time. The $57,000 would be "restored" to create the original account amount of $146,000. If the original policy amount had been increased several times under the inflation option, the policy typically would be restored to the face amount that existed at time of claim.

Bed Reservation Benefit

A person in a nursing home, assisted living facility, or a hospice facility may need to be hospitalized for several days due to a medical condition. If the facility he lives in charges to hold the bed until his return, the policy can reimburse the insured up to a specific number of days, usually with a maximum limit of 21 to 31 days, or sometimes a specific dollar amount. This allows for continuous care and ensures that an insured will have a bed at the same facility, providing a consistency of treatment that is important. Otherwise, the insured runs the risk of having to change facilities if no beds are available after the hospital stay is completed. With popular facilities that usually have a waiting list, this is a real possibility and a helpful provision to rely on.

Cognitive Reinstatement

Traditionally, insurance policies, by law, have a 31-day grace period beyond the premium due date. This allows the insured to make a late payment without any interruption or change in the coverage. Long-term care policies have extended grace periods. If it is satisfactorily demonstrated that the missed payment was due to forgetfulness or even a cognitive impairment, reinstatement of the lapsed policy can be made several months after policy lapse. The payment of back premiums is required to reinstate the policy. This allows individuals a maximum range of flexibility under which to continue the policy in good faith.

This provision may also be written in conjunction with a *third party notification* provision under which an individual, often a family member, receives lapse notices. This ensures that another individual can inquire about the missed payment and keep the policy in force. Because of requests by different states, this is now featured more prominently on applications.

Pre-Existing Conditions

There are situations that are specifically excluded from claims consideration under a long-term care policy. Today states require that a complete list of policy exclusions, including pre-existing conditions, be displayed on any sales material that is published. A pre-existing condition is one that is not disclosed on the policy application and for which the person received treatment or medical advice within a specified period of time (usually six months) before the policy went into effect. This means that if the individual was aware of a medical condition and treatment or advice was sought in the months prior to obtaining the long-term care insurance and did not disclose this condition on the application, it is considered pre-existing and there is no coverage. If the pre-existing condition is disclosed on the application and the policy is approved with or without restriction, it is no longer considered a pre-existing condition.

Other more common exclusions from coverage are:

1. War, or act of war, declared or not declared.

2. Intentionally self-inflicted injury or attempted suicide.

3. Injuries sustained while attempting to commit or committing a felony.

4. Services rendered for treatment of drug, alcohol or chemical dependence.

5. Non-organic brain disorders. (Alzheimer's is an organic brain disorder.)

6. Care covered by any state or federal workers' compensation, employer's liability or occupational disease law. (In tax-qualified plans, care

provided by Medicare, although the policy could pay in part if Medicaid reimbursement is lower than the actual expense.)

7.   Care provided by a member of the insured's family.

8.   Care received for which a charge would not have been assessed except for the presence of insurance, such as a free service provided by a church organization for which no obligation to pay would be the normal course of affairs.

9.   Care provided outside the United States, U.S. possessions or Canada.

10.   Care provided free of charge in a federal governmental facility, such as in a Department of Veterans Affairs facility.

Each policy may have other exclusions and should be evaluated on its own merit to see if it is legitimate. Many policies today have few exclusions.

Care Advocates/Coordinators

Today's long-term care policies are doing more to provide education for those needing care and (especially) their families. The need for long-term care services often involves difficult decisions. Moreover, the care itself may be complex, with a number of health professionals participating in the delivery of these services. Many policies now reimburse the consultations a family and claimant have with a qualified professional like a registered nurse or social worker. Claims are coordinated by a specific claims counselor. Fees for program counselors that furnish information on a number of aging issues (even in advance of a claim) may be reimbursed. While not potentially significant in cost to the insurer, these programs are valuable for the insured and family and can help to ease the burdens of long-term care decision-making.

Spouse Discounts

Many companies offer a 10 to 40 percent discount (and sometimes higher) if both spouses apply for long-term care insurance. The reasoning behind this offer is a clear relationship between the amount of time spent in a nursing home and marital status. In 2000, about 30 percent of non-institutionalized older persons lived alone (7.4 million women, 2.4 million men). Over half (55 percent) of older non-institutionalized persons lived with a spouse (10.1 million or 73 percent of men, and 7.7 million or 41 percent of women).[7] Most companies who offer this provision will let one spouse keep the discount even if the other is turned down for coverage because of health reasons. Other carriers will permit a spouse (or married) discount even if only one of them applies.

In addition, carriers are now introducing companion discounts, if the people certify that they have been living together for a specified period of time (such as three years or longer). Many older adults (often widows and widowers) live together, but opt not to marry for financial reasons. Insurers will still likely reap the benefit of informal care delivered by the companion, thus the discount. This would also apply to same sex companions, for the identical reason.

Policy Exchanges

Policy upgrades offered when an insurer upgraded a policy provision are generally off limits for pre-1997 long-term care insurance policies as it might render the entire policy or the new feature non-tax-qualified. So, while some older policies do not have some of the newer, more expansive policy provisions, changing or replacing them may not necessarily be prudent if it jeopardizes its tax status and other provisions of the policy are better than what is available today under a tax-qualified status. Careful evaluation should be done when reviewing these older plans.[8]

Most tax-qualified plans today have an exchange provision converting them to the older non-qualified language should clear direction ever be received from the Treasury Department regarding the taxation of long-term care policies that do not conform to HIPAA legislation. (For more details on tax-qualified plans, see Chapter 13.)

Non-Forfeiture Benefits

This is a recent addition to many companies' policies. The NAIC added a mandated non-forfeiture provision to its policies in 1993. This feature requires insurers to preserve some of the policy benefits even if the insured stops paying premiums. HIPAA legislation also addressed the non-forfeiture feature of long-term care policies. Today, policies offer non-forfeiture benefits on an optional basis. This feature can add a substantial amount of cost to the overall premium in exchange for having a "paid up" policy should the insured have the plan for a certain period of time and then stop paying premiums.

In life insurance, after a certain number of years, the premiums paid have achieved some ownership or vesting in the policy. In long-term care, the insured can elect to take a paid-up policy where the money paid in has been calculated to refigure the benefit level to allow coverage to continue for the same length of time with the same elimination period at a reduced daily benefit amount. In a "pool of money" concept, the amount of the maximum total benefit is refigured at either a multiple of the daily benefit amount or the total amount of premium paid for the policy, whichever is greater.

This provision ensures that premiums paid have some significance if the insured should decide to stop paying the premium. Otherwise, although the money was paid and the protection was present, the insured has little to show for that investment when premium payments cease.

In its recent amendment to the original LTC Model Policy, the NAIC has added a "contingent nonforfeiture benefit" that can be elected by the insured in lieu of accepting a premium rate increase, or if the rate increase exceeds a certain percentage. (More on this is in Chapter 14.)

Medical Help Benefit

Some policies will reimburse all or a portion of the cost to maintain a medical help system in the home. For some individuals who prefer home to a nursing facility, this is an extra feature that can provide the necessary emergency means of contacting someone should the need arise. There are numerous stories of people found hours and days after a medical emergency because they were unable to reach a phone to call for help.

Premiums

The cost for a long-term care policy fluctuates between insurers, issue ages, and benefit levels. This makes it difficult to compare premium cost between two plans.

For example, two quotes are ordered from two different insurance companies. The premium for one plan is $1,000 annually, for the other plan, $1,350 annually. The differences in the coverage of the two plans must be reviewed before recommending the lower premium plan. It may be that the $1,000 plan does not include inflation protection. Or, the $1,350 plan allows the insured to receive care in virtually any setting while the $1,000 plan limits coverage to a nursing facility or in the home.

There are some basic assumptions regarding premiums in general. Individuals in their 40s and 50s can expect to pay relatively low premiums for long-term care coverage. Typically, people in this age group will not file a claim for some time. The premiums for new business applications begin to accelerate each year, starting around age 60. Rates can be dramatically higher for those buying coverage in their 70s and 80s.

The relationship between premium and age underscores the need to plan ahead and consider coverage in pre-retirement years. Since premiums can be increased by the insurer in the years after purchase, a premium starting out low will be less affected by any change.

For example, if a prospect was paying $405 for a policy and the insurance company raised the rates by ten percent, the increase would be $40.50 annually, for a new annual premium of $445.50. If a prospect was paying $1,086, the increase would be $108.60 annually, for a new annual premium of $1,194.60. For a $4,372 annual premium, the rate increase would be $437.20 annually, for a new annual premium of $4,809.20. The chart below illustrates the rate increase relationship.

Premium	Rate Increase	Dollar Increase	New Premium
$ 405.00	10%	$ 40.50	$ 445.50
$1,086.00	10%	$108.60	$1,194.60
$4,372.00	10%	$437.20	$4,809.20

In addition to age, other factors can affect the amount of policy premium:

Elimination Period – the shorter the elimination period (0, 15, 20 days), the higher the premium.

Benefit Period – the longer the period of time benefits are paid, or the higher the lifetime maximum benefit in a pool of money plan, the higher the premium.

Daily Benefit – the higher the daily benefit, the higher the premium.

Gender – insurers generally charge the same rate for male and females (some states require this), so this is not usually a factor.

Health Risks – some insurers have tiers of risk classification and those applicants with health conditions may pay a higher rate than those who are relatively healthy.

Optional Benefits – if additional features, such as inflation protection and return of premium are selected, the cost of the policy will be higher. See Chapter 16, "Optional Benefits."

Earlier policies often had rate bands for certain ages and the premiums automatically went up when one moved from one rate band to another. The grouping of ages were typically 40-49, 50-54, 55-59, 60-64, 65-69 and so on. For example, if a policy was purchased at age 47, the premium would automatically change at age 50, again at age 55, at age 60, and so on. This increase was in addition to any other rate increases the insurer levied based on overall claims experience.

The NAIC (and many states) outlawed this rate banding practice for comprehensive long-term care policies several years ago. Now, when a policy is purchased, the only rate increases filed by the insurer will be based on claims experience. These increases may happen periodically or they may not happen at all.

Moreover, some insurers offer a period of rate guarantee, meaning during this time, rates cannot be increased under any circumstances. These offers range from three to twenty years. The longer the rate guarantee, the higher the premium amount. These rate guarantees may have a short shelf life as the confidence in long-term care pricing is still not considerably high. In addition, the NAIC has started formalizing the maximum percentages that rates may be increased by age (See table in Chapter 14), so carriers may be unwilling to rule out a premium increase for any specified length of time.

Managed Care

Managed care has invaded the world of long-term care insurance. While its influence on health insurance is unmistakable, managed care's effect on long-term care coverage is in its early stages.

Some carriers are beginning to introduce plans that have familiar managed care wrinkles. Initially, they contracted with a nationwide long-term care provider (usually in the home health field), to offer lower cost alternatives to claimants. For policies paying out under a "pool of money" concept, this was particularly important. If the claimant works with a preferred provider, for example, the usual long-term care service charge is discounted. Lower policy reimbursement means the "pool or money" can last much longer, extending the length of time benefits could be paid.

Some of the managed care influences have already been noted. The idea of a care coordinator or a patient care advocate for the family is typical of bringing patients and family through a continuum of care, where all phases of medical services delivered are supervised to avoid duplicative expenses while maintaining a high level of quality.

Products with coverage that varies in and out of a network setting are now starting to emerge. Use the nursing home preferred provider and obtain a discount or higher level of benefit payment. Utilize the services of a preferred alternate care facility and save out-of-pocket claim costs. Select a preferred home care provider and reimbursement levels increase accordingly. This is managed care, and as the costs for long-term care continue to escalate, the need for this type of cost containment will be inevitable. Some insurers have started now before claims losses start to accelerate.

Uniform Licensing of Facilities

While HIPAA standardized language for benefit triggers under a LTC policy, the states still have a vast number of rules governing the licensing and certification of long-term care providers. For example, the definition of a nursing home can vary because of requirements such as the number of beds, type of care provided, and required staffing, such as licensed nurses. The laws of the state in which the product is issued govern the terms of the product.[9]

The problem arises when someone takes a policy out in a particular state, with specifically drawn language, and then moves to a state that may have more or less liberal guidelines for certification of a facility or provider. Which language governs? The original policy, or the rules of the state in which care is received? This can be especially important when an individual moves from his current residence state to be closer to children when a long-term care event occurs, not an uncommon situation.

Most carriers will let the individual receive the benefit of the less restrictive language, be it the state law or the policy provision. You should check with your insurer, however, to be sure this is correct and to find out what to do if you do move from one state to the other after the purchase of your long-term care insurance policy.

Policy Review

Here is a checklist of questions for reviewing the basic policy design when evaluating a long-term care insurance program:[10]

1. What long-term care services are covered? Does the policy cover skilled, intermediate care, custodial, home health care, and adult day care and respite care?

2. When do benefits start? What elimination period choices are available?

3. How long will the policy pay benefits? How is the pool of money maximum amount calculated? Are home care benefits paid on a daily, weekly, or monthly basis?

4. Will the policy pay for care in all settings? Nursing homes, one's own home, assisted living facilities, adult day care centers?

5. What is the minimum and maximum daily benefit that can be purchased? Is the daily benefit reimbursed on an indemnity or incurred expense basis?

6. How are pre-existing conditions defined? What are the specific policy exclusions?

7. Is the policy tax-qualified?

8. Is the policy guaranteed renewable? Are there any rate guarantees?

9. Does the contract include waiver of premium? When and under what conditions does it start?

10. What is the spouse and companion discount?

This brief checklist can help you identify the key features of the policy for your clients and ensure that you are keeping up to date with the latest policy trends in the long-term care marketplace. In addition, be sure the company for your client is one that has a strong financial rating and some years of experience in this market. Long-term care insurance policies are enjoying unprecedented persistency levels, meaning very few people are lapsing their plans. They realize that the older one gets, the closer one is to potentially needing the policy. This makes the financial longevity of the insurer that much more important. It is probably best if the insurer has other lines of business from which assets are derived. Diversification of portfolio means that a downturn in any one line is likely to be made up by surplus from other lines.

Long-term care providers helped form policy language in the late 1980s-early 1990s, most of which still exists today, and that aided in the recognition by outside analysts of the quality of the coverage offered for consumers. It will be the government that will make the next move in putting its stamp on long-term care insurance products.

Chapter Notes

1. Frederick Schmitt, "HIPAA Expects Long-Term Care Sales to Rebound," *National Underwriter*, Life & Health/Financial Services Edition, May 13, 1996, p. 11.

2. Frederick Schmitt, "LTC Insurance Sales Rebounded in 1995," *National Underwriter*, Life & Health/Financial Services Edition, May 26, 1997, p. 3.

3. Source: HIAA Research: Who Is Buying Long-Term Care Insurance

4. Barry J. Fisher, "Sorting through the clutter of long-term care insurance policies," *Broker News*, October 2000, p. 10.

5. Source: Alzheimer's Association, 2003

6. Glenn E. Stevick, Jr., "Choosing an LTCI Product," *Advisor Today*, January 2003, p. 18.

7. Source: Administration on Aging, "A Profile of Older Americans: 2002"

8. Paul S. Bunkin, CLTC, "Hidden Traps in Old Policies," *Advisor Today*, November 2002, p. 26.

9. Jim Connolly, "LTC Sellers: More Uniform Licensing Of Facilities Would Help Sales Grow," *National Underwriter*, February 11, 2002, p. 25.

10. Steve Wnuk, "How Do You Spell Long-Term Care? OPPORTUNITY," *Health Insurance Underwriter* (February, 1998), p. 19.

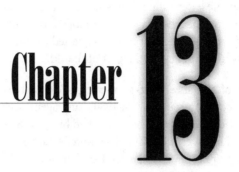

Chapter 13

Phase Three: Tax-Qualified vs. Non-Tax Qualified Plans

"Politics is the art of looking for trouble, finding it whether it exists or not, diagnosing it incorrectly, and applying the wrong remedy."

– Ernest Benn

"If you can't convince them, confuse them."

– Harry S. Truman

The HIPAA Cometh

By 1996, product development in the long-term care market had evolved through several policy generations. There was no resemblance between the initial policies introduced back in the mid-to-late 1960's covering some nursing home expenses and the products of the 1990's which provided numerous reimbursements in virtually any long-term care setting.

What the products lacked was a place in the Internal Revenue Code. Simply, there was no formal clarification of the tax consequences of long-term care. Were benefits payable under these policies taxable to the claimant? Could employers deduct any long-term care premium contribution made on behalf of employees? Nobody knew.

Yes, there were private letter rulings that seemed to indicate an IRS tendency to give long-term care policies the same tax favorability as health insurance, but those letters applied only to the taxpayer that requested clarification. They were not indicative of any broad policy on the part of the IRS.

Despite this lack of guidance, long-term care policies were sold. Employer-provided long-term care began in the late 1980's, and agents were advising that deductibility of premium was sure to be sanctioned by the IRS. Moreover, some agents recommended long-term care's inclusion in Section 125 cafeteria plans, guessing that if long-term care was treated as health insurance then this product could certainly be part of a Section 125 menu.

There were many attempts at tax clarification of long-term care insurance in the two decades leading up to 1996. Numerous legislative proposals were put forth in Congress, most suggesting that long-term care insurance be treated as health insurance for the purposes of taxation. All of these bills died natural deaths. Either Congress did not get around to it in a given year, or the proposal was tacked on to other legislation which was either rejected or tabled.

The insurance industry regularly lobbied the federal government to define long-term care expenses and insurance in the tax code. Send a message to the American public, we said, about taking financial responsibility for this problem. Encourage the consumer to consider long-term care insurance as a solution to this potential difficulty.

There are times when we should be careful what we wish for. In 1996, Congress finally passed legislation on the taxability of long-term care insurance. It was folded into broad legislation primarily regarding health insurance that was initiated by Senators Nancy Kassebaum (R-KS) and Ted Kennedy (D-MA). This seemingly incongruous pairing of two legislators of different perspectives was Congress' way of attaining bipartisan support for health legislation that was "on the ropes" after the Clinton health plan debacle of 1993-94.

On the surface, Congress appeared to give the insurance industry everything they wanted on long-term care taxation – and more. Tax clarifications in this legislation were, as follows:

- Premiums are deductible to individuals as a medical expense for those who itemize, subject to age and premium limitations.[1]

- Benefits received by a claimant are tax-free to the recipient, subject to some per diem limits to be indexed annually.[2]

- Employers who pay premiums on behalf of an employee are entitled to deduct those premiums as a business expense, just as they do for health and disability insurance.[3]

- Premiums paid by an employer on behalf of an employee will not be treated as compensable income.[4]

These rules were well received. Actually, the individual premium deductibility was a bonus. Contrast these new rules for long-term care insurance with disability income coverage. With disability income, if a tax deduction of the premium is taken, benefits when received will be taxable to the recipient. With long-term care, if either the individual is able to utilize the premium deduction or the employer buys long-term care coverage for employees, there is still no taxable effect on the benefits when they are paid. Premium deductibility and tax-free benefits together? Surprise!

Naturally, there was a catch for individual premium deductibility. The taxpayer had to itemize medical expenses to claim the premium as a deduction. This meant expenses had to exceed 7.5 percent of one's adjusted gross income.[5] According to the Internal Revenue Service, less than 10 percent of taxpayers are able to itemize medical expenses. Even if the individual is able to itemize, there are some limits,[6] although these are indexed annually:

Attained Age	Limitation (1997)	Limitation (2003)
Less than 41	$ 200	$ 250
41 - 50	375	470
51 - 60	750	940
61 - 70	2,000	2,510
71+	2,500	3,130

The likely deductions were probably going to occur for individual taxpayers over age 65, who had Medicare out-of-pocket expenses for prescriptions, higher LTC premium deductibility limits, and lower incomes from which to calculate the 7.5 percent.

For those under age 65, premium deductibility plays better as a sound bite than in reality. But so what? This was a throw-in anyway. What everyone wanted – and received – was the tax-free distribution of benefits. If you could deduct the premium, too, you were a leg up on the IRS. Agents would have to deal with high expectations from prospects regarding tax deductibility. The news that they probably aren't one of those able to deduct the premium would probably not play well in the hinterlands, but it would place agents in front of potential buyers. If the agent properly demonstrated a need for the coverage, many more sales would be made than existed currently.

Self-employed individuals, long overlooked for health insurance premium deductibility, were now able to add long-term care insurance to their ever-increasing percentage of premium deductibility that reached 100 percent in 2003. Long-term care insurance premiums for the sole proprietor, partner, or S-Corporation owner and their spouses were still subject to the age-based tables above, but this was at least an improvement over the previous decades where this type of personal deduction would likely not have existed. It has at least opened up a new market of long-term care prospects for the insurance agent.

This part of the HIPAA legislation regarding long-term care seemed to send a clear message to the American public with its tax incentives and favorable treatment. Long-term care, the Act said, should be everyone's personal responsibility.

Left at that, the industry would have been elated. Products had been improved, with assistance from long-term care service providers, and the market was growing daily with individual prospects in need of protection. Insurers were becoming more comfortable with the risk as it was presently known, and some state education requirements with regard to long-term care were signaling agents to learn this product well before presenting it to the consumer.

But tax clarification is never simple, as our convoluted tax code has often proven. The HIPAA legislation went much further than anyone expected. More rules were added to "define" long-term care insurance for the purposes of standardizing what long-term care expenses (including distributions from a long-term care insurance policy) would qualify under this new tax status. These rules were:[7]

1.   *Per diem cap.* Here, the IRS capped the amount of long-term care expenses that are deductible at $175 per day or $63,875 per year in 1997, to be indexed annually (it is $220 per day or $80,300 per year in 2003). Indemnity long-term care insurance products that pay daily benefits regardless of the actual expense incurred will create a taxable event for policyholders who purchase daily benefits in excess of the per diem limit of (currently) $220. The exception to this will be if actual long-term care expenses exceed this amount. If a policyholder owns both a per diem and expense-incurred contract, the $220 per diem amount will be reduced by the amount of benefits paid under the expense-incurred contract. Since per diem contracts are paid without regard to actual expenses, the IRS wanted to cap the total

daily benefit that could be received in the event this amount exceeded expenses incurred.

2.   *Cafeteria plan.* Long-term care insurance is *excluded* from a Section 125 cafeteria plan. Contrary to some insurance agents' earlier beliefs and despite its favorable tax treatment as a health insurance product, employees would not see the benefit of adding long-term care insurance to their flexible benefits menu.

3.   *Medicare coordination.* Long-term care policies paying on an expense-incurred basis are allowed to coordinate their benefits with Medicare to avoid duplicative reimbursement. This overrides a Health Care Financing Administration initiative calling for long-term care insurance to be considered primary and pay first before Medicare. Now, Medicare will pay and the policy benefits will be reduced accordingly.

4.   *Non-forfeiture benefits.* Insurers must offer a non-forfeiture benefit for plans to be considered as qualifying for favorable tax treatment under this legislation, if the policy has no cash surrender value in the event of policy lapse or death. Some insurers already had this provision included in their contracts.

5.   *Benefit triggers.* In order to deduct either the expenses incurred or receive tax-free benefits under an insurance policy, the claimant must be *chronically ill.* The legislation defines a "chronically ill" individual as one who is certified by a licensed health care practitioner as:

     a)   being unable to perform, without substantial assistance from another individual, at least two out of six activities of daily living (ADLs) due to a loss of functional activity that will last at least 90 days in length;

     b)   requiring substantial supervision to protect the individual from threats to health and safety due to a severe cognitive impairment; or

     c)   having a similar level of disability as determined by the Secretary of the Treasury in consultation with the Secretary of Health & Human Services.

The six activities of daily living are eating, toileting, transferring, bathing, dressing, and continence.

After a review of these benefit triggers, it became clear that insurers who had enhanced their long-term care products to provide a triple-trigger option of qualifying for benefits would have to re-file their policies. Simply, these plans no longer conformed to this federal legislation. What happened?

Insurers' triple-triggers were (See Chapter 12):

1.   inability to perform 2 of 5-7 ADLs;

2.   suffer a cognitive impairment; or

3.   doctor prescribed due to medical necessity.

Under HIPAA, the law expanded the ADLs to six but added a 90-day requirement to the first trigger, placed the word "severe" in the second trigger, and eliminated the "medical necessity" trigger entirely, replacing it with a yet-to-be-defined trigger that would be drawn up in collaboration between the Treasury and HHS departments.

Essentially, the new law trimmed the eligibility options from three to two. Moreover, one of the two triggers left standing was significantly modified with a 90-day expectancy requirement. The elimination of "medical necessity" from the benefit triggers was particularly bothersome, since its inclusion was due primarily to provider input about the gaps left by using only the first two triggers for legitimate claimants. Now, in one sweep, this product development work was nearly eradicated.

Repercussions

The insurance industry was stunned by this news. The cheers concerning tax favorability had barely subsided when this new definition of long-term care silenced the celebration. Questions immediately ensued such as how much time will it take to prepare, price, and file one of the new tax-qualified plans?

Insurance agents specializing in long-term care were angered by this turn of events. Having fought for competitive products and pricing for so long, one congressional act had undone that hard work in short order. The loss of "medical necessity" rankled even the most loyal agent. There had been some industry rumbling that this trigger was the most problematic for insurers. It left the potential claims loss ratio wide open for these products since physician certification of a long-term care need might be generally easy to obtain. Some agents saw the HIPAA legislation as a Faustian bargain between the federal government and insurers to eliminate this popular benefit trigger.

It is unlikely that the medical necessity trigger was on the chopping block when HIPAA passed in 1996. Claims results were still in their infancy and it was premature to draw conclusions about the potential claims results under this eligibility option. Some insurers were even angrier about its loss than their agents who sold their policies.[8] They saw the loss of "medical necessity" as unfair, but were even more upset about the new 90-day requirement under the ADL trigger.

This language revision made it imperative that a licensed health practitioner certify the loss of 2 of 6 ADLs as likely to last at least 90 days for benefits to be payable. This effectively eliminated any short-term claims for long-term care services. Some insurers revealed that they had a significant number of LTC claims lasting less than 90 days.[9]

Insurers who offered elimination periods of less than 90 days were also in a quandary. Does this 90-day certification effectively dispose of elimination periods of 0, 15, 20, 30, 45 and 60 days, among others? Further, what if an insurer began paying benefits after an elimination period of 30 days based on a 90-day certification, but the claimant recovered after 70 days? Do the benefit payments have to be repaid by the insured?

The setting of ADLs at a total of six also defied state legislation in at least three jurisdictions – Kansas, Texas and California, the latter two requiring a listing of at least 7 ADLs. Would the states revise their laws to accommodate the new federal legislation even though it appeared less beneficial to the consumer?

Questions, questions. What did the terms "substantial supervision" and "substantial assistance" mean? What constituted a "severe" cognitive impairment? When will the third benefit trigger be defined?

Congress did anticipate one problem with this legislation. Most insurers would not have long-term care insurance policies that conformed to this new law. Premium tax-deductibility was effective beginning in January of 1997, but tax-qualified plans wouldn't likely be available until the spring of 1998 at the earliest. These difficulties were addressed as follows:

1. There was a "grandfathering" period where any long-term care insurance contract sold would be considered "tax-qualified" if it was purchased and put in force prior to January 1, 1997.[10] More important, this included all the plans sold prior to HIPAA's enactment in August 1996.

2. Long-term care policies issued on or after January 1, 1997 could be written on the old basis until the new tax-qualified plans were approved for that insurer in the insured's state. The insured had one year – until January 1, 1998 – to exchange this old policy for a new tax-qualified plan.[11] The insured must be guaranteed the ability to make this exchange. If a claim occurred after the policy was purchased but before the exchange, the benefits would still be considered tax-free. This applied to policies issued after January 1, 1997 and for claims beginning prior to January 1, 1998.

This "grandfathering" had multiple effects. First, insurance agents went into "fire-sale" mode, selling as many of the triple-trigger plans as possible to insureds that wanted the seemingly better policy and favorable tax treatment. This motivated many prospects that were hedging about long-term care insurance into action. Second, after January 1, 1997, long-term care prospects felt like they could wait until the tax-favored plans were available. After all, why buy a policy you'll have to exchange later anyway? The problem, of course, was the potential loss of insurability before the tax-qualified plans were approved in a given state. If the individual could currently qualify for coverage, it made more sense to obtain it – even on the old policy form – and convert it later. Most insurers were trying to make this process as easy as possible for the insured. An example of a "Certificate of Exchange Privilege" can be found in Figure 13.1.

FIGURE 13.1

Certificate of Exchange Privilege

Presented to _____

For tax years beginning on January 1, 1997 or later, long-term care policies that meet the requirements of the Health Insurance Portability and Accountability Act of 1996 qualify for favorable federal income tax treatment. _____ Insurance Company has already filed in your state a long-term care policy that is intended to be tax-qualified, but approval is still pending. *The policy we can currently offer you does not meet the requirements of this federal act. But when the tax-qualified policy is approved in your state you may exchange this policy for a new tax-qualified plan.*

> **FIGURE 13.1 (continued)**
>
> The premium for the tax-qualified policy received in the exchange will be based on your current age and will not require further underwriting.
>
> In order to meet the guidelines in the new federal legislation, our new tax-qualified policy will have different provisions than your current policy. _____ Insurance Company will provide specific information regarding those differences at the time of the exchange offer.
>
> ## For specific tax advice, contact your accountant or tax advisor.
>
> *I have read this Notice and I understand that the policy for which I am applying does not meet the requirements of federal law for favorable tax treatment. I also understand that I may exchange the policy for a tax-qualified policy provided that one is approved in my state.*
>
> _____   _____
> Signed (Applicant)   Date

The Essential Question

But the overriding question everyone had was "What about the tax status of plans written after January 1, 1997 that don't conform to the new legislation and are not exchanged for plans that meet these new specifications?" That was a difficult question to answer and one that the Treasury Department consistently ducked in post-HIPAA questioning.

Some analysts maintain that the status of these "non-qualified" plans was the same as it was prior to HIPAA – uncertain. Private letter rulings before HIPAA were primarily favorable towards beneficial tax treatment. Why wouldn't this still be the case?

The quick answer to this question was that prior to HIPAA nothing was clarified about the tax treatment of long-term care insurance. Now, there was clearly a policy form that would achieve a positive tax result. An IRS representative deciding the tax fate of a non-qualified long-term care insurance plan could point to the tax-qualified plan as the one singled out by HIPAA for tax-friendly treatment. Insurers and policyholders cannot plead ignorance or point out that the IRS has nothing on its books about long-term care, except a few private letter rulings.

However, some analysts thought the lack of Treasury Department clarification meant that HIPAA's primary purpose was to create a safe harbor for tax-qualified plans, and not to render pre-HIPAA plans as entirely taxable coverage.[12] HIPAA had not, in its language, drawn a distinction between pre- and post-HIPAA long-term care insurance policies. The issue remained unclear.

Insurers initially began to line up on either side of the argument. Some insurers felt strongly about not selling non-qualified plans at all in the event of adverse tax consequences for the policyholder. Other insurers who are still championing the benefits of non-qualified plans believed that tax-qualified plans hurt the consumer and insurers only marketing HIPAA-approved tax-qualified plans were denying better coverage to the consumer.[13]

Whereas some insurers were positive about HIPAA, citing tax favorability, fewer agents were supportive of the legislation. They bemoaned the loss of medical necessity and the new 90-day certification and argued that seniors were worse off after HIPAA than before any clarification had been made. As tax-qualified plans began to emerge from the insurers' shelves, the expected lowered premiums (since benefit triggers were reduced) didn't materialize. Thus, it seemed to agents that consumers were basically paying the same price for more restrictive (in their view) coverage.

That the Treasury Department was slow to comment and respond to these questions made the issue more difficult. Consumer questions to agents and insurers have gone unanswered. Policies were sold – especially in the last four months of 1996 during the grandfathering period – but 1997 results slowed as everyone waited for more clarification. The legislation that was supposed to shed light on long-term care insurance had smothered it in darkness.

The Treasury Department Speaks

In mid-1997, the Treasury Department finally broke radio silence. In IRS Notice 97-31[14] interim guidelines were provided to clear up the questions the HIPAA legislation had provoked.

HIPAA was supposed to clarify not only long-term care insurance taxation, but primarily to provide guidance for those individuals who were self-insuring their long-term care expenses. As we know, there were far more people in this situation than those that had purchased insurance and they, too, had been in limbo as far as understanding what the tax ramifications were for their dollars spent on long-term care expenses.

One must also remember that the legislative climate in Washington in 1996 was focused on a balanced budget. Spending legislation had to be accompanied (and still does) by details of where the dollars would come from and there was a great reluctance to do anything that might derail the balanced budget express. HIPAA gave a number of opportunities for a long-term care expense tax deduction and in so doing was reducing the revenue opportunities for the Treasury Department. It was therefore expected that they would try to curtail their losses if possible.

Short-term medical expenses of the chronically ill and the simplicity of a physician's certification were seen as tax deductions that could be abused. "Chronically ill," to the IRS, implied a longer term of illness. Short-term claims and even doctor-prescribed services didn't fit neatly into the "chronically ill" definition. Moreover, ease of qualification for the deduction meant potential significant revenue loss and thus guidelines were imposed to attempt to ensure that only expenses for the truly chronically ill would be deductible. By avoiding "medical necessity" as a qualifier and adding a 90-day certification requirement, Congress was able to reduce the potential deductions and reduce the revenue loss, arguably making it easier to get the bill passed.

Insurance policies, which weren't necessarily the intended target of these rules, were unfortunately lumped together with personal long-term care expense deductions. HIPAA was complex enough, so the rules for insured and self-insured situations were equalized. As a result, the new benefit triggers that define long-term care insurance were less liberal than those triggers that were then available in long-term care policies.

But the Treasury Department was not likely to change the HIPAA rules at this point. Instead, they offered clarifications to the law:[15]

1. "Substantial assistance," part of the ADL trigger, means either hands-on assistance or standby assistance. "Hands-on assistance" is defined as the physical assistance of another person without which the individual would be unable to perform the ADL. This is consistent with insurers' interpretations. But it was "standby assistance" that was an unexpected break. This is defined as the presence of another person within arm's reach of the individual that is necessary to prevent, by physical intervention, injury to the individual while the person is performing an ADL. An example of this is a person who is ready to catch an individual if he or she falls while getting out of the bathtub. Or, as being ready to remove food from someone's throat if the indi-

vidual chokes while eating. These situations will qualify an individual as being unable to perform the ADLs of bathing and eating. That people did not necessarily need physical assistance with an ADL was a welcome liberalization and conceivably could make it easier for an insured to meet the 90-day certification requirement.

2. The 90-day certification requirement must be made at time of claim. Any licensed health care practitioner can make the certification, including social workers with the proper credentials. The health professional is merely giving an educated opinion that the two ADL losses will likely last at least 90 days. If the disability turns out to be shorter, benefits paid would not be affected. This breathed new life into the shorter elimination periods.

3. Severe cognitive impairment, the second trigger, meant a loss or deterioration in intellectual capacity that is (a) comparable to (and includes) Alzheimer's disease and similar forms of irreversible dementia, and (b) measured by clinical evidence and standardized tests that reliably measure impairment in the individual's short-term or long-term memory, orientation as to people, places, or time, and deductive or abstract reasoning. Substantial supervision also needed clarification under this benefit trigger. It was defined as meaning continual supervision (which may include cuing by verbal prompting, gestures, or other demonstrations) by another person that is necessary to protect the severely cognitively impaired individual from threats to his or her health or safety (such as may result from wandering). These definitions could now be added to the tax-qualified policies. These clarified terms weren't, at any rate, significantly different than the pre-HIPAA claims handling of cognitive impairment claims. Now, at least, tax-qualified policies had a means to define these new terms to ensure conformity with the tax code.

4. Questions surrounding the issue of changes to grandfathered policies arose during the four-month fire sale of pre-HIPAA long-term care policies that would be grandfathered in on a tax-favored basis. The big questions was if a change is made to one of these grandfathered policies after January 1, 1997, would it remove the qualified status from the policy? The Treasury Department's answer was "yes."[16] If a material change was made to an existing policy, it will be considered issuance of a new contract. One type of material change is the alter-

ation of the timing or amount of any item payable by the policy-holder, the insured or the insurance company. While a change that resulted in an increase in benefits for the insured is arguably the target of this guideline, the Treasury Department seemed to be taking the position that even changes that result in the same or less benefits still constituted a material change and the probable loss of tax-favored status. This seemed unfair to someone who, for example, wished to reduce the daily benefit from $125 to $100. This would be considered a material change and unless the policy itself conformed to HIPAA language, tax-favored status would be lost. Reaction to this was heated, and organizations and individuals began pressing the Treasury Department for a definition of "material."

Finally, the Treasury Department did issue clarification in December 1997 of what constituted a "material change" to long-term care policies that could jeopardize a policy's grandfathered tax-qualified status. This was intended to let policyholders, agents and insurers know the alterations that could be made to an existing policy *without* changing its tax-qualified status. These exceptions were:

1. premium mode changes;

2. class-wide premium increases or decreases for a guaranteed renewable or non-cancellable policy;

3. after-issue application of a spousal discount or the policyholder's exercise of any other right provided in the contract in effect on December 31, 1996;

4. benefit reductions if requested by the insured;

5. continuation or conversion of coverage following an individual's ineligibility for continued coverage under a group contract;

6. addition, without an increase in premium, of alternate forms of benefits that may be selected by the insured; and

7. purchase of a rider increasing benefits of a grandfathered policy if the rider alone would be considered a qualified long-term care insurance contract.

The first five exceptions are self-explanatory. The sixth, addition of alternate benefits, has to do with the "alternate plan of care" provision under the policy (See Chapter 12). If the insured elects an alternate plan of care that is not specifically defined in the policy, it is allowable without consideration that a material change has been made. This could mean receiving a different type of service than those listed in the policy or receipt of any services in a setting not defined in the contract.

The last exception has to do with increasing coverage under a "guaranteed insurability" type of provision where the insured can increase coverage without any evidence of insurability. This exception means that a separate policy would not have to be issued, although any benefit increase has to be subject to the new plan parameters (including 90-day ADL certification) sanctioned under HIPAA. It may ultimately be easier for the insurer to issue a new policy, but the outlet exists to add new coverage by rider to a grandfathered plan without hurting its tax status.

5. Form 1099-LTC was the Treasury Department's non-verbal answer to the pre-HIPAA plans that don't conform to the new long-term care definitions. The Treasury Department has said that it was Congress who was silent about "non-qualified" plans by not addressing their specific status in the HIPAA legislation, The inference being that it is Congress who should address the oversight. The Treasury Department merely had to work with the legislative hand it was dealt. So, they introduced Form 1099-LTC, a current copy of which is included in this chapter. Instructions to insurers are to file the form when paying any benefits under any long-term care insurance policy. Policyholder taxpayers are instructed in their copy that this is important tax information being furnished to the IRS. If the insured is required to file a return, there are sanctions for not reporting this income. The form points out that amounts paid under a qualified long-term care insurance plan are excluded from your income. However, if payments are made on a per diem basis, the amount excluded is limited ($220 per day in tax year 2003 and indexed annually). While no reference is made to non-qualified long-term care coverage, the inference from the form is that only amounts distributed under qualified plans are excludable from income. There is even a corresponding form (8853) that owners of tax-qualified LTC plans can submit with their return, negating the 1099-LTC form. Non-qualified plans have no such corresponding form.

Form 8853 (2002)   Attachment Sequence No. **39**   Page **2**

Name of policyholder (as shown on Form 1040)	Social security number of policyholder ▶

Section C. Long-Term Care (LTC) Insurance Contracts. See **Filing Requirements for Section C** on page 6 of the instructions before completing this section.

If more than one Section C is attached, check here . . . . ▶ ☐

16a Name of insured ▶ .... **b** Social security number of insured ▶ _____

17 In 2002, did anyone other than you receive payments on a per diem or other periodic basis under a qualified LTC insurance contract covering the insured or receive accelerated death benefits under a life insurance policy covering the insured? . . . . ☐ Yes ☐ No

18 Was the insured a terminally ill individual? . . . . ☐ Yes ☐ No
    Note: *If "Yes" and the only payments you received in 2002 were accelerated death benefits that were paid to you because the insured was terminally ill, skip lines 19 through 27 and enter -0- on line 28.*

19 Gross LTC payments received on a per diem or other periodic basis. Enter the total of the amounts from box 1 of all Forms 1099-LTC you received with respect to the insured on which the "Per diem" box in box 3 is checked **19**

    Caution: *Do not use lines 20 through 28 to figure the taxable amount of benefits paid under an LTC insurance contract that is not a qualified LTC insurance contract. Instead, if the benefits are not excludable from your income (for example, if the benefits are not paid for personal injuries or sickness through accident or health insurance), report the amount not excludable as income on Form 1040, line 21.*

20 Enter the part of the amount on line 19 that is from **qualified** LTC insurance contracts . . . **20**

21 Accelerated death benefits received on a per diem or other periodic basis. Do not include any amounts you received because the insured was terminally ill (see page 7 of the instructions) . **21**

22 Add lines 20 and 21 . . . . **22**

    Note: *If you checked "Yes" on line 17 above, see* Multiple Payees *on page 7 of the instructions before completing lines 23 through 27.*

23 Multiply $210 by the number of days in the LTC period **23**
24 Enter the costs incurred for qualified LTC services provided for the insured during the LTC period (see page 7 of the instructions). . . **24**

25 Enter the **larger** of line 23 or line 24 . . . . **25**
26 Enter the total reimbursements for qualified LTC services provided for the insured during the LTC period **26**

    Caution: *If you received any reimbursements from LTC contracts issued before August 1, 1996, see page 7 of the instructions.*

27 Per diem limitation. Subtract line 26 from line 25 . . . . **27**

28 **Taxable payments.** Subtract line 27 from line 22. If zero or less, enter -0-. Also include this amount in the total on Form 1040, line 21. On the dotted line next to line 21, enter "LTC" and the amount **28**

⊕   Form **8853** (2002)

Proponents of non-qualified plans contend that it can't possibly be the intent of Congress or the IRS to tax a benefit which merely serves to reimburse the insured for the cost of long-term care services, especially if the insured does not take any kind of premium deduction up front.[17] It's difficult to disagree with this statement but why then the need for the 1099-LTC form at all? If no distributions from a long-term care insurance plan are to be taxable, the form does not seem necessary. From the "non-qualified" corner, though, comes the obvious thought that if Congress intended to tax non-qualified plans, why didn't the legislation address it?

If it is ultimately Congress' intention for people to buy only qualified contracts, this will emerge in a later technical corrections bill. Trying to guess what
Congress was thinking is as easy as dancing with jell-o. They may have overlooked this issue entirely. They may have known what they were doing but
thought it easier to deliver the message in a smaller, less publicized bill later. They
may have been addressing concerns about self-insured taxpayers that would
potentially deduct long-term care expenses and didn't think about the effect on
the insurance industry. Congressional leaders have already begun receiving letters from constituents regarding this non-qualified situation and will likely have
to respond at some point.

In 1998, regional IRS offices had no consistent policy with regard to taxing
non-qualified LTC policy benefits. Some IRS officials insisted they would consider the policies to be "health and accident plans" and treated accordingly, which
would be favorable to the policyholder. By 2002, private letter rulings going out
to individual policyholders of non-qualified LTC plans were being told if they did
not take a premium deduction up front, benefits would not be taxable.

When pressed for a formal Revenue Ruling on the matter, the IRS backed off.
They have advised at least one agent organization based in the D.C. area not to
petition for the formal ruling, because "you would not be pleased with the
result." Where the Treasury Department is at the present seems clear. They are
perfectly happy to issue favorable private letter rulings, and not enforce the taxation of policy benefits currently paid out under non-qualified plans, but they
refuse to close the door on the possibility of future taxation. With the 2003 federal budget in a shambles once again, this is a prudent thing for them to do. They
may need this revenue some day, and it would likely only happen if consistently
large deficits surfaced again. So, the risk remains (for taxation), but presently the
IRS has turned the other cheek – for now.

The National Association of Health Underwriters reports only two cases they
have been made aware of where the IRS is trying to tax LTC benefits paid out.
Curiously, in both cases, the policies were issued prior to January 1, 1997. This
should settle the tax question quickly, since those policies were grandfathered in
to the law. Apparently, at least one of the policies is an indemnity plan where
benefits were paid directly to the individual's bank account and then transferred
to the provider of services. This shouldn't matter, but it has stalled the case for
the moment from resolution.

The Market

Following HIPAA, insurers initially split on the tax-qualified/non-qualified issue. Here is a sampling of what some carriers were offering, post-HIPAA, in 1997:

- Nine insurers selling both qualified and non-qualified plans.

- Six companies selling only non-qualified plans.

- Twenty-two carriers selling only qualified contracts.[18]

Early on, it was obvious the majority of companies had decided to work only with qualified plan contracts. The tax status for these plans was known and therefore placed all parties to the agreement on safe ground. Some carriers adding benefit enhancements to the new qualified contracts, while still including all the language required by HIPAA. One carrier added the term "mobility" to its "transferring" ADL for purposes of better defining it for coverage purposes. A lack of mobility, the insurer contends, could quickly qualify a person for benefits because a loss of bathing and transferring would be immediately evident. Yet another carrier expanded home care coverage to pay for multiple services on a given day that would otherwise have exceeded the daily benefit.

Still another carrier actually introduced a new, non-qualified plan in mid-1997, despite the controversy surrounding the policy's taxation. State insurance departments, not concerned about possible tax consequences, approved the product for sale in many jurisdictions. As long as agents continued to explain the possibility of taxation and had appropriate waiver forms understanding this possibility signed, non-qualified plans continued to be sold. Many agents still believe that non-qualified plans continue to be of interest to consumers, despite the potential adverse tax consequences.

Product development activity was high in the couple of years that followed HIPAA, and most of it focused on tax-qualified plans. Only a few carriers still offer both, with conversion privileges either way in the event of final Treasury Department clarification. One insurer that offers both showed that 90 percent of their business was tax-qualified LTC coverage. Whether it's agents concerned about their E&O situation if non-qualified plans are ever taxed, or consumers gunshy about having to potentially deal with the IRS in the future, or some combination of both, it's clear that currently, tax-qualified plans dominate the current long-term care market.

Effects on the Market

The truth is that the long-term care insurance product is needed. Even qualified plans, despite their shortcomings, still provide valuable protection in many long-term care situations. The new definition of "standby assistance" seems sure to assist in getting claims certified. Rather than go without, these plans do furnish asset and retirement income protection. Even "taxed" non-qualified benefits (the worse case scenario) provide more dollars than not owning any coverage at all.

Both tax-qualified and non-qualified proponents have argued long and hard for their side of this issue. The discussion about the differences between TQ and NTQ plans essentially comes down to three components: (1) the 90-day ADL loss requirement; (2) medical necessity; and (3) taxation.

90-day requirement. This is the time frame Congress placed on tax-qualified plans' ADL losses to ensure that the long-term care being received was truly a long-term situation. This effectively eliminates short-term claims under TQ policies. But is this care covered elsewhere? Medicare and private health insurance both have coverage for short-term situations that might involve long-term care services. Short-term claims like this are usually temporary problems – a broken hip, even a heart attack, might see the claimant back on his feet within three months. This is not what LTC policies are for, especially if the coverage is already picked up elsewhere. Typically, the person that needs custodial care (assistance with ADLs) and not skilled care, is more likely a long-term situation than a short-term one. Insurance is generally intended to be responsible for the large catastrophic bills, not the smaller ones, but we have oversold the value of this and other health-related type coverages so that the consumer is conditioned to expect coverage in virtually every situation.

The real problem that has surfaced with the 90-day requirement has been the challenge to that certification by insurers' claim departments. Once a health practitioner of some kind signs off on the 90-days, that should be sufficient, but a few carriers have wanted second opinions. Fortunately, this is not a widespread practice yet, but it is a concern for those holding TQ plans.

Medical necessity. The loss of this provider-aided definition has created a clear advantage for non-qualified plans. There are three triggers for benefits in a non-qualified plan and only two (at present) in a tax-qualified plan. The question then becomes how significant could the medical necessity trigger be at claims time? The definition, you will recall, was inserted to cover those individuals who needed long-term care assistance but did not consistently meet the requirements of the first two triggers.

Many of those who utilized the medical necessity trigger were the most frail of claimants. It wasn't that they couldn't perform the activity of daily living, they simply needed some help with it. They may also need help with Instrumental Activities of Daily Living. Under TQ plans today, the loss of an ADL is considered if a person needs supervision with that ADL (standby assistance). This is not hands-on help per se, and many frail elderly could qualify for benefits under a TQ plan due to this policy language. But these are people who are likely not going to get better. Their situation is, in fact, long-term, and thus is in keeping with the spirit of TQ plans.

Medical necessity will undoubtedly help qualify a person for claim benefits in situations where TQ plans will not. Whether this is a good thing or not depends on how this ultimately impacts loss ratios. If claims experience is poor, NTQ plans may find rate increases to be plentiful. It is interesting that there is very little premium difference (5-10 percent) between TQ and NTQ plans at this point. Will NTQ plans ultimately cover more because of medical necessity? Eventually, we will know the answer.

Taxation: As noted earlier, the IRS is refusing to issue a Revenue Ruling on the subject of taxation of a non-qualified plan. My advice is to write for a Private Letter Ruling that the policyholder can keep with the policy.

Perhaps the fastest growing segment of the market today is in employer-sponsored plans. Here, to obtain the deduction and favorable tax-status, TQ plans must be used. This is quite clear in the law.

It is also interesting that all legislative proposals in Congress that pertain to long-term care insurance (above-the-line premium deduction for individuals, Section 125 inclusion) only pertain to TQ plans. NTQ plans are never mentioned in any of these potential legislative enhancements. This seems like a message of sorts to us in the industry, that we will always be fighting an uphill battle for recognition of NTQ plans. That the vast majority of insurers sell only TQ plans also indicates where most of the insurance industry stands on the matter.

Naturally, some other questions remain, namely:

What is the third trigger mysteriously worked into the law as "to be determined" at a later date by Health and Human Services and Treasury? If this third trigger is clarified as "medical necessity," that may clear up a lot of the fuss.

Why not allow long-term care insurance to be included in a Section 125 (flexible benefit cafeteria) plan allowing premiums paid by the employee to be paid on a pre-tax basis? If dependent child care and supplemental health plans like accident and cancer insurance are allowed inside a Section 125 plan, why discriminate against long-term care insurance? If the law arguably is to encourage personal responsibility, the cafeteria plan deduction could give even more access to long-term care insurance through TQ plans, the governement's preferred funding method. Of course, this Section 125 inclusion will be even harder to get now with the federal budget in fiscal crisis yet again. Congressional leaders have made it known that Section 125 inclusion is a revenue deflator, and unless funding possiblities are found, not likely to happen.

When will these questions be answered? Maybe never, or not in our lifetimes, but continued diligent efforts on the part of agents and consumers lobbying their Congressional representatives may speed up the process.

Personally, I think the agent has a duty to offer both TQ and NTQ plans to their clients and prospects. They should be educated to help them make a thoughtful decision on the coverage to buy. While there may be as much disparity between the plans as we think, clearly there is a difference, and we owe it to consumers to completely inform them of their options as they look to fund their future long-term care needs.

Chapter Notes

Source material used was from: The Health Insurance Portability and Accountability Act, the Internal Revenue Service, and the Treasury Department. Special thanks to the National Association of Health Underwriters and their LTC Working Group, who has pursued matters relevant to the TQ-NTQ issue faithfully and fervently since 1996.

1. IRC Section 213(d)(1); HIPAA '96 Section 322(c).

2. IRC Section 7702B(a).

3. IRC Section 7702B(a)(3).

4. IRC Section 7702B(a)(3). See IRC Section 106(a).

5. IRC Section 213(a).

6. IRC Section 213(d); Rev. Proc. 97-57, 1997-52 IRB 20. "Favorable Tax Treatment for Long Term Care Signed into Law," *LTC Update* (September, 1996), p. 1.

7. See generally IRC Section 7702B.

8. James Heyer, "Were Seniors Better Off without HIPAA?," *National Underwriter*, Life & Health/Financial Services Edition, October 13, 1997, p. 37.

9. *Ibid.*

10. HIPAA '96, Section 321(f)(2).

11. See HIPAA '96, Section 321(f)(3).

12. Craig R. Springfield, "Some Unanswered Non-Qualified LTC Tax Questions," *National Underwriter*, Life & Health/Financial Services Edition, April 28, 1997, p. 8.

13. Joe Niedzielski, "LTC Tax Issue Splits Industry," *National Underwriter*, Life & Health/Financial Services Edition, October 6, 1997, p. 62.

14. Notice 97-31, 1997-21 IRB 5.

15. *Ibid.*

16. See generally Prop. Reg. §1.7702B-2.

17. Steven Brostoff, "HIAA Wants IRS to Clarify 'Qualified' LTC Rules," *National Underwriter*, Life & Health/Financial Services Edition, July 28, 1997, p. 1.

18. "Individual Long-Term Care Plans," *Life Insurance Selling* (December, 1997), p. 129.

Chapter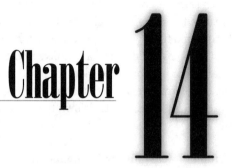

Today's LTC Products: Back to the Future

"Experience is that marvelous thing that enables you to recognize a mistake when you make it again."

– F.P. Jones

"History is more or less bunk."

– Henry Ford

Heading into 2002, the long-term care market was, relatively speaking, in decent shape. Sales were picking up, there was very little in the way of insurer disaster stories with the product, the number of consumers who should be seriously considering purchasing this coverage was increasing, and a growing number of agents were starting to take this market seriously.

A year later, products were being pulled from sale, new, higher priced plans were replacing them, the lifetime benefit period appeared doomed to extinction, reinsurance for this product line was drying up, and several large LTC insurers had their blocks up for sale.

Clearly, a health-related insurance market just can't stand prosperity.

What in the world happened?

While there have been some recent difficulties in the market, it has primarily centered on the tax-qualified versus non-qualified discussions. Some agents are still in a post-HIPAA funk, and there will always be a need for more agents to be telling the LTC story, but many producers had settled into a comfort zone, whether selling tax-qualified or non-qualified plans, or both. A couple of major insurers had exited the long-term care market over the past few years, but other insurers acquired their business to increase their own market share, and no one seemed to miss a beat.

Educational opportunities were growing by the month to help ensure that agents were up to date on how to properly sell long-term care. States were enacting suitability standards to be on the safe side, further channeling producers towards the appropriate potential insureds for this coverage. Product development had slowed, allowing agents and consumers time to catch their breath and take stock of what was out there to purchase. Consumers, in post-9/11 sober moods, spent some serious time reviewing their financial planning situations and long-term care (among other) business increased as a result. Some stability had finally settled in to this market.

But a year after 2002 dawned with bright hopes for the long-term care future, someone turned the lights out on the party. By New Year's Day 2003, so many changes (and not positive ones for the consumer or agent) were coming so fast that agents went into fire sale frenzy again, convincing fence-sitters that this coverage was never again going to be as low-priced or as liberal as it is now.

Why the Jekyll and Hyde act? We've seen this before in the health insurance and disability income market, this overreaction in both good and bad times. Long-term care had yet to experience this roller coaster ride in a meaningful way. The "one ADL" qualifying for benefits from the early 1990s was an example of outreaching during good times, or in this case, before any bad claims news turned up, but we may be able to mark that down to an overzealousness on the part of a carrier or two. At the time, the key to long-term stability for LTC was that, unlike those other lines of business, nobody followed the Product Pied Piper. Most carriers understood that a one ADL trigger was too easy to qualify for a claim, making it difficult to price a product one didn't really know much about pricing in the first place.

We seemed to come through those early 1990s stages of policy liberalization thanks in part to the mess handed down by Congress in the form of the Health Insurance Portability and Accountability Act in 1996. Say what you want about the TQ-NTQ controversy, defining "chronically ill" in a policy helped keep insurers heads out of the product development clouds, and a more sane approach to insuring this market for the long haul seemed to come into focus.

There are reasons for the sudden turnaround, and only time will be able to judge whether carriers (and regulators) have overreacted or not, and whether it will ultimately stifle growth in LTC insurance. This chapter will trace the path of these changes, and point agents and consumers toward the future in this anything but "business as usual" market.

A Rosy Future, or Ignorant Bliss?

Most agents and carriers seemed to agree (always a small miracle) on one thing two years ago: long-term care sales could be better. Yes, new business was increasing every year, but not in the substantial chunks it should be considering the availability of favorable products, the number of existing clients that hadn't yet contemplated the financing of long-term care, consistently positive consumer press, and a clear blueprint for employer-sponsored sales given the highly auspicious tax environment.

Education was thought to be the key to success. Enough agents weren't promoting the product it was thought, so perhaps increased training opportunities was the right answer to bolster production. Better trained agents would likely sell more coverage. A typical call to arms in the industry press read, "What is needed, the veteran (LTC) marketers urge, are more LTC marketers educating the public about the risks associated with LTC and convincing them of the need to insure against those risks."[1] More marketers would only be found through more education about the LTC need.

Other analysts saw the lack of realized market potential differently. Weiss Ratings, Inc., a provider of consumer shopping guides for long-term care insurance policies and typically a hard judge on the insurance industry, seemed to feel the stunted market growth was due more to confused consumers who were looking at solving a fundamental funding problem with complex policies and inexplicably large variations in premiums. Weiss complained that insurers, for example, could not agree on a standard method of satisfying the elimination period.[2]

Actually, premiums among the major, highly rated carriers (with one exception) were within reasonable striking distance of each other, especially in the tax-qualified market. With policy language also being relatively similar, it was often coming down to the consumer's relationship with the agent that was finally closing the sale. Most of these top insurers were considered good buys – common sense benefits at fair prices – and everyone at the top was enjoying increased market share.

There were some product language differences, and elimination period and waiver of premium had the most significant fluctuations. But these provisions were explainable, and consumers are savvier today than they were twenty years ago. They are better educated, have done more research themselves, ask better questions, and understand most of the basic policy features.

In a January 2002 analysis of the long-term care market, Fitch IBCA, Duff & Phelps, called LTC an "industry in transition." They were surprised that long-term care insurance has taken this long to become "mainstream," but its time, it appeared, had finally arrived. While noting that the top ten LTC insurers wrote 83 percent of the business in 2000, they expected sales to continue to be concentrated among these giants as there were high barriers to entry into this marketplace. The report warned that if a company grew too fast or if LTC became too large a part of their total business, then this would be viewed as a credit negative. A well-managed LTC division is credit neutral given the long tail on the business and limited data.[3]

The Fitch report went on to say, "The profitability and viability of LTC writers is hard to predict. While some agree that actuarial assumptions are well documented and nursing home care estimates are better documented than first thought, the main problem lies in the lapsed time between the policy inception date and the time in which benefits may be paid. Moreover, the fact that the products are untested in a mass scenario and with an average duration of stay possibly extended due to medical technology makes the long-term care risk unpredictable at this point. Technology may also work in favor of LTC providers, reducing the likelihood of strokes or other disabling diseases. New medical advances may make it possible for individuals to remain independent despite being disabled. Fitch expects the next decade will bring with it continued change and uncertainty in the way long-term care is bought and sold."[4]

Well, there is certainly nothing there we didn't already know. Any insurance line is a risk. Some analysts compared long-term care to disability income, and I think it's a mistake to associate their claims situations. Yes, a disability event has to occur, but the ultimate measurement of that medical situation is far different. Long-term care has an ADL (or cognitive) trigger to it, quite unlike an "ability to perform occupational duties." LTC insureds will likely qualify for their product in a more disabled state, thus probably shortening the claims duration. One top

LTC insurer admits that their longest claim in more than three decades barely exceeded six years.

We are still several years away from being able to judge this market accurately. In the meantime, the essential question was still being asked in 2002. Why aren't LTC sales growing faster? One researcher characterized consumer attitudes as a "mix of ignorance, anxiety, wishful thinking and inability to plan." A consumer journalist countered that LTC products were just too expensive, especially for seniors, and rising drug costs were competing with the discretionary dollars to purchase LTC. Younger people remained concerned over what long-term care would even look like in 20 or 30 years when they were more likely to need it and expressed more concern about potential rate increases as a reason to duck the purchase of this product for now.[5]

Contrast this with HIAA's virtually annual LTC summary in 2002, which stated that the study "proves there is a market out there, it's growing, it's strong and it has a lot of potential growth areas. The products are getting better and premiums are not as high as people think."[6]

Insurers were also upgrading their existing products to keep pace with the times. Not wanting to penalize a policyholder who took coverage out before some of the recent LTC innovations, most carriers, with little fanfare, simply took more action under their "Alternate Plan of Care" policy benefit. It was here that assisted living facility claims were being paid on older policies that did not contain any reference to this newer institution. Stand-by assistance was also added routinely to older policies as a liberalization.[7] In this way, insurers were intent on giving current clients the benefit of an evolving industry whose even better technology and trends may lie ahead.

Given this atmosphere, one might easily say long-term care had a rosy future. Or, in the words of a Milliman USA actuary, "is ignorance bliss?" Three forces were coming to collide to yield the sudden market transition we are now in: (1) NAIC's new Rate Stability Amendment to the Model Policy Act began to be adopted by states; (2) a September 2002 Society of Actuary Intercompany Study on long-term care policy issues; and (3) the post-September 11th reinsurance blues, which is not a song by Bob Dylan.

Poetry in Motion

Insurance regulators were probably first to whistle everyone out of the pool. In February 2003, I sat in the office of Oklahoma Insurance commissioner

Carroll Fisher, himself a former insurance agent and Past President of the National Association of Health Underwriters. On his desk was a request from a LTC insurer for an 88 percent rate increase on an existing policy line. And this, he told me, was representative of the type of request that was in virtually every state insurance department, and had been for some time. While many of the top carriers were holding onto the cards they were dealt, apparently a number of others were folding their hands.

Concerned with (especially) the impact of such jumps on elder LTC policy-holders (Oklahoma does a terrific job at helping out their older residents with insurance questions and education), the NAIC had already begun suggesting ways to squash this premium trend before it became any larger in size. Perhaps you could chalk up these initial rate increase problems to company's under-pricing to attract market share. Or were there other, more basic forces at work, such as the original estimates by actuaries simply not holding up for this product? Folks like Carroll Fisher had two tasks at hand: find the right answers to the pricing problem, and come up with a solution to prevent this from becoming a plague in the future.

The Amendments to the NAIC Model Policy Act are intended to accomplish these objectives. These are:[8]

Elimination of the 60 percent loss ratio requirement and the establishment of a new 85 percent requirement. This means insurers will have to demonstrate true adverse claims circumstances to achieve a successful rate increase. No longer can the rate increase be split between exceeding loss ratios and administrative costs (previously at 40 percent of the rate calculation).

1. A requirement that rates be actuarially certified, meaning the actuary anticipates the premiums filed to be adequate for the life of the policy, even under "moderately adverse" conditions.

2. Insurance applicants confirm by signature that they understand rates could go up.

3. Insurers must disclose their past rate history to potential applicants on all long-term care products they have sold for the previous decade.

4. Insurers whose rate increase receives approval, but later monitoring reveals the increase not to be justifiable, will have to refund the policyholders accordingly.

5. Authorization for an insurance commissioner to bar from the state for five years a carrier that exhibits a pattern of rate increases.

6. Should rate increases exceed certain cumulative limits (see Table below), the insurer would have to (a) offer the policyholder a reduced benefit that would eliminate any future rate increases, and (b) offer a non-forfeiture benefit that the insured could accept in lieu of a rate increase. This is called *contingent nonforfeiture*.

FIGURE 14.1

Age at Policy issue	Increase triggering nonforfeiture	Age at Policy issue	Increase triggering nonforfeiture
29 & under	200%	72	36%
30-34	190	73	34
35-39	170	74	32
40-44	150	75	30
45-49	130	76	28
50-54	110	77	26
55-59	90	78	24
60	70	79	22
61	66	80	20
62	62	81	19
63	58	82	18
64	54	83	17
65	50	84	16
66	48	85	15
67	46	86	14
68	44	87	13
69	42	88	12
70	40	89	11
71	38	90 & over	10

What's obvious here is the attempt to discourage from the marketplace those insurers who will come in, under-price their LTC product, collect premiums, and then file for substantial rate increases that will probably discourage many people (especially older policyholders) from keeping their policies. Thus the insurer makes their profits and does not have to deal with claims losses later. It's an abhorrent practice, long prevalent in the health insurance industry, and long-term care is an easy target because of the nature of the disability-based product where claims experience takes time to be felt, and the guaranteed renewable policy provision that gives the insurer the option to raise rates (unlike DI's non-can provision).

Can it work? Certainly it explains the sudden pricing changes recently. Some insurers pulled products faster than radio stations yanked Dixie Chicks records. Currently, fifteen states have adopted these regulations.[9]

Can actuaries certify their rates are not likely to increase? They'd probably rather bet five years' salary that they can strike out Barry Bonds. There are so many moving parts to the pricing equation beyond claims such as rates of investment return, lapse percentages, underwriting costs, among others. And, with contingent non-forfeiture in place, the sky is no longer the limit for these subsequent increases. At issue age 65, a policyholder will know that if rate increases cumulatively exceed 50 percent, the carrier has to give them other choices.

Companies will now have to get the rate right up front. But they must also be careful to still price the product competitively enough so that someone buys the policy. With many claims unknowns still ahead, this is a tightrope act for personnel who instinctively find this kind of pressure threatening.

The NAIC is only one of the forces shaping the LTC product and market future. One can understand their situation. How else do they deal with 88 percent rate increases?

A September 2002 Society of Actuaries Intercompany study on LTC (and Milliman USA guidelines) also sent insurance executives to their medicine cabinets for more Valium. Here are some trends noted:[10]

1. Voluntary lapse rates for policies with unlimited lifetime benefits are lower than those for policies with limited benefit amounts, suggesting that those who buy unlimited benefit plans value the financial and psychological security that comes with such a benefit and are less than inclined to give up the protection provided by the plan.

2. Mortality, according to the 1983 Group Annuity Table (83GAM), one used frequently in LTC pricing and the prescribed valuation mortality table, overstates active life LTC insurance mortality. This indicates that policyholders are staying around longer than 83GAM predicts, and that more of these folks will reach claims paying age.

3. Insured claim incidence is declining gradually, consistent with published trends in general population morbidity. Over the past two decades, the prevalence of deficiencies in activities of daily living has been declining in the elder population. This is often attributed to

advances in medical technology. There is considerable disparity in opinion among industry professions whether this trend will continue, and, if so, to what extent; therefore an assumption of continued morbidity improvement in the future should be approached carefully.

4. Across different underwriting styles and ages at issue, the morbidity savings attributable to being married averages closer to 40 percent in the early policy duration, significantly higher than the typical 20 percent premium discount offered married couples currently.

5. Reasons for closed-out claims: 65 percent – death; 26 percent – recovery; 9 percent – benefit expiration.

6. Alzheimer's claims are the most expensive, most frequent and most longest-lasting, and they are also trending higher. Many carriers did not routinely perform screening for early signs of cognitive difficulties until the late 1990s, and this has clearly had an impact on the number of Alzheimer's claims.

You can see the items that probably jumped off the page for the pricing gurus. First, lapse rates are part of the overall premium formula. There is an expectation that some policyholders will not make it to claim time, and the attrition rate is vital to determining what your claims rates and reserving are likely to be. But, lo and behold, insurance agents were actually selling this policy well. Insureds understood that the longer they held the policy, the closer they were to using it. Selling LTC insurance as a family and asset protection vehicle emphasizes the likelihood of a lengthy window between date of application and date of need.

So, more people than expected were keeping their policies. LTC insurance enjoys an incredible persistency rate. Worse, for actuaries and insurers, the more expensive plans with lifetime (unlimited) benefits were carrying much higher than expected retention. This meant, for many companies (despite the lack of useful claims experience and, as noted above, improving morbidity), their policies were under-priced as submitted. People weren't dying fast enough, either, based on assumptions, so those people enjoying the fruits of longevity were also contributing to better than expected lapse ratios.

Finally, Alzheimer's claims are the scariest for LTC claims people. These conditions can go on and on for a considerable period of time. With more individuals hanging on to their lifetime benefit periods, especially those whose contracts also included simple or compound inflation, the numbers started overloading the actuarial slot machine. In Las Vegas, you could just call the cashier. Who do you call in an insurance company?

Don't call the investment department. Another part of the policy pricing equation is an assumption for investment returns; making money on the premiums collected to help meet future claims. Granted, risk-based capital requirements instituted after the Mutual Benefit/Executive Life meltdowns over a decade ago, limit the insurers' investments to safe money, the kind that doesn't earn much. So how could they over-estimate that number? Well, anyone that has a money market checking account has seen the interest rate decline over the past few years to miniscule numbers. Welcome to an investment manager's world. Safe money has eroded in returns, well below normal expectations. Anytime Alan Greenspan goes on TV to announce The Fed just lowered the interest rate again means your LTC (and other insurance policies) are under-priced some more.

This leads us to problem #3. Reinsurers, a small number even in good times for the LTC industry, took a licking in the September 11 tragedy. While most kept on ticking, there was a concerted effort to rewind the watch, and evaluate all blocks of potential disaster on their books, currently and into the future. While one could not have likely forecasted September 11, a study of what was being reinsured, weighed in with the NAIC and SOA reports, meant it was suddenly "High Noon" for long-term care. Compounded inflation, combined with lifetime benefit periods, were viewed as potential Titanic scenarios. State laws required compounded inflation to be offered to clients, so that feature couldn't be dismissed. But nothing mandated lifetime coverage, and the reinsurance market for this coverage began drying up quickly.

Therefore, for the last year or two, insurers have been sitting on the following information: better than expected lapse rates (but no celebrating), lower investment returns, new actuarial certification of premium rates, higher loss ratio requirements, maximum percentages for rate increases by age, probable self-insurance on their LTC business, and a bleak forecast for policyholders that are diagnosed with Alzheimer's disease. If you put this to music, it would likely be a funeral dirge.

Carriers reacted quickly, some with the artistry of synchronized swimmers, others with all the subtlety of a buffalo stampede. But act they did, and products have been reshuffled and re-priced in short order. One insurer in Florida raised their premiums on their new product an average of 22 percent in light of these developments. Another carrier's new product pricing went, in the words of one agent, "from Wal Mart to Saks Fifth Avenue."

Ironically, one of the age groups hit the hardest would be younger buyers. Bargain prices have abounded for those under age 50, but now insurers are more sensitive to the impact of inflation increases on long duration policies. Thirty years can mean an incredible increase in insurer liability, as these carriers should have known all along. For example, a $150/day plan purchased today at age 45, with a 5 percent compounded inflation rider and a 5 year benefit period increases total policy liability from a manageable $273,750 to $1,183,132 in thirty years.

This benefit potential shouldn't come as a surprise. Inflation (often compound) riders are routinely sold to younger buyers. Otherwise, the policy loses substantial impact in a few years. It doesn't take a lot of effort to convince consumers of the importance in keeping their daily benefit indexed. The main question for many is will 5 percent compounded increases be *enough*?

Predictably, under this banner of bad news, underwriting tightened, too.[11] Better risk selection also helps claims loss ratios, so the likelihood of an attending physician statement and at least a phone assessment went up accordingly. There has also been an underwriting thought process that evaluates certain medical conditions as to whether the person is more likely to die shortly after a disabling medical event, or be a long-term claimant. Errors in mortality judgment, as noted earlier, may well change that type of thinking.

In Florida, the adoption of NAIC Rate Stability included a paragraph about the 90-day certification of ADL loss under tax-qualified plans. It read, "When a licensed health practitioner has certified that an insured is unable to perform activities of daily living for an expected period of at least 90 days due to a loss of functional capacity and the insured is in claims status, the certification shall not be rescinded and additional certifications shall not be performed until after the expiration of the 90 day period."[12] This would effectively end that post-claims practice of challenging the 90-day certification on ADL loss, but it once again is forcing insurers to do it right the first time. LTC sales should come with a posted warning sign now: Rougher underwriting waters ahead.

Reinsurance hasn't played that critical a role to date, with estimates ranging from 3 to 10 percent of the present LTC business being reinsured.[13] But it will make a difference in the future, and features like lifetime coverage may be a casualty of this higher involvement. Prices will have to be as finely tuned as they can be up front, maintaining a balance between what is insurable and what is salable.

Thus, 2002 was quickly becoming far from a year to remember. As one LTC specialist put it, "Insurance stocks are depressed (as are most), budgets are being trimmed, and, due to corporate pressure from above, various LTC insurance manufacturing leadership teams are being asked to produce sales and bottom line results that are hardly realistic, given the current environment."[14] It's enough to chase LTC producers back into the disability income market.

As the LTC market moves, poetry in motion, some folksy advice is being launched on what to do if your policy undergoes a rate increase. By January 2003, six of the top 10 carriers (over 80 percent of the business) had hiked prices, with a seventh on the way.[15] The prevailing wisdom was for policyholders to hang on to their plans if they could. Older policies may contain some more liberal phrasing than current counterparts, and today's higher rates in new product filings could mean that even with the jump up in price, the old policy may still be a better deal than a new one. There are benefit reductions one can take, too, like a longer elimination period, shorter benefit period, lowered daily benefit level, or changing inflation from compound to simple. Decreases in coverage would not affect a grandfathered tax-qualified plan.

Not surprisingly, much of the media seemed to miss this trend, too. "CBS Market Watch" released a story in November 2002 noting the rising costs of LTC insurance, expecting premiums to soar by as much as 100 percent in 2003 as insurers confronted falling sales, rising claims and weak investment returns. One insurance executive remarked, "An actuary's motto: When in doubt, price the hell out of it."[16] It seemed we had come back full-circle to the days of yore, when these new policies appeared without any real data to help price them. We're now in the insurance industry version of "Back to the Future."

The truth is nobody has the crystal ball for this line of business. The future of long-term care is hardly a known quantity. Some insurers have chosen to believe worse-case scenarios, and one can hardly blame them based on the pricing errors brought to light even in these early stages. Some carriers took even more drastic measures on the heels of these studies and NAIC actions – they bid a fond farewell.

Exit – Stage Right

The noted third-party industry analyst, A.M. Best, issued a Special Report on long-term care in December 2002 in which they opened with, "The impact of Penn Treaty American Corp.'s problems and temporary exit from the insurance market, followed by Conseco Inc.'s well-publicized difficulties, has had an impact on the long-term care insurance industry. Previously, these companies were the second and third-largest writers of new long-term care business. The problems experienced by both companies demonstrate that being a large company does not always guarantee success."[17]

Jane Bryant Quinn had noted the Conseco problems months earlier in a column entitled, "Is Your Insurance Safe?" In the article, Quinn makes it clear she is still a fan of LTC insurance ("Believe me, you're going to want to pay privately for care, and LTC insurance is one way of doing it."), but points out that "your policy has to come from a successful company" and that "insurers with profit problems in LTC will probably raise premiums for its existing policyholders as we've seen at Conseco Senior Health," and "these hikes will get harder to pay the older you get."[18] In December, Conseco, Inc. filed for Chapter 11 protection, becoming the third largest bankruptcy on record, behind Worldcom and Enron.[19]

Penn Treaty put their sales on hold in 2001 and went out and raised capital and a new reinsurance arrangement with an offshore company, Centre Solutions (Bermuda) Ltd.[20] They're back for now, and the question is will agents feel comfortable that financial lightning won't strike twice here. It may not help that in Florida (one of their largest sales states) a class action lawsuit was filed in January 2003 on behalf of Florida residents who purchased LTC insurance from Penn Treaty beginning in January 1997. The complaint alleges the use of "low ball pricing" and the promise of stable rates to lure unsuspecting consumers into purchasing coverage, then dramatically increasing the rates.[21]

In 2002, Hartford Life sold its group long-term care insurance to MedAmerica, exiting the long-term care business entirely. They claimed the book of business wasn't large enough to have an economy of scale and didn't believe they were likely to gain a stronghold in sales.[22]

Finally, Employers Reinsurance Corp., one of the larger long-term care reinsurers, voluntarily left the market, and LTC insurers were left with one less outlet for their business.[23]

As the late author Douglas Adams said, "Goodbye – and thanks for all the fish."

We're used to exits in the health insurance-related marketplace. If agents and insurers based career and market decisions on these departures, we'd all have joined the Peace Corps by now. There has been, is, and always will be volatility in this type of marketplace. The most successful insurers to date are the ones that know how to positively deal with negative information. Only the strong (hearted) survive. But the sun will continue to come up on a market that is only growing larger every day.

As if we needed some encouraging news that we are doing the right thing, Life Plans, Inc. in October 2002, published a study advising that the private long-term care insurance policies that are already in place could save Medicare and Medicaid about $30 billion. The researchers found that private LTC coverage saved an average of $1,668 in out-of-pocket expenditures per month for insureds who used home care, and $2,458 per month for insureds who needed nursing home care. Private LTC coverage also reduced the probability that an insured would become poor enough to qualify for Medicaid nursing home assistance to 3 percent, from 9 percent.[24]

There's no reason not to be a believer in the power of this product and its need. The federal government is convinced the private market is the funding answer to this problem, and demonstrated it with the new Federal LTC plan.

Reinventing Government

In April 2001, a group called the Citizens for Long-Term Care (CLTC), not to be confused with the Certified in Long-Term Care (also CLTC) designation program, or Stephen Moses' Center for Long-Term Care Financing (CLTCF), called for a new national policy for the financing of long-term care, based on principles of social and private insurance. The coalition, made up of 63 long-term care providers, consumers, insurers and workers agreed that there must be a new social insurance benefit that finances a minimum floor of financial protection combined with a program of incentives for the early acquisition of private insurance."[25]

What's interesting is that there is already a private-public alliance in four states (Partnership Programs) and they have been suspended by the Federal government for several years, even though a number of other states are ready to launch similar initiatives. Bills have been pending in Congress for some time trying to break this deadlock.

Even more interesting is that currently the Federal government does not share the coalition's enthusiasm for a national LTC plan. The new Federal Long-Term Care Insurance Program, created in 2000 by the Health Security Act, launched its first salvo in 2002. The nation's largest employer decided to go the private route, contracting with a joint partnership of MetLife and John Hancock to provide a product and underwrite, issue, and administer the policies.

As with the Federal Employees Health Benefit Program, there was to be no agent involved. The program did contract some agents to do educational seminars throughout 2002, when open enrollment was in effect. The Feds placed the potential audience for this product, offered to employees, retirees, veterans, and their spouses and other family members at about 20 million people.[26]

Much of the information and education for this product was published on the web site for the Office of Personnel Management (OPM). Curiously, the web site encouraged Federal LTC Plan eligibles to shop around the private market for LTC coverage, suggesting that there were better buys to be had out there. The web site primarily featured four packaged plans to choose from, although any participant could design their own program within plan parameters. The Fed LTC Plan offered the eligible individuals (and family members) a substantial group discount, but calculations and comparisons with the private market seemed to indicate that younger people could do better elsewhere, while older people seemed to be getting a good price break. There was very little underwriting for employees, while retirees and family members had to answer questions.[27] In addition, the home health care benefit was pegged at 75 percent of the daily benefit amount, whereas the private market would let the individual buy up to 150 percent for this same coverage.

The last six months of the year was the opportunity for eligible participants to enroll. The resulting education and publicity from this Federal initiative was, while difficult to accurately measure, surely a lift for private LTC insurance as well, ironically during a year where the news in the backroom was getting progressively worse.

By February 2003, the results were in. More than 265,000 applications had been received, and (surprise) many of them were still in an underwriting logjam. When the risk evaluation dust finally settles, Long-Term Care Partners (the MetLife – John Hancock co-venture) expected to have 215,000 policyholders. Not bad for six months work. The enrollees were split evenly among two groupings: employees, members of the uniformed services, and their spouses in one, and retirees, their spouses, and other qualified relatives in another. Of approved applicants, 54 percent were female. The average age of an active civilian enrollee is 51; the average age of the active uniformed services person is 45; the average retiree age is 65 for civilians and 63 for uniformed services. Not surprising (considering no agent was involved) was the news that 70 percent of the applicants opted for one of the four prepackaged plans. The most popular was a $100/daily benefit, 90-day elimination period, 3-year benefit period, with compounded inflation. Overnight, the Fed LTC plan was the largest employer-sponsored LTC plan in the U.S.[28]

This program couldn't have come soon enough for veterans. In January 2003, the Veterans Affairs Department decided to suspend health care enrollment for some higher income veterans who don't have military service-related ailments or injuries. This enrollment suspension applied to individuals who were already in the lowest priority range for benefits.[29] These are the people that should be considering the private market for long-term care anyway. But it's a precedent that could have farther reaching effects and an indication that government funding of health care (including long-term care) is more of an endangered species than an inevitable solution.

The Market Has Issues

OK. So the long-term care market has issues. Who doesn't? Health products have long been the shifting sands of the insurance industry. There will always be peaks and valleys here, and currently it seems that free-fall reigns.

But after all the news in 2002, and carrier reaction in early 2003, I believe the market seems poised to move ahead. Sure, insurers are going to send some scouts out first, but they'll eventually yell "all clear ahead" and sanity will return to this market. The need isn't going to change. Private long-term care insurance will remain a viable funding solution. The higher premiums may eliminate some prospects, but those with assets (and families) to protect will find a way to pay for this peace of mind, with a little help from the agent field force.

The larger concerns remain the continued fiscal pressure on Medicaid, and the chaotic world of the long-term care provider. Liability insurance is killing the businesses that care for the aged. These huge expenses have created a cycle of destruction, where corners are cut, staffing is short, care problems emerge, and property and casualty insurance costs continue to escalate, further spinning this doomed treadmill. The Medicaid program cannot continue to support people who are able to "artificially" qualify for benefits. As noted in an earlier chapter, Medicaid qualification has reached the point of extending coverage to folks who could have (and probably should have) purchased long-term care insurance. This easy access has made private insurance an afterthought, if indeed anyone is thinking about it at all. Less people covered in the insurance risk pool defies the law of large numbers and could ultimately hurt the private market. A shortages of providers – either facilities or personnel – is also going to make long-term care a seller's market, raising provider costs well past the current inflation trends for which today's policies are designed.

A recent actuarial study showed that much of the increased government funding for senior care between 1995 and 2001 has actually gone for lawyers and other litigation expenses and not towards improved patient care for seniors. This is a result of skyrocketing costs of general liability and professional liability claims against long-term care providers, who rely on federal dollars to help cover patient care costs for three-quarters of America's frail elderly and disabled residing in nursing homes.[30]

The market in general needs fixing – not just reducing the potential for future large rate increases – and national LTC coverage, as the federal government will tell you, is not the answer. But agents and consumers would be wise to continue monitoring industry trends as they market, sell and buy long-term care insurance.

Two major trends support increased volume potential in long-term care insurance: (1) recognition that LTC insurance must be a standard part of retirement planning, and (2) emphasis on "aging in place," a circumstance that requires extensive home and community services.[31] Millions of Americans await the planning call.

Finally, the NAIC will continue to be the watchdog for the private market. They are already into a LTC reserving project that will both review the current requirements in the Health Insurance Minimum Reserves Model Regulation for possible changes, and develop longer term actuarial standards to ensure there is proper reserving. The project is due to be completed in 2004.[32] The greater the longevity of this market, the more confident actuaries and insurers will be of their numbers. This is only a matter of time. When that level of experience is reached, we can all concentrate again on getting back to the future of the LTC business.

Chapter Notes

1. "LTC Insurance Grows in Popularity," *Advisor Today*, May 2001, pg. 31.

2. Source: Weiss Rating, Inc., "Long-Term Care Premiums Vary Widely; Policies Too Complex," June 4, 2001.

3. Jim Connolly, "Fitch See Long Term Attractiveness in LTC Market," *National Underwriter*, January 28, 2002, pg. 25.

4. Fitch, IBCA: "Long-Term Care: An Industry in Transition," reprinted in *HIU Magazine*, March 2002, pg. 47+.

5. Stephen Piontek, "Why Isn't LTC Growing Faster?" *National Underwriter*, February 11, 2002, pg. 24.

6. Marcella de Simone, "LTCI Policyholders Tripled In 10 Years," *National Underwriter*, March 11, 2002, pg. 26.

7. Claude Thau, "Surveying Industry Practices On Changes To In-Force LTCI Policies," *National Underwriter*, April 8, 202, pg. 26+.

8. Source: National Association of Insurance Commissioners, 2002.

9. Linda Koco, "An Actuary Certifies – But Then What?" *National Underwriter*, February 17, 2003.

10. Amy Pahl, FSA, "Managing LTC Insurance: Is "Ignorance Bliss?" *Disability Newsletter*, Milliman USA, published April 2003.

11. Marlene Y Satter, "The Long View," *Investment Advisor Magazine*, September 2002.

12. Source: Florida Statute 4-157.119.

13. Jim Connolly, "As The Long Term Care Market Grows, So Will Reinsurers' Role," *National Underwriter*, February 17, 2003, pg. 8+.

14. Peter S. Gelbwaks, "2002 Saw Some Rough LTC Patches, But It Had Bright Spots, Too," *National Underwriter*, December 23/30, 2002, pg. 17.

15. "What to Do if Your Long-Term Care Insurance Rate Increases," *Business Wire*, January 21, 2003.

16. "Long-Term care premiums soar amid slumping sales," *CBS Market Watch*, November 2002.

17. "Concerns Remain Regarding the Long-Term Care Market," *A.M. Best*, Special Report issued December 9, 2002.

18. Jane Bryant Quinn, "Insurance: Is Yours Safe?" *Newsweek*, September 2, 2002, pg. 47.

19. Jim Connolly, "Agents Have Questions on What Conseco Bankruptcy Means For Clients," *National Underwriter*, December 23/30, pg. 53+.

20. "Penn Treaty Reinsures New LTC Policies," *National Underwriter*, Online News Service, January 10, 2003.

21. Source: Law Firm of Forizs and Dogali, P.L., Ocala, Florida, January 14, 2003.

22. "Hartford Life to Exit Group Long-Term Care Market," *Best Wire*, May 1, 2002.

23. "Concerns Remain Regarding the Long-Term Care Market," *A.M. Best*, Special Report issued December 9, 2002.

24. Allison Bell, "LTC Policies Now In Place Could Save U.S. $30 Billion," *National Underwriter*, October 14, 2002, pg. 18.

25. Mary Jane Fisher, "Coalition Calls For National Policy To Fund Long-Term Care," *National Underwriter*, April 16, 2001, pg. 30.

26. David B. Hillelsohn, "Federal Long-Term Care Insurance: Ready or Not," *HIU Magazine*, February 2002, pg. 11.

27. Lee R. Parsons, "Federally Endorsed Long-Term Care Insurance," *HIU Magazine*, January 2002, pg. 32.

28. Source: Long-Term Care Partners, LLC, "Federal Long-Term Care Insurance Program Announces Open Season Preliminary Results," February 13, 2003.

29. Suzanne Gamboa, "V.A. Stops Enrolling Higher Income Vets," *Associated Press*, January 17, 2003.

30. "New Study Reveals Federal Tax Dollars Meant for Senior Care Instead Diverted to Trial Lawyers," *PR Newswire*, May 7, 2002.

31. Jack Crawford, "LTC Insurance Premiums: How To Respond To Future Changes," *National Underwriter*, October 28, 2002.

32. Jim Connolly, "LTC Reserving Project Starts At NAIC," *National Underwriter*, March 17, 2003, pg. 49.

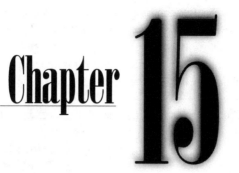

Chapter 15

Stand-Alone vs. Life Insurance-Based Approach

"For every problem, there is one solution that is simple, neat and wrong."

–Henry Louis Mencken

Long-term care insurance offers choices for people when a disability occurs. This flexibility helps tailor a specific care program to the individual needs of the claimant. Funding choices in the long-term care insurance market should also be flexible and offer the consumer choices in how long-term care expenses can be paid for.

Stand-alone long-term care products have long dominated the long-term care market. The policy is sold separately from other insurance, and addresses the need for financial support should a chronic illness occur. The insured pays an annual premium or, depending on budgetary concerns, semi-annual, quarterly, or monthly premiums.

The older one is, the greater the premium outlay. Rates start to accelerate past age 55. For those individuals addressing their long-term care needs at age 60, 65, 70, or older, the cost for this protection can be substantial. While the need still exists and the asset and income protection remains important, many people forego the proper insurance solution due to the high price of solving their problem.

There are premium options in long-term care insurance policies today that allow for a finite period of premium paying. These limited pay plans allow LTC coverage to be paid up, for example, in ten years or at age 65. This is a way to avoid paying premiums forever, and to avoid future rate increases, but it is also requires substantial dollar outlay in the years premiums are paid.

There are modifications that can be made to the coverage to tailor the policy to the individual's budget. Lowering the daily benefit, extending the elimination period, reducing the benefit period, or deleting the inflation protection are all examples of altering the solution to reach premium affordability. These choices can be difficult ones to make, but people who believe some coverage is better than none at all make these changes every day.

One question that seems to arise often during the course of this financial planning is the fate of the premium should policy benefits never be used. There will certainly be people who purchase long-term care coverage who will die without a long, chronic illness. Stand-alone policies have generally not provided a satisfactory answer to this question. There are some policies that provide a return of premium feature. Chapter 16, "Optional Benefits," furnishes descriptions of the type of choices available. However, this policy benefit is either a hard-sell to a prospect since premiums are not returned unless the person surrenders the policy or dies, or it adds substantial cost to a premium that may only be barely affordable as it is. There are individuals who decide to gamble on their chances of needing long-term care assistance, rather than lay out significant funds that they (or their heirs) may never see again.

Stand-alone long-term care insurance works well for many consumers. But there are answers to the questions posed above that other prospects can take advantage of in their quest to protect their retirement income and assets.

Life Insurance and Estate Planning

Most insurance agents are trained initially in the presentation and sale of life insurance. Like most workers, agents are comfortable with what they have learned first – in this case, life insurance. Whether term, interest-sensitive whole life, universal life, or variable life, these are all means of solving an income need should someone die.

Long-term care insurance and other health-related products have long been a secondary market for most agents. But there is a need for long-term care insurance, and how well the agent analyzes and solves the long-term care need for his client depends on the agent. There are those who learn how to provide this protection, others who refer their client to someone who does, and still others who do not address the need at all.

This means that long-term care insurance, potentially a key tool in pre-retirement estate planning, may be overlooked because the agent is not comfortable working with it as a stand-alone product. However, what if there was a life insurance vehicle that could also provide long-term care benefits? With an increasing number of financial planners adding long-term care to their regular list of planning recommendations, a product that solves dual needs may be a proper choice for some consumers.

This strategy could persuade more agents to bring up the subject with their clients. Agents specializing in estate planning typically work with products that help consumers either accumulate wealth or protect it. Long-term care insurance typically falls into the latter category, but combining this coverage with a life insurance product gives the client a vehicle that can help to accomplish both objectives.

One of the recurring complaints about stand-alone long-term care insurance is that it does not provide a safety net for those who do not use the coverage (or use very little of it). Today's consumer is more market-savvy, hunting for the best return on his money. The dollars spent on a long-term care policy provide peace of mind that accumulated wealth will be protected from these medical expenses. But, for some, this is not enough.

Moreover, agents frequently work with older clients who have the need but not the steady cash flow with disposable dollars to pay long-term care insurance premiums. These people may have large deposits in extremely safe (and low-interest earning) investments like CDs and money market savings accounts. What if the agent could simply move some of this cash into a product that furnished long-term care protection and potentially earned a higher interest rate, all in a tax-sheltered vehicle?

Death and taxes are the given assumptions in estate planning work. But a disability can disrupt the excellent planning that may have been done on a client's behalf. If the industry could structure long-term care protection inside a plan that life insurance agents understood better, more consumers might find this critical coverage a part of their estate planning.

Life Insurance-Based LTC

When one presents long-term care protection to a consumer, there is a discussion of the various alternatives to financing this need. (See Chapter 9, "A Long-term Care Sales Presentation.") Self-insuring the risk with available cash and assets is a gamble if the long-term care costs are high and the need lasts for a lengthy period of time. Medicare provides very little in the way of nursing home care, slightly more for those receiving home health care. Medicaid is for those individuals who have already spent down their assets. And, stand-alone long-term care insurance is fine if you ultimately need care. If you do not, the premium spent is not generally recoverable. Moreover, your premiums could increase over time.

These last lines are not usually part of the sales presentation. But they can be if the agent also works with a life-insurance based long-term care program. This program is available and many agents are using it to satisfy long-term care insurance needs. It is an easier concept for many to work with since it has a familiar base – life insurance. Building a presentation around a product that an agent was schooled in from the outset has helped provide a substantial amount of long-term care coverage to consumers than might otherwise have happened.

Agents have considered a life insurance-based approach to long-term care needs when clients do not want to: a) commit to paying ongoing premiums; (b) risk losing money if their needs change; and (c) pay taxes on any existing assets that might be used.[1]

Let's look at a client who has $250,000 in liquid assets. The client takes $100,000 of it that has been languishing in two CDs paying 3 percent interest. This leaves $150,000 left for the client to continue investing in whatever vehicles are satisfactory. The $100,000 is placed in a single-premium life insurance contract that generates a $200,000 death benefit and a $400,000 long-term care "pool of money." In addition, the $100,000 premium is earning interest at a higher guaranteed rate than 3 percent and is accumulating on a tax-deferred basis. This money is available for emergencies if needed, just as it was in the CD.

So, the client still has $250,000 working for him. But now, there is a death benefit and long-term care coverage, depending on the need. No extra outlay has been made, simply a shifting of assets to provide necessary protection. The pool-of-money long-term care concept is available under the stand-alone product, except now the client has a death benefit should he die prior to using the long-term care coverage. If the client eventually decides to surrender the policy, the money is returned along with earned interest. The interest is not taxable until the surrender, letting more money work for the client than a conventional investment. For the elderly, the low risk associated with investment in a life insurance policy that also handles their long-term care needs can be appealing. Even younger buyers may see this as solving two needs with one funding solution – the kind of simplicity and efficiency that has appeal.

I have heard a number of veteran long-term care insurance agents denigrate this type of long-term care sale. Why? Long-term care market penetration is not that great. Not everyone is attracted to the stand-alone product approach. This does not mean the long-term care insurance need disappears. If it can be handled through a life insurance-based product and the client likes it for all the reasons outlined above, then this vehicle should be used. You cannot shoehorn a client into the only product at your disposal. People have different preferences and the more diversity brought to a problem's solution, the greater the chance of helping more individuals.

The life insurance and long-term care insurance markets have experienced virtually no growth since 1996. It is believed that this is due to many insurers who have offered this policy decreasing their marketing efforts, leaving the market, or pulling this product choice from the sale shelf.[2] But, for some prospects, some insurance agents, and some insurance companies, this remains a fundamentally sound way to solve a long-term care need.

How Do These Products Work?

The plans are generally funded with one single premium payment, although there are other alternatives for premium paying. The lump-sum solution is ideal, as pointed out previously, for the individual that has a lump sum of money that is doing little to accumulate wealth.

There are agents that have worked with their clients to invest this money into an annuity, with the interest generating enough money to pay for a stand-alone long-term care policy every year. The principal essentially stays protected and may even generate additional value, plus long-term care coverage is secured, all by simply transferring the asset to a different vehicle. However, the problems of not using the policy benefits and potential rate increases still exist.

With a life insurance-based product, the money is transferred in a single premium payment to the policy. This single payment buys a death benefit and a long-term care insurance benefit, plus gives the client access to the accumulating money. If funds are needed for an emergency that remaining assets are insufficient to handle, these dollars can be withdrawn. This will reduce the death and long-term care benefits accordingly, but the money is there to assist the individual.

If a woman, age 69, deposits $50,000 into this policy, her benefits might be calculated as follows, based on a 6.25 percent credited interest rate:[3]

Year	Age	Account Value	Surrender Value	Estate Benefit	Long-Term Care Benefit
1	70	$49,551	$50,000	$91,400	$182,800
2	71	50,867	50,000	91,400	182,800
3	72	52,189	50,000	91,400	182,500
4	73	53,526	50,526	91,400	182,500
5	74	54,880	51,880	91,400	182,500

The $50,000 payment buys a death benefit of $91,400. In this particular example, a long-term care pool of money of twice the death benefit is generated. The cash value is less than $50,000 in the first year due to policy expenses and commissions, but begins to accumulate above $50,000 in the second year. This particular plan, however, guarantees the client's return of principal, so $50,000 is available in spite of surrender charges (less any withdrawals that were made).

Long-term care benefits are paid out over a two-year period, whether for a nursing facility or for home care. A lower payout can be made for adult day care. The client may have the chance to add an option that extends benefit payments longer than two years. In addition, some policies carry an extra death benefit payable at the insured's death even if all long-term care payments have been made. This is often calculated as 10 percent of the original death benefit. In the example above, if the $181,200 has been paid out for long-term care, a $9,140 death benefit still remains to function as a burial expense plan.

Another carrier has established a joint product that provides coverage to both husband and wife. For example, a male and female, both age 65, decide to transfer $100,000 into a joint whole life product. Based on a 6.75 percent credited interest rate, here are the benefits generated:[4]

Year	Age	Cash Value	Surrender Value	Death Benefit	LTC Max. Benefit	Mtly LTC Benefit
1	66	$106,059	$100,000	$231,208	$231,208	$4,624
2	67	112,275	101,048	234,656	231,656	4,693
3	68	118,621	107,945	239,616	239,616	4,792
4	69	125,095	115,087	242,684	242,684	4,853
5	70	131,670	122,453	246,223	246,223	4,924

This product generates identical death and long-term care benefits, which increase as the cash value accumulates. The long-term care benefit is paid out as needed, up to 2 percent of the accumulated death benefit each month if the individual stays in a nursing facility. In the first year, $4,624 ($154 per day) is 2 percent of the $231,208 maximum long-term care benefit. At that rate, it would take 50 months to pay the entire benefit out, slightly more than four years. Home care is reimbursed at half that level each month, or $2,312 per month ($77 per day).

Like the previous product illustrated, this plan guarantees return of principal in the first year. After that, the return could be higher, so the client at least knows the original investment can be recovered. Once again, if the insured does not need long-term care coverage, there is a sizable death benefit available that could help with estate taxes or other life insurance income needs.

As with the previous plan, extended long-term coverage can be added for an extra charge. Under this joint approach, the policy's death benefit functions as a second-to-die plan, with the face amount payable after the second death. However, either or both spouses can access long-term care benefits.

Under a third scenario,[5] a life insurance policy accepts a single premium and later, if a long-term care need arises, pays out the entire death benefit in four equal semi-annual installments. For example, a $40,000 single premium deposit into a universal life plan for a 65-year-old male will generate $97,000 in death benefit. This is the amount available for the four payments should the individual qualify for long-term care in the first policy year. Thereafter, the benefit will adjust upwards based on interest rate accumulations.

The typical agent compensation is similar to an annuity or single-premium life insurance. Being able to reposition assets rather than having to modify long-term care insurance needs to fit a budget can make this an easier sale while achieving similar protection results.

The single-premium whole life product lost much of its marketing edge in 1988 when the federal government introduced the concept of a modified endowment contract. Policies issued after June 20, 1988 must meet a "seven-pay" test to be labeled as life insurance instead of a modified endowment. The seven-pay test requires a certain level of premium be paid for a certain level of policy death benefit. A policy that does not pass the test is subject to less favorable taxation on policy distributions than one that does pass the seven-pay test. One aspect of this less favorable taxation is that policy withdrawals made before age 59½ are subject to a 10 percent premature distribution penalty tax.

A single premium life insurance policy is not likely to pass the seven-pay test, subjecting withdrawals to the 10 percent penalty. However, many clients who purchase a life insurance-based long-term care insurance product will be over the age of 59½. Still others are unlikely to need long-term care prior to this age, making the policy a good buy for those who wish to finance their long-term care needs this way. In addition, the agent has answered the questions about return on investment and potential premium rate increases.

As mentioned, these policies have begun introducing other premium payment methods for those who like the death benefit safety net, but do not have a sufficient lump sum deposit to make into the plan. Annual premiums and even more frequent premium payments can be elected. Other payment scenarios include a 10-pay program where all the premiums are paid in the first ten years. The policy is then considered paid up. It is like taking the single premium payment and spreading it out over ten years.

HIPAA

The Health Insurance Portability and Accountability Act of 1996 had a dramatic effect on stand-alone long-term care insurance. Similarly, this legislation also affected long-term care coverage that was purchased inside a life insurance product.

From a tax-free distribution standpoint, payments made under this life insurance-based plan carry favorable tax status if the policy benefits conform to the HIPAA language. The plan must, therefore, be a qualified long-term care product. Eligibility for benefits is limited to the dual choice of inability to perform 2 of 6 ADLs or a cognitive impairment. In addition, daily benefit payments must not exceed the per diem amount of $220 per day (in 2003) if the incurred costs are lower.

Prior to HIPAA, distributions made under these plans for long-term care expenses carried a two-part consequence. One portion of the payment came from the net amount at risk that was tax-free. The other part of the distribution was from cash value and was taxable to the extent of the gain.

As an example, assume a client paid a $25,000 single premium, and at the time of entering a nursing home had a $100,000 death benefit and a $40,000 cash value (a $15,000 gain over the $25,000 single premium payment). If payments made to the nursing home were $20,000 for the year, the tax consequences before and after HIPAA are illustrated below:[6]

Before HIPAA:
>$8,000 of $20,000 comes from cash value and
>is fully taxable to the extent of the gain

>$12,000 remaining comes from the life insurance
>net amount at risk and is tax-free

After HIPAA:
>$20,000 entire amount is not taxable if policy is a
>qualified long-term care plan

The best of HIPAA, of course, confirmed the tax-free distribution of long-term care proceeds. The policy, however, must be tax-qualified to receive this favorable treatment. The insurers marketing this life insurance-based product all filed new tax-qualified plans much as carriers selling stand-alone long-term care plans have done. Tax-qualified plans specifically fall under the HIPAA guidelines. Non-qualified plans will continue to pay out as before HIPAA, with the appropriate taxation of the cash value gain. Those policies put in force prior to January 1, 1997, were grandfathered in as tax-qualified plans.

These policies are being reviewed by the NAIC. There is some question about what becomes of a long-term care portion (often a rider) of a universal life policy if the plan does not have sufficient cash value to remain in force.[7] In an era of declining interest rates, this is a distinct possibility. There may be some guaranteed floor of benefits that will need to stay intact, regardless of what happens to the life insurance. Consumers and their agents should monitor their policy's annual statements to track the values in their plan to be sure it is adequately funded.

Life insurance-based long-term care insurance is a product that answers some clients' questions about premium safety nets and a return on investment. It is a policy many life insurance-trained agents feel more comfortable presenting. It has achieved tax-qualified status under HIPAA. It is an important alternative method of financing long-term care health insurance costs.

Chapter Notes

1. Nicholas Orobello, "The Combination Sale: Solving Two Needs With One Product," *Life Insurance Selling*, p. 44.

2. Source: HIAA, Long-Term Care Insurance in 2000-2001, published January 2003.

3. Illustration furnished courtesy of First-Penn Pacific and based on its MoneyGuard Plus product.

4. Illustration furnished courtesy of Golden Rule Insurance Company and based on its Asset Care I product.

5. Linda Koco, "Clarica Broadens The 'Living Benefits' Scope of UL," *National Underwriter*, November 19, 2002, p. 12.

6. "New Health Insurance Bill Includes Asset-Care Tax Benefits," *Financial Services Review*, Golden Rule Insurance Company, Volume IV, Number 2, p. 1.

7. Jim Connolly, "Market Changes Pushing Update of LTC Model Act," *National Underwriter*, March 24, 2003, p. 30.

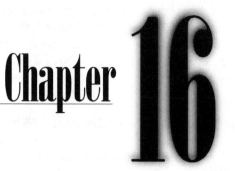

Chapter 16

Optional Benefits

"No one ever went broke underestimating the taste of the American public."

–Henry Louis Mencken

"Inflation is the one form of taxation that can be imposed without legislation."

–Milton Friedman

One of the many tasks of the insurance agent when working with a client is to structure the proper planning program that will specifically meet the individual's financial and emotional needs. It may mean modifying coverage to suit a budget to pay premium. Or it might mean working around existing financial alternatives already in place.

There are times when an agent must look beyond the scope of the basic policy to answer particular needs. During the fact-finding and presentation interviews, the agent will be listening to what the prospect has to say. This feedback will indicate what the client is trying to accomplish in addressing protection against potential long-term care expenses. This discourse may require the agent to use optional benefits to supplement the basic insurance plan for additional coverage.

The basic long-term care policy does a reasonable job of providing comprehensive coverage. There are additional benefits, however, that can enhance the base coverage and tailor a long-term care program to an individual's specific needs. The optional benefits available in a long-term care policy are few but can be considered extremely important.

Base Coverage or Optional Rider?

The essential features of a comprehensive long-term care policy were discussed in Chapter 12. The most common provisions found in these contracts were defined and detailed. It is important to note that while most policies build these features into the base plan at one cost, other products may offer these features as optional benefits.

The structure of a long-term care portfolio varies from company to company. Tax-qualified plans may have equalized the policy benefit triggers, but the balance of features may vary in location. For simplicity, most plans have loaded the key features into the base plan, making them comprehensive plans. But others strip down the base plan to provide minimum coverage at an affordable cost. Then, through the use of optional benefits, the policy can be built with as few or many of the features as the client wants or needs.

For that reason, benefits like *home health care* and *alternate care plans* may not be a part of the base plan. If not, these extra options must be reviewed thoroughly and the client given the opportunity to add them.

Home health care benefits must be offered to a client. While this is a requirement for comprehensive long-term care plans, the coverage may not be part of the base coverage. If it is a rider, it is almost essential to add it. Nursing homes still carry a stigma for many adult Americans and less than 20 percent of long-term care services, as previously noted, are delivered in this environment. The home is the ideal, if not always the practical, place to care for a loved one.

Still, agents should be careful about their presentation of home care benefits. While the daily benefit level should be set at least the same as that reimbursable for nursing home care, a substantial need for home health care may be more costly than a stay in a facility. The more care needed, the more varied the specialists, the greater the number of visits necessary, the higher the daily costs. For that reason, some insurers are allowing a higher percentage purchase of daily benefits for home care, up to 150 percent of the facility care amount.

In addition, check to see if the home health care benefit is calculated on a daily, weekly, or monthly basis. Remember that the weekly or monthly calculations are a significant advantage at claim time as it coordinates better with the way home health care agencies schedule their visits. The ability to have higher pools in weekly or monthly amounts may be an "enhanced" rider that has to be added to the policy as an optional benefit.

There will be more pressure on home health care benefits depending on the future of home care under Medicare. This government program is whittling away at its home care reimbursements, which represent a major (and growing) part of the Medicare budget. Since the Balanced Budget Act of 1997, Medicare has reigned in these freewheeling costs, making the home care benefit of a private insurance policy even more valuable. Agents need to discuss this with the client and set the home care benefit as high as possible, based on policy limits and affordability. If offered as an optional rider, the agent must stress its importance during the sales presentation.

Many carriers have generally added *alternate care benefits* to the basic policy provisions. The primary purpose of this feature is to provide benefit reimbursement in non-traditional settings, such as assisted living facilities that were not mentioned until recent policy versions. This benefit also allows the Claims Department to keep up and utilize current and emerging long-term care treatment trends, as this industry, and its technology, is still evolving.

Most policies offer this as part of basic coverage, but, if not, they generally have this feature available as an option. It gives clients (and their families) and insurers' care coordinators additional treatment choices to consider when the need arises. Having these alternatives available can help to ensure that the best decision will be made on behalf of the chronically ill adult.

Inflation Protection

Inflation is a given. It is easy for consumers to see the impact of it on their policy benefits that may not pay off for a number of years. The younger the buyer, the more important this coverage enhancement becomes.

Between 1985 and 1995, nursing home prices increased annually at an average of 9.7 percent. This is significantly higher than the Consumer Price Index, which has consistently been under 5 percent for years. For example, in 1995 general inflation increased by 2.8 percent while nursing home prices moved ahead by 8 percent.[1]

Nursing home cost inflation is the easiest to measure. A one-year stay in 1996 cost $30,000. This grew to $55,000 annually in 2000, and to over $60,000 in 2002. By 2030, a year in a nursing home could cost well over $200,000.[2]

Insurance policies of every type have alternatives to keep benefit levels from eroding due to inflation. Long-term care insurance is no different. The best time to buy a long-term care policy, from a premium and an insurability standpoint, is when a person is in his 40s and 50s, even though it may be many years before benefits are actually needed. For most people, the inflation option is essential. This is especially true for younger buyers, whose chosen benefit levels will be eroded by inflation when they reach the time to make a claim.[3]

Inflation is a wild card in benefit design. When will the client need care and what will it cost them?[4] A young couple in their 30s documented their search for the right long-term care benefit design and policy in a *Wall Street Journal* article. Regarding inflation they wrote, "We were easily persuaded that one choice, though costly, is a must-have: automatic inflation protection, generally compounded at 5 percent a year. Take a look at the math: With the compound inflation option, a $140 daily benefit would be worth $371.46 a day in 20 years. Even a simple inflation option would increase the benefit to $280/day."[5]

Older individuals (age 70+) might consider this alternative for providing inflation protection: buying a much larger daily benefit amount than the average local cost of a nursing home at the time application is made. For example, if the current average nursing home rate in the area is $150 a day, the purchase of a $220 a day benefit (the per diem cap in 2003 under HIPAA) will provide some protection against rising long-term care costs for a few years. Order product quotes showing inflation options with $150/day, and a $220/day plan with no inflation and compare the price. The higher daily benefit may be a more economical way to approach inflation protection.

If added as an optional benefit, the inflation rider will automatically increase the benefit amount by a specific percentage each year. This percentage, for most companies, is fixed at five percent. The NAIC has required that this option be offered two ways: (1) increases made on a simple basis, or (2) increases made on a compounded basis. This has an effect on both the daily benefit and the premium for this option. Figure 16.1 illustrates the effect of the inflation rider for a $100 a day benefit.

FIGURE 16.1

Policy Year	Daily Benefit (no inflation)	Simple 5% Inflation Rider	Compounded 5% Inflation Rider
1	$100	$100	$100.00
2	100	105	105.00
3	100	110	110.25
4	100	115	115.76
5	100	120	121.55
6	100	125	127.62
7	100	130	134.01
8	100	135	140.71
9	100	140	147.75
10	100	145	155.13
11	100	150	162.89
12	100	155	171.03
13	100	160	179.59
14	100	165	188.56
15	100	170	197.99
16	100	175	207.89
17	100	180	218.29
18	100	185	229.20
19	100	190	240.66
20	100	195	252.69

While differences in the daily benefit increases are more obvious in the later years, a couple of dollars difference in the early years can make a substantial difference in the daily benefit. Figure 16.2 illustrates the differences in an annual payout based on 365 days.

FIGURE 16.2

Year	5% simple	5% compounded	Annual Difference	Cumulative Difference
1	$100	$100.00	-0-	-0-
2	105	105.00	-0-	-0-
3	110	110.25	$ 91.25	$ 91.25
4	115	115.76	277.40	368.65
5	120	121.55	565.75	934.40
6	125	127.62	956.30	1,890.70
7	130	134.01	1,463.65	3,354.35
8	135	140.71	2,084.15	5,438.50
9	140	147.75	2,828.75	8,267.25
10	145	155.13	3,697.45	11,964.70
11	150	162.89	4,704.85	16,669.55
12	155	171.03	5,850.95	22,520.50
13	160	179.59	7,150.35	29,670.85
14	165	188.56	8,599.40	38,270.25
15	170	197.99	10,216.35	48,486.60
16	175	207.89	12,004.85	60,491.45
17	180	218.29	13,975.85	74,467.30
18	185	229.20	16,133.00	90,600.30
19	190	240.66	18,490.90	109,091.20
20	195	252.69	21,056.85	130,148.05

These numbers show the difference between the simple and compounding effects on increasing the daily benefit. Though the simple inflation rider provides adequate protection, the compounded inflation rider provides better coverage, and keeps the policy benefit closer to the current annual nursing home inflation rate. Compounded inflation is the most popular rider purchased.[6]

However, the premium cost for the rider may influence the option selected.

A simple inflation rider will increase the premium by 20 to 30 percent or more. The compounded inflation rider option will likely double the simple inflation rider premium.

While the compounded inflation rider is the ultimate protection, every client should seriously consider adding at least the simple inflation rider. While it will increase the cost somewhat, this is more than balanced by the resulting increase in protection when the policy benefits are needed. While the cost of the compounding inflation rider is prohibitive for some, the simple inflation rider (as illustrated in Figure 16.1) is still considerably better than leaving the daily benefit on a level basis.

There may be a few inflation riders available that increase daily benefits based on the Consumer Price Index (CPI). With the CPI consistently under five percent in the last few years, and well under the nursing home inflation measurements, the CPI increases will not effectively keep pace with long-term care inflation. It is still better, however, than buying a level daily benefit without an option to increase the daily benefit amount.

Unlike the cost of living options available under disability income insurance policies, the inflation rider for long-term care insurance increases the daily benefit each year the policy is in force. For disability insurance, the insured must be on a claim first before any increases are made. A 50-year-old who purchases a long-term care policy with an inflation benefit rider, and who does not use the benefits for 20 years, will have 19 increases in the daily benefit amount before a claim is filed.

Guarantee of Insurability

The guarantee of insurability option (GOI) increases the daily benefit at specified option dates. Also called the guaranteed purchase option, the increases can be significantly larger than the increases under the inflation option.

For example, the insured may have the option to increase a $150 daily benefit level by $25 a day or $50 a day every two or three years. This increase can be taken in one step, bringing the daily benefit to $175 a day or $200 a day. A five percent simple inflation rider would increase the daily benefit to $165 a day by the third year. The guarantee of insurability option has a more notable immediate effect on the daily benefit increase.

In addition to larger daily benefit increases, this option requires no evidence of insurability. Once the original policy is issued, there are no health questions involved when an increase in the daily benefit occurs. As the insured grows older, this option becomes more and more important.

However, unlike the cost for inflation protection that is included in the annual premium, the cost for the GOI increases, when exercised, is based on company rates and the attained age of the insured. The additional benefit amount is subject to new rates and the original benefit remains as issued and rated.

The insured can waive the option to increase the daily benefit, but usually only once or twice in the lifetime of the policy. If, for example, an increase is scheduled every three years, the insured can exercise the option at that time or waive this right. Once you have exceeded the number of waives you are allowed under the rider's terms, you forfeit the right to any future increases. In addition, these increases are not available past a certain age, usually age 80 or age 85.

The guarantee of insurability option can be an alternative to the inflation protection rider or the purchase of a higher daily benefit than needed at time of application. It may be a more cost-effective way to handle the rising cost issue, at least initially.

It is important to remember that if a client owns a long-term care insurance policy with this optional feature purchased prior to January 1, 1997, exercising this option may result in a disqualification of the policy as a tax-qualified plan. All policies placed in force before January 1, 1997 were grandfathered into the law without regard to their benefit triggers and how they were defined.

This gives these policies increased value at present. But Treasury guidelines state that a material change to the policy will change the tax status of the policy unless it has the HIPAA-specified language. Increasing the policy's daily benefit with this option will be considered a material change, unless the additional benefits are issued under satisfactory language that conforms to the tax-qualified definitions. To avoid any confusion, some insurers will issue the increase as an additional policy, rather than alter anything about the present plan.

NOTE: Some life insurance policies are getting a new wrinkle – an ability to purchase long-term care insurance on a GOI basis. These options, added to life insurance coverage, guarantee that these policyholders can buy a comprehensive individual long-term care policy at one of several future dates. It is primarily designed for younger clients who are not yet ready to buy long-term care insurance but who wish to protect their future ability to do so.[7]

Nonforfeiture Benefit

This book has already noted the availability of life insurance-like nonforfeiture benefits in long-term care policies today (Chapter 12), as recommended by the NAIC. Contingent nonforfeiture benefits (Chapter 14) were also noted as required in policies written in those states that have approved the NAIC's Rate Stability amendments to the Model Policy Act. The nonforfeiture benefit may also be offered as an optional benefit for an additional price.

This feature protects the consumer if the long-term care policy is lapsed by providing a benefit of a minimum amount or 100 percent of the sum of all premiums paid, or to have the policy stay in effect (on some coverage basis) for life. Many financial planners urge clients to forego this option because it can add as much as 40 percent to the premium without a corresponding increase in the value of the coverage.[8] This option is rarely sold, and with the inclusion of contingent nonforfeiture in some policies, may be even less necessary to consider.

Return of Premium

A few insurers offer a return of premium benefit to give individuals something in exchange for the premiums paid – especially policy benefits that were never utilized. The drawback to this option is that the policy must be surrendered or the insured must die before the premium (or a percentage of it) is returned.

The amount of premium returned may vary depending on the language of the rider. Some insurers return all of the premiums paid beyond a certain date less any policy benefits utilized. Others may pay a stipulated percentage (30 percent, 50 percent, or 80 percent) depending upon the year the insured surrenders the policy or upon the insured's death, less any claims benefits paid. Still others simply return the premium paid, after a specified period of time, without regard to any claims that might have been paid.

Examples of each type are:

#1:   Annual premium: $1,125
        Policy kept for 11 years before surrender
        Claims = $4,175
        Calculation: $1,125 x 11 = $12,375 - claims ($4,175) = $8,200

#2:   Annual premium: $1,125
        Policy kept for 11 years before surrender
        Claims = $4,175
        Percentage returned in year 11: 80%
        Calculation: $1,125 x 11 = $12,375 x 80% = $9,900 -
            claims ($4,175) = $5,725

#3   Annual premium: $1,125
        Policy kept for 11 years before surrender
        Claims = $4,175
        Calculation: $1,125 x 11 = $12,375 (claims not considered)

The additional premium for this option is exceptionally high (50 - 100 percent or more of the base policy cost) and may not be worth the money. An insured may be better off to take the extra dollars that would have been used to purchase this option and invest it in another vehicle that earns interest rather than let the insurer hold it for future payout.

Moreover, to collect the money, the insured would have to surrender the policy. This would leave him without coverage at an age when benefits may soon be needed. If the insured is changing insurers for some reason, there could be some return of premium from the original policy that can be applied to the new plan. However, any substantial return of premium would accumulate only after the policy has been in force for a number of years. Changing policies and paying a significantly higher premium due to an age change makes little sense despite a return of premium. The insured may be better off buying additional coverage than investing in this option.

In addition, the insured who is concerned with a return on investment should policy benefits not be used might consider the life insurance-based long-term care insurance approach. (See Chapter 15, "Stand Alone versus Life Insurance-Based Approach," for more details.)

Spousal Benefits

Long-term care policies today try to encourage joint purchase of coverage by a husband and wife. There are discounts usually offered if both buy policies. As was noted in an earlier chapter, actuaries have placed the savings to insurers when spouses purchase coverage at around 40 percent, due to the hands-on presence of an actual caregiver at home. Thus, encouraging married couples and companions to apply makes good business sense. Moreover, one of the products discussed in Chapter 15 was a joint whole life plan with long-term care coverage built into the policy.

Some insurers place more specific spouse features into their optional benefit packages for those that wish to add the coverage to their base policy. These usually take the form of "shared benefits" and "survivorship" coverage.

Shared benefits: There are several types of shared benefit approaches. The first is one long-term care policy with two insureds accessing the policy benefits. The second is a spousal transfer concept, where two long-term care policies are purchased, but each spouse can access the other's should one's benefits run out.

The third is to have two long-term care policies and a shared benefit rider that either spouse can access.[9]

The latter approach is generally an alternative to lifetime coverage, and is often used as a more economical way to increase potential coverage for either or both insureds. The spouses purchase identical coverage, such as a $500,000 pool of money and then add the rider that gives them another $500,000 in coverage that either or both could access when their coverage is exhausted.

Survivorship coverage: This rider pays off any future premiums for one spouse after the other has passed away. They both must buy long-term care coverage from the same insurer and each policy must contain the rider. If so, after a specified number of years (usually from seven to ten years), should a spouse die, the remaining spouse is not required to ever pay premiums for the long-term care policy again. This can ultimately represent a substantial savings, and since historically the male spouse often dies before the female, it is quite feasible that the woman could outlive spouse for a substantial number of years. Having a paid-up long-term care policy can ease future financial concerns.

Other features may be available and should be reviewed with a husband and wife. One is a joint waiver of premium where if one insured is receiving benefits, the premium is waived for both. Other plans may pay for caregiver training on behalf of the healthy spouse.

End of Life Care

In 2002, the states were graded in an analysis by Last Acts, a coalition headed by former first lady Rosalynn Carter, as to how they handle end of life care for the terminally ill. The result: poor grades for most states in areas such as advance directive policies, palliative care, hospital end-of-life services and pain management, and hospice use. In any given state, at least one in four nursing home residents is experiencing pain for at least two months without appropriate pain management.[10]

Long-term care insurers are incorporating end-of-life care to their policies. Most include hospice care coverage, and all utilize the alternate plan of care benefits to handle various pain management situations. At least one long-term care carrier provides an end-of-life care rider as an optional benefit where daily benefit amounts double upon diagnosis of a terminal illness, allowing claimants to financially access better quality care during this last part of life.

While HIPAA has limited the benefit trigger language that could distinguish long-term care policies, innovative carriers will work on the balance of the product to add extra benefits that could prove beneficial to your clients. Agents should review the carrier's information carefully to see what is available before soliciting clients.

Managed Care

Although this benefit is not an option, it is worth mentioning because there are only a few insurers using this concept. A long-term care claim can be a fairly complex matter. This is partly due to a variety of services and treatments provided by a number of different health care personnel.

A treatment plan may consist of a skilled nursing facility stay, follow-up treatments at home, or adult day care. To coordinate these types of care and effectively manage the claim to maximize recovery at the most efficient cost, insurers are turning to claims managers and care coordinators (sometimes third party) who can meet or talk with the insured's physician to map out a plan of care.

Flexibility is the buzz word in long-term care today and the inclusion of coverage for alternate plans of care in the basic long-term care policy makes the managed care approach more sensible. Carriers are now more likely to assign care coordinators. Care coordinators are health care professionals who play an integral part in assessing needs and ensuring that treatment prescribed is as closely aligned to policy benefits as possible. The initial assessment done for the insured is typically part of today's long-term care claim procedures.

Managed care eliminates the multitude of claim forms that the insured (or a family member) must provide the insurer. It is also clear from the beginning what the treatments consist of, when they are scheduled, and the cost. The treatment plan can be modified as necessary depending on the course taken for recovery.

Some companies attempt to establish a claims file long before any benefits are needed. For example, my mother's long-term care insurer, CNA, contacted her in the second year of the policy to obtain some basic information about her that would be forwarded on to a claims manager if and when a claim occurred. Her past medical history, any current medications, her personal physician and other health preferences are already noted within her claim file to make it easier to discuss treatment plans with her doctor. Also, it does not require my mother's input, which she may or may not be able to give at time of claim.

Some insurers have set up relationships with nationwide nursing home and home health care agency chains to obtain preferred rates for their long-term care charges. Use of these facilities (an option) may have an advantage for the claimant if the daily benefit level normally would not be high enough to cover the usual costs of care. The insured can review a booklet listing the carrier's preferred providers of long-term care services, just as one reviews the same information about his health insurance program today.

Toll-free numbers are usually available to any policyholder for advice or counseling on any long-term care issue or for recommendations on a facility. Managed care is an integral part of health insurance today and is becoming an important part of long-term care insurance. Look for more product wrinkles using managed care components in the months ahead.

As you can see, the optional benefits available with a long-term care insurance policy can help tailor the plan to the specific needs of an insured. Any or all of these features can take on significance in this important part of pre-retirement estate planning. By listening to the individual or couple, the planner can perhaps match interest or need to a specific optional benefit. Agents and consumers should at least be aware of their existence, and how each can enhance the basic protection purchased.

Chapter Notes

1. "How to Judge a Policy," *Consumer Reports* (October, 1997), p. 40.

2. Source: American Council of Life Insurers.

3. Ralph D. Leisle, "Use Inflation Option With Most LTC Insurance Plans," *National Underwriter*, February 12, 2001, p. 11.

4. Stephen N. Mathieu, CFP, CLU, "Financial Products to Fund LTC," *National Underwriter*, July 1, 2002, p. 14.

5. Kelly Greene, "Cutting Through The Confusion," *Wall StreetJournal*, March 24, 2003.

6. Barbara Stahlecker, CSA, "LTC 101: Cost of Living Riders," *HIU Magazine*, October 2002, p. 78.

7. Linda Koco, "New Wrinkle on Guaranteed Purchase Options: Offer it for LTCs," *National Underwriter*, August 6, 2001, p. 20.

8. Jeanne Sahadi, "Playing the odds on long-term care," *CNN/Money Magazine*, August 26, 2002.

9. Marilee Driscoll, "Shared Benefit LTC Policies: Their Time Has Come," *National Underwriter*, September 2, 2002, p. 32.

10. Patricia Guthrie, "End-of-life care lags in Georgia," *Atlanta Journal & Constitution*, November 19, 2002, p. D1.

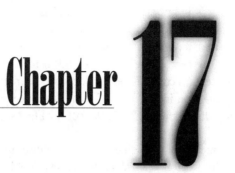

Chapter 17

Alternate Long-Term Care Financing Options

"Sure, I'm for helping the elderly. I'm going to be old myself some day."

– Lillian Carter, in her 80s

While most of the product discussion to date has centered on individual long-term care policies sold on a stand-alone basis, it is important to note that there are other ways to finance the long-term care risk. These additional methods give consumers other choices in meeting their long-term care needs. A look at life insurance-based approaches to long-term care was discussed in Chapter 15.

In this chapter, the focus will be on the various hybrids of long-term care coverage that are marketed today. An outline of the most common benefit provisions for an individual long-term care policy appears in Chapter 12, "Provider-Aided Design." Group coverage marketed through employers, a long-term care market ripe with opportunity, is covered in Chapter 19, "Group Long-term Care Insurance."

Living Benefits

For years insurance companies focused on death benefits and how important it was to protect against premature death, estate tax, and debt settlement as well as to provide income for the surviving family members. While most people know that life insurance is an important financial tool, many dreaded reviewing these plans since the central issue was about death. There also was an emphasis on cash values which were receiving only four percent interest while the market rate was closer to 15-20 percent. In the late 1970s, the life insurance industry was hit hard with huge losses and competitive products on the market. The shift to pure death benefit protection in the form of term insurance began in earnest. This shift significantly altered the premium flow of the life insurance industry.

Ironically, at the same time, a growing realization concerning the impact of substantial advances in medical science started to take hold. Life spans were increasing with regularity. Many people were living into their 80s, especially women. The financial services industry not only had to deal with premature death, but was also confronted with people living longer.

The new era of living benefits was ushered in. This aspect of life insurance was appealing to the insurers – what life insurance can do during someone's lifetime (not just after) added a positive spin to the subject. It had the same attractive aspect that disability income offered – providing income during the lifetime of the policyowner. With mixed reviews on universal life insurance to ponder, the industry set about adding features to the life insurance policy that highlighted living benefits as a new approach in sales.

The idea of emphasizing living benefits played well with customers. They preferred to focus on accumulation of value for use at a later date by the *policyholder* and not the beneficiary. Protection of that accumulation became a second focus in which the consumer also showed interest.

The first living benefits idea launched successfully was the accelerated death benefit concept.

Accelerated Death Benefits

The living benefits approach was based on the universal complaint of life insurance policyholders: that those who suffered from a catastrophic or terminal injury or illness struggled physically and financially while a substantial death benefit was in force but inaccessible. While there was easy access to the cash value (if the policy was not term insurance), the amount was not nearly as high as the actual face amount of the policy.

An accelerated death benefit gives the policyholder access to at least a portion of the death benefit before he dies. The money can be used for a variety of expenses before death actually occurs. Included in these expenses are nursing home stays and home health care expenses.

The accelerated death benefit was a policy option that was first added to life insurance policies at an additional premium charge. Today, few, if any insurers charge for this benefit until the policyowner exercises his or her right to withdraw the money. At the time of payout, an administrative fee is assessed to process the paperwork and pay out the lump sum amount. Almost all life insurance policies today have this type of option, and most specifically mention use of proceeds for long-term care services.

Initially, certain terminal or catastrophic illnesses such as a stroke, renal disease, and heart failure qualified for accelerated death benefits. However, most insurers today have broadened their categories to include a stay in a nursing facility or, in some cases, any type of long-term care expense.

The popularity of accelerated death benefits has grown dramatically. The growth of the viatical settlement industry has set competitive standards for insurers, many of whom have responded by liberalizing their accelerated death benefit provisions. Most insurers offered it to existing as well as new policyholders and may well have added the option to existing policies since there is no additional premium needed for this feature. Today's new product offerings usually find an accelerated death benefit option as a regular policy feature.

Some insurers place a limitation on the amount of the withdrawal, varying from 25 to 50 percent, while other companies allow a higher amount (up to the entire face amount). For example, a policy with a $250,000 face amount and a 50 percent accelerated death benefit will permit the early withdrawal of $125,000 to be used for medical and other expenses due to the illness or condition that precipitated the need to exercise this provision.

The accelerated death benefit can be used, depending on the amount of benefit allowed, to fund long-term care expenses. But at what cost to other income needs that life insurance was intended to satisfy? If the policy was purchased, for example, to specifically pay estate taxes and a mortgage balance, and to provide income for the family, there may be little or no money available to handle these financial concerns if the accelerated death benefit option is exercised to pay for long-term care expenses. If long-term care expenses *were* budgeted into the face amount calculation, then it is another way to meet long-term care needs. Agents assessing total financial needs can keep in mind long-term care expenses as part of an accelerated benefit when determining policy face amount, if not addressing the long-term care need in another manner.

In theory, long-term care expenses may be more likely to become necessary later in life, perhaps at a time when life insurance needs are dwindling. While one cannot count on that when planning, it is important to remember in later years if the client encourages a reduction in life insurance face amount for these reasons, yet has done nothing about financing long-term care needs.

The passage of the Health Insurance Portability and Accountability Act of 1996 (HIPAA) also provided needed tax clarification for this type of benefit payment. If the triggers for payment of the accelerated death benefit for long-term care expenses match the language required by the law (see Chapter 13 on tax-qualified plans), the benefits are paid tax-free. The agent and consumer should check the policy language carefully to ensure the "chronically ill" provision conforms to HIPAA's requirements.

This should not necessarily be considered a substitute for long-term care insurance. Read the accelerated benefits feature carefully to ascertain the flexibility involved in using the death benefit to cover long-term care expenses. If the accelerated death benefit provisions are adequate, increase the death benefit by an amount that can help pay at least a minimum of long-term care expenses. Like regular long-term care benefit design, this can be calculated by multiplying the local annual long-term care costs by at least four years, the minimum recommended term to adequately fund most long-term care situations.

Long-term Care Riders

Accelerated death benefits are not the only type of coverage that can be used on life insurance to meet long-term care expenses. Today, there are a number of long-term care riders that are offered as living benefits on life insurance policies. These riders are usually different than the life insurance-based long-term care coverage reviewed in Chapter 15. However, the principle is the same. Since the agent is reviewing pre-retirement estate planning with the client, if both living and death needs can be met using the same policy, this convenience may be attractive for the consumer.

Historically, consumers have not considered buying long-term care coverage before age 65. They typically associate the long-term care need with post-retirement concerns. However, by the time the coverage is sought, the premiums may be too high or the coverage unattainable due to health conditions. As noted earlier, buying long-term care coverage before age 65 results in a lower cost and (perhaps) ease of insurability due to medical history. Consideration of a long-term care rider added to a life policy would accomplish this early purchase objective.

As noted, the need for a larger face amount in a life insurance policy usually diminishes with time – children grow up and move on, the mortgage is almost paid off, and other debt is reduced. With a potential long-term care need looming, the use of the larger death benefit can be applied to long-term care expenses. If forced to rely on cash value, the money available may not be adequate to pay for the cost of these services.

Some long-term care riders allow direct access to the policy face amount at a stipulated percentage each year. Typically, the rider pays two percent of the face amount of the policy each month for long-term care expenses. For example, a $200,000 policy would yield a $4,000 monthly payout for long-term care expenses, or approximately $133 a day. Payments continue until a policy payout limit is reached (50-100 percent of the total face amount). When the entire face amount is paid, it would take 50 months at two percent. With nursing home costs averaging closer to $168/day, a policy face amount of around $250,000 would generate this daily amount.

Initially, this type of rider paid a flat percentage of the face amount out each month for a nursing home stay only, but now most non-nursing home long-term care services are eligible for this type of funding. A policy might offer a different percentage of monthly payout depending upon the type of long-term care service needed. For example, a nursing home confinement yields four percent of the policy face amount each month for up to 25 months, while the standard two percent payout is made for home health care or adult day care expenses. Using the example of a $200,000 policy, the nursing home pay-out would be $8,000 per month or $266/day, while the pay-out for home care would be $4,000 per month or $133/day. The agent and client should be careful in the amount selected, because the nursing home rate in this example would exceed the $220/day per diem cap (in 2003), resulting in possible tax consequences unless actual LTC expenses were higher. Similarly, home health expenses could be even greater than nursing home fixed daily costs, depending on the care that is needed. The selection of the amount should be consistent with planning done using a stand-alone long-term care policy.

This option can also be enhanced by allowing an extension of benefits. In one insurer's version, after the 50-month period of paying two percent of the face amount exhausts the policy death benefit, an extension of benefits creates a continuing monthly flow of the same benefit amount for another 50 months or as long as needed. In effect, this option creates a second face amount to be similarly paid out at the conclusion of the first payout. The products discussed in Chapter 15, "Indemnity versus Life Insurance-Based Approach," have the options to extend out the length of payments. The cost to do this is relatively low since the initial payout period would have to be exhausted first before carrying over into the benefit extension time frame. Still, with more and more people able to function (although not independently) due to advances in medical science, this option helps to reduce the likelihood of outliving the benefits.

A second version of this rider functions similarly to a stand-alone individual long-term care policy, paying a separate daily benefit with an elimination period and benefit period. This option has its own pool of benefits and the face amount of the life policy remains untouched. The cost is much higher than the version which reduces the face amount, but it allows both types of coverage – life insurance and long-term care – to be independent of each other while encompassing all the benefits under one policy.

The tax treatment of this early payout of life insurance benefits is covered under the HIPAA legislation. Language in the long-term rider must conform to the tax-qualified requirements of defining "chronically ill" to achieve the tax-free distribution.

A convenient way to obtain long-term care insurance and at the same time incorporate it into someone's financial plan is a long-term care rider in a life insurance policy. Young buyers are targeted for this type of insurance because it allows insurers to effectively spread the risk because it is more likely that the elderly will utilize this coverage in greater numbers. The ease of purchase, low cost, and better chance of eligibility make this option potentially attractive to future long-term care insurance buyers.

As noted in Chapter 15, the NAIC is exploring the alternatives that insurers should be required to offer if the cash value of a life insurance policy is no longer adequate to continue the policy in force. This would, in place of a specific requirement, cause the long-term care coverage to lapse, too.

Finally, the new 2001 CSO tables will be available shortly. The 2001 CSO Mortality Table is a "valuation mortality table," meaning its primary purpose is to determine the mortality risk when calculating insurance company reserves. As such, the table will only affect riders that have mortality risk. This includes term insurance riders, annuity riders, disability income riders, and long-term care riders.[1]

Annuities

The growth in annuity sales for the past several years has been phenomenal. While long-term care sales have also enjoyed growth, it pales in comparison to the annuity results. Yet, often the prospect for annuities is also a potential customer for long-term care insurance. The opportunity for cross-selling would seem to be a natural.[2]

Many deferred annuity policies now contain a provision similar to the life insurance riders noted above, that allows the annuitant to withdraw funds, avoiding any applicable surrender charges or penalties, to pay for long-term care services. Access to this money, which could represent a significant amount of retirement assets, may meet most of the long-term care costs on an immediate basis depending on the amount of the annuity. If the annuitant needs care in a nursing home and there is little chance of recovery or release from the facility, these proceeds might be more appropriately used to fund the long-term care need rather than funding retirement needs.

Many agents and financial planners recommend variable annuities because of this product's tax deferral and potentially substantial interest rate. The interest earned may be withdrawn to pay the premium for a long-term care policy. This alternative preserves the original asset, creates an alternate funding vehicle for a long-term care policy, and still results in a large asset that can be used to meet a variety of other needs, including retirement funding.

One such variable annuity provides: (a) nursing home/critical illness waiver of surrender charges that can be triggered by the annuity owner or the spouse, even if the spouse is not a party to the annuity contract; (b) an elder care resource that offers referral and consultation service for the annuity owner and any family member; (c) discounts on long-term care services through preferred long-term care providers; and (d) a credit to the annuity value should the owner need long-term care.[3]

Variable products may not be considered suitable for the older client, so caution should be exercised in discussing this option with a potential long-term care insurance buyer. If interest on the principal of an investment is sufficient to pay long-term care premiums, fine. But is there room for the interest generated to decrease and still pay the premium? Is there enough margin in the interest received to cover any rate increases that might be levied by the insurer on the long-term care policy? Be sure everyone is satisfied with the answers to these questions before proceeding.

But annuities with some provision enhancements should long-term care arise is only part of this type of alternative financing vehicle. Today, more carriers are developing a new hybrid product similar to life insurance-based products – annuity and true long-term care coverage wrapped together. One indication of the higher level of interest in these types of products is that in June 2002, the Treasury Department and Department of Health and Human Services sponsored a forum in Washington, D.C. on these hybrid annuity-long-term care concepts and drew attendees from the NAIC, AARP, and the Urban Institute, among others.[4]

One such hybrid has an individual investing money into a fixed deferred annuity, say $150,000. This purchases an additional face amount for long-term care coverage equal to $300,000, payable over a specified period of time like five or six years. Charges are deducted each month from the accumulating annuity value to pay for the long-term care coverage, which has benefits and provisions in accordance with tax-qualified plans. If the individual is disabled and needs long-term care services, he will begin drawing money from the annuity portion of the policy first, and then ultimately from the long-term care coverage once the annuity proceeds are exhausted.

In other words, he is paying for long-term care with his own money first. This makes the underwriting of this risk almost on par with annuities (at least in terms of quick issue) because the insured is actually self-insuring initially. So, instead of just buying an annuity, the individual is actually creating a long-term care benefit at the same time. For individuals who can move an asset around, directing it toward this type of program, it represents a unique way to finance long-term care needs. Showing a consumer this type of illustration and measuring net return (current rate less long-term care charges less taxes on these charges) may well be the best financial alternative for the person.[5]

There are still some questions that need further clarification from what we already know:[6]

1. If the long-term care portion of the long-term care annuity represents a tax-qualified long-term care insurance contract, what part of the premium is deductible?

2.   If a long-term care benefit payment affects the annuity portion of a contract (e.g. account value), how is the benefit payment treated for tax purposes?

3.   What are the consequences of funding long-term care coverage from the annuity portion of a contract?

4.   How is the line to be drawn between the long-term care and annuity portions of the contract for purposes of the tax law requirements applicable to each, such as the definition of a tax-qualified long-term care contract and the distribution-on-death rules applicable to annuity contracts?

5.   Can long-term care-annuity combos be used in connection with qualified retirement plans, and, if so, what issues exist in that context?

Insurers selling these programs have different interpretations about these questions, and you should check with them as you consider these products. Still, it may make sense to utilize these plans for certain clients, and the two concepts, although inversely related, would seem suited to being handled under the same umbrella. Since discussions about annuities often focus on retirement, what better time to talk about the serious threat of long-term care that can affect retirement income and assets?

State Partnerships

In the May, 1991 issue of *The Disability Newsletter*, the following statement appeared at the conclusion of an article on long-term care insurance:

Many people believe that the private sector will not be able to fill the entire void (for long-term care), and that the only means to address all consumer needs is some sharing of coverage between the public and private sectors. As such, the most popular scenario for the long-term care market is that sometime in the late 1990's, the public sector will become more active in providing long-term care coverage to our society.

This prediction came almost on the eve of the state of Connecticut's newly announced public-private concept of funding the long-term care need and saving the state's Medicaid program in the process. The rest of this forecast has not materialized. The ill-fated, sweeping overhaul of the nation's health care system led by Hillary Rodham Clinton's task force was "faced down." The reality of long-term care costs and coverage for this need was all but eliminated by the final proposed version. Current Medicare and Medicaid reforms are almost certain to result in less spending on long-term care expenses, not more.

Back to Connecticut. Their program represented a public and private sector cooperation that reached new heights with programs designed to encourage consumers to purchase long-term care coverage rather than rely on Medicaid funds after assets are either spent or transferred. In 1987, the Robert Wood Johnson Foundation funded a study done by the state of Connecticut to assess the chances of a collaboration between insurers, consumers, and the state to solve both the financing of long-term care and the preservation of a Medicaid program that was teetering on the edge of extinction. The result was the creation of the Connecticut Partnership for Long-term Care.

This partnership resulted from efforts put forth following a conclusion that the chances of the insurance industry or the government shouldering alone the burden of providing long-term care coverage for a continually aging U.S. population was unrealistic. Private insurance would be appropriate and affordable for some, the study concluded, but would not ease the strain on the Medicaid budget created by the growing need for long-term care funding for poor Americans.

Connecticut's purpose, as then stated by Kevin J. Mahoney, project director for the Connecticut partnership, was to provide people with the chance to plan ahead to meet long-term care needs without impoverishment, and to rein in Medicaid expenditures, which threatened to spiral out of control.

On August 28, 1991 Connecticut received formal approval from the federal government for its Long-term Care Partnership program. This was a much needed endorsement because the partnership would affect Medicaid rules. The program involved the sale of a specified state approved policy form sold by insurers, which provided long-term care coverage in a lump sum amount. Upon entry into a nursing home, costs would be reimbursed from this lump sum amount until the individual recovered or the funds were exhausted. The key point here is that for every dollar of coverage paid under the policy, the insured could protect a similar dollar amount in assets that would not need to be spent or transferred to become eligible for Medicaid.

For example, a $50,000 policy paying benefits in full would enable the individual to shield an additional $50,000 of assets from Connecticut's current Medicaid rules (assets of $2,000 are allowable) without divesting assets in other ways – an obvious advantage for residents of Connecticut. The state benefits, too, because the $50,000 policy benefits must be exhausted first (including any assets over and above $50,000) before any Medicaid funding is needed. Some people will not outlive the policy benefits and thus will not file for Medicaid. Here are examples of asset sheltering:

	Personal Assets	Long-term Care Insurance Payouts	Medicaid Countable Assets
Person #1	$ 65,000	$ 65,000	-0-
Person #2	250,000	250,000	-0-
Person #3	500,000	250,000	$250,000
Person #4	500,000	-0-	500,000

Each of these individuals represents a different scenario.

- Person #1 has used the entire policy benefit and completely preserved the $65,000 assets owned without transfer. Without the partnership allowing a dollar for dollar exclusion, the assets would have had to be exhausted.

- Person #2 also accomplished the same goal but with a greater benefit need and a matching policy benefit.

- Person #3 purchased a lump sum amount below the fully countable assets. If the entire $250,000 lump sum is spent and a need for benefits still exists, $250,000 of assets preserved and $250,000 is subjected to payout (unless already transferred) before application for Medicaid can be made.

- Person #4 chose not to participate in the partnership, leaving the full $500,000 asset base potentially exposed to Medicaid countable assets.

Since the start of Connecticut's private cooperative effort, a number of Connecticut residents have elected to purchase long-term care coverage through this partnership program. In the first version of the policy, a 65-year-old buying a $50,000 policy would pay a premium of approximately $960 a year. Currently, there are several insurers participating in the Connecticut Partnership program offering residents a variety of carriers to choose from. A variety of long-term care services are covered in the current policy version available. Plans have been re-filed to conform to HIPAA regulations to ensure tax-free distribution. The policies are available through an insurance agent.

The partnership allows for preservation of wealth – and the Medicaid program. Three other states have received funding and have started their own partnerships – Indiana, New York, and California. At least 19 other states have passed resolutions or actual legislation that would enact state partnership programs. Unfortunately, there is a federal impediment to kick-starting these programs. The Omnibus Budget Reconciliation Act of 1993 contains a provision that prevents additional states from launching long-term care insurance partnership programs on a favorable basis.[7]

California's plan imitates Connecticut's plan, but New York's plan has even more liberal provisions, and Indiana's plan has a hybrid form of partnership. Listed below are the policy types:[8]

Connecticut and California: Dollar-for-dollar model. Policies must cover at least one year at issue and pay a minimum daily benefit. Once policy benefits are exhausted, every dollar paid out by the insurer will be deducted from resources counted for Medicaid eligibility.

New York: Total assets model. Policies must cover three years of nursing home care, six years of home care, or a combination of the two. Once policy benefits have been exhausted, protection is granted for all assets, but an individual's income must be devoted to the cost of care.

Indiana: Hybrid model. Policies must cover at least one year and pay a minimum daily benefit. The value of coverage purchased, and later used, determines the method used for calculating asset protection in Medicaid eligibility. If the amount purchased is equal to or above a set amount for the policy effective year, total asset protection is applied. If the amount purchased is less than the set amount, the dollar-for-dollar method is used. Regardless of the method used, an individual's income must be used for the cost of care.

By the end of 2001, nearly 80,000 long-term care policies have been sold through these partnerships (New York had the most). The average age of the purchasers of these policies was 63. Over 800 people had qualified for benefits and 21 had exhausted their benefits and accessed Medicaid. This has been a cost-saving measure for these states.

The essential drawback of the plans is what happens if the purchaser moves to another state. The policy is still valid, but the Medicaid protection is not. Insureds would have to move back to their partnership state to achieve the Medicaid protection. This is inconvenient at best if, for example, the person moved to Florida or Arizona to retire. In 2001, Indiana and Connecticut enacted a reciprocity agreement that would allow policyholders to carry their Medicaid Asset Protection coverage from one state to the other.[9]

These plans have proven that the public and private sectors can work together to provide this important protection. To preserve Medicaid, alternate long term financing must happen. Far too many people spend all of their assets and then move to Medicaid for future care. There have recently been partnership bills introduced in Congress. In 2003, H.R. 1406 was introduced by Rep. John Peterson (R-Pennsylvania). This bill would allow long-term care partnership programs to be offered on a favorable basis in all states, bringing affordable access to long-term care insurance to millions of Americans.[10]

The future of partnerships could increase the public's exposure to private long-term care insurance. If the government is truly sending a message of personal responsibility through HIPAA and the new Federal long-term care plan, this is a great start down that road.

Viatical Settlements

A number of long-term care policies contain benefits payable while receiving hospice care. Hospice care is provided for those with terminal illness. Medicare provides substantial coverage for hospice care.

Terminal illness can also necessitate the need for long-term care services as part of treatment. As mentioned earlier, accelerated death benefits can be used to fund some of these expenses in the last days and months of life.

Viatical settlements are another method used to obtain funding to pay long-term care costs. Derived from the word viaticum, meaning communion given to Christians who are dying, a viatical settlement arrangement calls for an exchange.[11] The terminally ill patient transfers ownership in a life insurance policy in return for a smaller amount of cash. The individual receives the much needed cash and the company bestowing the dollars receives the policy death benefit upon the death of the insured at a substantial high rate of return.

Typically, the individual receives 60 to 80 cents (and possibly higher) on the dollar for the policy.

Most commonly, people with AIDS have sought viatical settlements to help fund their final months and expenses. Cancer and Alzheimer's patients have also received dollars under this type of program.

State regulators, while acknowledging that this source of funding of medical costs has been beneficial to many, are trying to find a balance between desperation and greed. Too often, these policies are exchanged for far below their value, simply because the patient sees no other way to obtain money needed for living and health care expenses. Several states have passed regulations concerning the registration of viatical companies and their agents.

The public perception of viatical settlements is mixed. Those that need the money are obviously in favor of them and many have had the opportunity to "die with dignity." Others believe these organizations "rip off" needy individuals for more of the face amount than necessary since they know the seller of the policy proceeds is desperate. Writer Lawrence Block in his 1997 book "Even the Wicked" writes of a man who is buying up policies and then murdering the sellers to ensure a quicker payoff. Is this a new twist to a mystery plot or a social commentary on these types of policies?

At age 71, a retired lawyer in Miami was looking to improve his 5 percent return on his investments and, after being approached about an investment idea, he consulted with an insurance agent, did some research, and eventually put $175,000 into a viatical settlement deal. He was lured by the promised rate of return (from 20 to 40 percent) and the opportunity to help a sick person who needed money in the last days of life. It took the man less than two years to learn he had been defrauded in a viatical scam. His money is gone.[12]

The Securities and Exchange Commission (SEC) has examined these transactions at length to decide whether they should be registered securities. Typically, an organization has several outside "investors" putting up money to buy the policies. They then wait for death to occur to receive the return on their investment. Is it a security or not? Some organizations have voluntarily registered their product.

Florida passed the Viatical Settlement Act in 1996, giving the power of their regulation to the state insurance department. The act defined the role and the licensing requirements of both the viatical settlement provider and the viatical settlement broker.

In the meantime, the National Association of Insurance Commissioners (NAIC) developed a model policy for viatical settlements. But it was HIPAA that added further endorsement to the whole issue of viatical settlements. In this federal legislation, people are allowed to exclude from their income certain payments received in a viatical settlement. Until that time, viatical payments were taxable events.

As a means of funding long-term care services, viatical settlements may have some merit. There are a number of competent viatical firms today and, without a long-term care insurance policy, the financial alternatives available to individuals who need long-term care services are few. While disposal of the life insurance policy may defeat other financial objectives originally intended, a viatical settlement will mean cash when it's needed.

A person must apply for a viatical settlement (some applications are quite lengthy) and answer questions in regard to one's medical history. Obviously, the more advanced the illness, the more likely a settlement. Viatical companies do not need the money right away, but the longer the wait, the lower the investment return. Those individuals with high medical costs are likely to have long-term care medical expenses that need payment. Viatical funds can provide these dollars.

The American Council of Life Insurers expressed five concerns to the NAIC during its ongoing work on viatical regulation:[13]

- Clarify that it is a fraudulent action against an insurer to purchase, to induce, or to encourage any person to purchase a life insurance contract for the sole purpose of selling that contract to a third party as an investment in the insured person's life.

- Create a legally rebuttable presumption that if an assignment of a life insurance contract occurs within the contestable period as defined under the contract, there exists evidence of intent to assign the policy when it was originally purchased and therefore the assignment is void (and/or the contract can be rescinded for fraud).

- Require that viatical companies participating in these secondary market sales and purchases share all their underwriting information with insurers at the time a secondary market transaction takes place.

- Ensure that the secondary market companies are subject to any and all of the same state underwriting restrictions that insurance companies are subject to.

- Clarify that an action for fraud perpetrated on an insurer that occurred as part of a secondary market transaction is not limited by the policy's contestability clause.

Life Settlements

The viatical settlement business refers, in general, to the purchase of a life insurance policy from someone with less than a two-year life expectancy. The life settlement (or senior settlement) business refers to the purchase of a life policy from someone who usually has less than a ten-year life expectancy.[14]

At best, this is considered to be a sophisticated financial planning tool for older affluent individuals. It is generally for people over age 65 who have had a change in health but are not terminally ill. The policy face amounts that are purchased are typically much higher than that of viatical settlements. Life settlement financing generally comes from institutional buyers.[15]

Life or senior settlements seem to be a vibrant business with potential. According to Conning & Company, life settlement purchases in 1999 were about $1 billion in face amount, and they project a market potential of about $100 billion.[16]

But it's not just another Pleasant Valley Sunday for these life settlement companies. The NAIC is hard at work on these transactions, too, continuing their campaign on some of the less desirable elements that wander into non-regulated areas like this. In a 2001 letter to insurance agents in the state of Kansas, Insurance Commissioner Kathleen Sebelius and Securities Commissioner David Brant wrote, "We want to make it clear that we consider a life settlement or senior settlement a viatical contract. The recent attempts by some members of the viatical industry to create products that no longer target life insurance policies of terminally or chronically ill individuals in no way changes the analysis applied to viatical investments." They defined a "viatical investment" as "any sale or offer to sell the death benefit or ownership, or any portion of the death benefit or ownership, of a life insurance policy or certificate, for consideration that is less than the expected death benefit of the life insurance policy or certificate." They went on to add that Kansas views its position as emanating from two state court decisions (in Oklahoma and Arizona) that these transactions are securities and will enforce it as such.[17]

Producers should be wary about working with these types of financial vehicles. While some feel that "life settlements are viable financial tools that liberate liquidity and value trapped within life insurance policies,"[18] some of the same questions that surround viatical settlements are still in play here. Some of the institutions involved are starting to accept that these are securities, so agents and consumers should beware of those that are not.

Miscellaneous Alternatives

Agents should be aware of as many of the alternative financing arrangements as possible. Their clients may not always qualify for long-term care coverage and some may not be able to afford the coverage necessary. Other arrangements represent outlets whereby consumers could access long-term care insurance.

Discount programs – At least one organization has a nationwide Preferred Provider Organization (PPO) of nursing homes and home health care agencies. Subscribers receive a discount card to utilize the services of these PPO members. If the need for care exists, the individual contacts one of the member providers, shows the card, and receives the discount. This is not really insurance, but anything that saves long-term care expense dollars might be useful to some clients. There is a small annual fee for the service, but the savings can add up (discounts are typically in the 20 percent range).

AARP – The long-running contract between AARP and Prudential (16 years) came to a close on December 31, 1997. Metropolitan Life replaced Prudential as the provider of AARP's long-term care insurance. Prudential had amassed about 70,000 policyholders that were given the option of transferring to Met Life's program. Refer to AARP's web site for more details on this program.

Banks: An uneasy alliance still exists between banks and insurance agents. Still, a bank's customers are often strong candidates for long-term care insurance. Banks have been fearful about giving agents access to their customers, yet the bank's representatives lack the necessary expertise to present long-term care insurance in a meaningful way.[19] Working closely with the bank's investment people, an agent can arrange seminars for the bank's account holders on the subject of long-term care. Joint presentations are often powerful, with the bank's representative being a familiar face and the agent an outside expert in the field. It can work, and if it helps more people secure this necessary future financing for long-term care needs, then it's well worth exploring.

Critical illness plans: Critical illness policies have still not been fully accepted in the United States even as they flourish elsewhere. The allure of critical illness insurance is that it generally pays a lump sum upon diagnosis of a covered illness. This can provide valuable dollars to people since, in any given year, individuals are three times more likely to be disgnosed with a critical illness than to die from those illnesses.[20] Since long-term care may be needed after any of these significant events, this is another possible funding source for these expenses. Money usually gives you choices, and the critical illness plans provide those dollars.

Advocacy Programs – The use of an advocate to assist a convalescing senior can help to reduce long-term care health costs. This could involve working with needy seniors by calling on them in their home, accompanying them to medical appointments and completing paperwork, assisting with errands, and linking the senior to primary resources available. Local Area Agencies on Aging are a great resource to find this type of help. Geriatric case managers can also be an excellent source for finding some help when the budget is extremely low and there is no long-term care insurance in sight.

Sub-acute insurance plans: The sub-acute genre of health services came to the forefront when Medicare hospitals started releasing patients as soon as their prospective payment money was up. These people were still too sick to go home, but not (apparently) bad enough for acute care in a hospital. Sub-acute care became the link that connected this Medicare limited hospital stay with services outside the hospital. Most of these people are on the road to recovery. If the sub-acute need will last less than 90 days, there is a strong likelihood that it will not be certified under a tax-qualified plan. Medicare is not paying and tax-qualified coverage is not reimbursing, so the creation of another insurance market was born. Sub-acute, or post-hospital stay supplemental coverage can help patients get reimbursed for this care. Sold typically in 90 to 180 day benefit periods, these plans help pay for the costs that have slipped through the coverage gap everywhere else.[21]

Having many options open to the client makes the agent more valuable as people do their pre-retirement estate planning. Depending on the health budget of the prospect, any one of the alternatives mentioned in this chapter could be a viable method for long-term care expenses.

Chapter Notes

1. Kent Scheiwe, "New CSO Tables Will Impact Riders," *National Underwriter*, September 2, 2002, p. 5.

2. Wilma G. Anderson, "Use LTC Insurance As A Springboard to Annuity and Other Sales," *National Underwriter*, May 28, 2001, p. 16.

3. "Hancock Introduces Industry's First Variable Annuity Suite With Protection for Long-Term Care Expenses," *Business Wire*, August 31, 1999.

4. "Craig R. Springfield and Chelsea K. Bachrach, "LTC-Annuities: Two Birds, One Stone," *National Underwriter*, September 2, 2002, p. 11.

5. Mike Sause, "Close Annuity LTC Combos," *Agent's Sales Journal, Florida Edition*, 1st Quarter 2003, p. 1.

6. Craig R. Springfield and Chelsea K. Bachrach, "LTC-Annuities: Two Birds, One Stone," *National Underwriter*, September 2, 2002, p. 11.

7. Janet Stokes Trautwein, "Partnerships Offer Common Sense Approach to Financing Long-Term Care," *Health Care News*, January 2003, p. 4.

8. Source: The Robert Wood Johnson Foundation, University of Maryland Center on Aging, 2002

9. Source: A.M. Best, "BestDayNews," July 18, 2001.

10. Janet Stokes Trautwein, "Partnerships Offer Common Sense Approach to Financing Long-Term Care," *Health Care News*, January 2003, p. 4.

11. Jane Bryant Quinn, "Middlemen Profit Most on Death Deals," *Daytona Beach News Journal*, 1995.

12. Carole Fleck, "Buying this insurance can leave you poorer," *AARP Bulletin*, September 2001, p. 3.

13. Source: American Council of Life Insurers, 2001.

14. Steve Leisher, "The Life Settlement Controversy," *Life Insurance Selling*, February 2003, p. 82.

15. Eileen Shovlin, "Clearing Up Common Misconceptions About Life Settlements," *National Underwriter*, December 10, 2001, p. 22.

16. Ron Panko, "Package Deal," *Best's Review*, August 2001, p. 103.

17. Source: Kansas Insurance Department, August 1, 2001.

18. Ava Harter, Esq., "Life Settlements Can Benefit All," *Life Insurance Selling*, February 2003, p. 59.

19. Ken LeClair, "To Sell Through Banks, LTC Agents Must Build Trust," *National Underwriter*, March 10, 2003.

20. Ron Panko, "Critical Mass," *Best's Review*, August 2002, p. 88.

21. Carroll Busher, "Your Senior Clients Might Want To Own Sub-Acute Care Insurance," *National Underwriter*, May 28, 2001, p. 22.

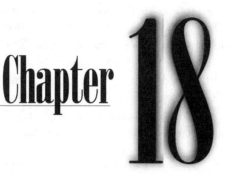

Chapter 18

Underwriting and Claims Experience

"You have to stay in shape. My grandmother, she started walking five miles a day when she was 60. She's 97 today and we don't know where the hell she is."

– Ellen DeGeneres

Long-term care insurance is still a youthful product. The pricing, under-writing and claims handling of most of the other plans sold by insurers have the benefit of decades of experience. Like most goods sold, optimum success is reached through an early trial and error process, followed by emerging patterns that are then analyzed to establish future procedures based on past results. Long-term care is still partially in the trial and error stage and starting to see some emerging patterns.

Long-term care is still a ground-floor opportunity for insurers that want to tap into a market that will continue to grow prospects at an incredible rate for the next two to three decades. Most of the nation's top insurers have discussed this market at one time or another when constructing their long-term goals and marketing objectives. Some have entered the arena with their own coverage version, others watch and wait on the sidelines to see experience results before jumping on stage, and still more have entered and left the market, unable to solve the mystery of how to successfully penetrate it.

As noted in Chapter 11, "Early Bad Press," carriers took a very conservative initial approach to this market. There were "gatekeepers" that served as claim sentinels, guarding the portfolio from exorbitant loss ratios by making qualification for benefits a formidable task. Prices tended to be on the high side, simply from lack of quantitative data rather than from an emphasis on profits. High-cost, low-benefit plans typically don't have long futures, and the market quickly evolved to a more reasonable coverage base with prices actually falling as insurers continued to crunch what numbers they could find.

Now, the long-term care product line is in a conservative, belt-tightening mode again as trends are seen for certain conditions that might have created better experience if underwriting was done in a certain way. This is the type of information that will dictate the next few years of underwriting guidelines.

This uncertainty as to pricing and experience is one of the reasons that less than ten carriers own the lion's share of the market. So, while 130 or so companies market long-term care insurance, only a handful are writing most of the business to date.

This means only a few carriers are developing a large enough sample of business to make some predictions about the future. This might be enough, however, if the information is properly processed, analyzed and made available to the industry at large.

Underwriting at Older Ages

One of the keys to a successful insurance product line is its underwriting. The underwriter has the task of sifting through an individual's paperwork and assessing the risk that person brings to the company. Separating out good risks from bad can only be effectively done when the underwriter understands what could trigger poor claims experience. Once these factors are identified, a more confident effort at underwriting review can be made.

The time has now arrived for insurers to begin understanding the risk at older ages. As this country continues its aging process, the number of viable older age prospects will continue to grow exponentially for products the insurance industry sells.

There are burial expense policies, annuities and lower face amount life insurance plans for people in their 70's and 80's to buy, but few venture to age

90. Fewer still market plans with sizable face amounts. Yet, the fastest growing population segment is that of the 80+ age group, many of who are still active, healthy and with several years of life expectancy probably left. Learning how to underwrite this older risk will be beneficial to life, annuity and long-term care markets.

This means studying the most likely health conditions and their treatments and seeing how older people cope with their medical difficulties. Most older people have at least one chronic condition and many have multiple conditions, according to a 2001 report on older Americans. The most frequently occurring conditions per 100 elderly in 1996 were arthritis (49), hypertension (36), hearing impairments (30), heart disease (27), orthopedic impairments (18), cataracts (17), sinusitis (15) and diabetes (10).[1] There is nothing here underwriters haven't seen before. The question is how do these impairments affect the elderly in relation to the benefits being purchased? For long-term care, does it affect the ability to perform activities of daily living (ADLs)? Are there medications and other treatments that minimize the effect of these conditions?

As always, the more information the underwriter has, the greater the ability to make a decision. The accumulation of information in long-term care begins, as it usually does, with the field underwriting of the agent.

Field Underwriting

Agents that are experienced in the disability income and health insurance markets already recognize the importance of accurate medical information. The typical long-term care application is detailed in its specific questions and so must the agent be when asking these questions to the prospective buyer.

Before any questions are directed to a prospect, the agent interested in the long-term care insurance market should review the underwriting guides of the carriers he or she will represent. Read these carefully. This will tell the agent about what medical conditions will disqualify a potential long-term care insurance applicant.

There will be some conditions that will vary as to how they will be handled by an insurer. Depending on the condition (or, as importantly, the combination of conditions), underwriting could range considerably on a prospect from declining to issue any policy to issuing the policy with an extra premium rating required.

The agent should list the conditions that are easily seen as red flags for an insurer. Some insurers have a quick list on the front portion of the application to see if the applicant answers "yes" to questions such as "are you in a wheelchair, are you currently on Medicaid, do you currently need help with any ADLs, are you using medical equipment like a catheter or respirator, or have you ever had Lou Gehrig's Disease, Parkinson's or Multiple Sclerosis? These queries are fairly obvious and indicate an individual who is not insurable for coverage.

Early signs of dementia are very likely declines since the cognitive impairment trigger is one of the key policy benefit qualifiers. Substantial heart history, limited activity, and a combination of two or more medical problems will present issue problems for agent and potential insured.

The agent can then pre-qualify interested buyers in the product. Most agents contact an individual about setting an appointment. If, as part of this process, they are doing some pre-qualification, it is a good idea to ask about any health conditions and, as important, listing the current medications being taken, if any. Many underwriting guides today list prescription drugs and their likely corresponding medical condition. This information can assist the agent in preparing the most accurate rate proposal for the prospect or identify a person who would obviously not qualify for long-term care coverage. The agent then needs to be prepared to discuss some alternative means of financing any long-term care need identified.

After reviewing the company underwriting guides, comparing and sorting out which carrier is more likely to issue a policy for someone with a certain medical question, the agent should then review the actual applications. What actual questions are asked? Again, the length and breadth of questions asked will not surprise those agents used to health insurance-related products. At this point, insurers are accumulating as much information as they can about the older risk. Given that they actually record the data and follow the results, the experience story this information will tell will continue to shape the size and scope of future underwriting.

Today's long-term care applications focus on both medical and lifestyle-type questions. On the medical side, the questions are divided into those that reflect recent history and those who's past presence can be indicative of future health problems. Some companies divide their application questions up into time frames, such as "have you ever had such condition" in the past 2, 5, 10 years or ever. This separates the more immediate relevant history from something that may have occurred several years ago. The longer back in time the question goes, the more likely any history of the condition will have an impact on the underwriting decision.

It is important to remember that this information is a primary medical underwriting tool as the applicant will not have to undergo a medical exam. The more thorough the agent is in the questioning, the better for all as it can speed up the underwriting process considerably.

The following are examples of questions asked that begin with "During the past 12 (or 24) months, have you ...

- used a cane, accessed home care services, used braces for the spine or lower extremities, or had any physical or rehabilitative services?

- have you been medically advised to have testing, treatment or surgery (excluding cataracts) that has not been performed?

- when you walk 4 blocks at a normal pace or climb a flight of stairs, do you experience difficulty such as shortness of breath, dizziness or leg cramps?

- experienced confusion, forgetfulness or memory loss, dizziness, fainting, weakness or fatigue, falling, unstable gait, or tremors?"

Examples of questions that seek to go back much farther for medical history (5 years or longer) begin with "Have you been diagnosed, advised or medically treated for any of the following?"

- aneurysm

- amputation

- alcoholism, drug or substance abuse

- angina

- atrial fibrillation

- bypass surgery

- emphysema

- diabetes

- hepatitis

- joint disorder or replacement

Other questions can be even more specific, such as:

- If you are age 80 or older, please list your physician's name and address.

- With whom do you currently live? Spouse? Family? Alone? Other?

- Have you ever been declined for a policy providing either nursing home or home health care benefits with another carrier?

These are only a few of the questions asked. Some applications are shorter than others, but all of them ask a number of medical questions most of which are focused on the older applicant. Questions such as do you suffer from osteoporosis and with whom do you live are not everyday insurance application questions. They are, however, pertinent for long-term care coverage.

Carriers are also looking for lifestyle clues to see who is a possible future candidate for a nursing facility. An insurer may ask for the applicant to describe in one's own handwriting what they do in a typical day. There may be questions about how active a lifestyle the person maintains. Do they still perform the basic instrumental activities of daily living like cleaning, shopping, money management or driving? This cumulative information provides clues about an individual's current daily existence. When you're measuring the ability to perform ADLs, these questions become important.

We have also discussed combo plans such as combining life insurance with long-term care, or annuities with long-term care. Annuities with long-term care do not change the medical underwriting for the worse since there is no reason to look at health history. The worse the health history, the easier the annuity issue. As noted earlier, when you have an annuity/LTC combo where the insured is accessing his own money first, the underwriting will be somewhat more liberal, as if there was a long elimination period involved.

Life insurance is a different vehicle and, in some cases, at odds with LTC underwriting. You can't just assume the underwriting is easier with life insurance. It may not be. For example, I recently had a client that had high cholesterol and blood pressure, both normal with medication and a stint surgically inserted near the heart. His LTC application came back in less than a week – standard, not preferred. The life insurance application took three weeks, and he was finally issued as a rated case.

The underwriter for long-term care isn't as concerned about the conditions that will test mortality, as this could mean short duration disability claims. On the other hand, conditions that could disable you will catch their eye, while the life underwriter may not be as concerned for their part of the risk.[2]

The field underwriter is also a sort of informal assessor of the health risk involved. They get to do what most underwriters cannot: see the applicant face-to-face. Generally, you can spot an underwriting risk for LTC by noticing frailty, obvious medications, how they respond to questions, etc. You can give an underwriter "sight" by relaying your observations on the "comments" section of the application.

Once the underwriter receives this information, either via the application or by attending physician statements, they can decide to either accept or pass on the risk.

Home Office Underwriting

Underwriting – art or science? Or both?

Certainly, there is a scientific body of knowledge accumulated about medical and other conditions that forecast the potential claims future of an applicant. With long-term care, this data is still being assembled. It's one thing to understand the nature and probability of disability, and still another to apply it to today's older client, who will be separate and distinct from the older risks of twenty years ago. For every little bit known, there are significant amounts more that remain unknown. Decisions made today consist of both hard data and gut feelings. The "gut" part is the art of underwriting.

A former mentor once told me that there comes a time for a good underwriter when he or she can get a "feel" for the risk of the applicant just by reading the information obtained in the underwriting process. It's like the hunches the good television detectives play when they develop a working knowledge of the case and its suspects. Underwriters experienced in reviewing long-term care claims are starting to develop the "art" side of the underwriting equation even as the science of assessing older age risks for long-term care is still progressing.

Companies that are looking to develop some experience on a block of business may decide to write some risks just to see what future claims results will be on a particular medical condition or class. For that reason, some insurers are issuing several rate classes on their long-term policies, based on the person's medical history. Aside from preferred and standard classes, there could be substandard tables an insurer is willing to write. Some carriers have multiple levels of risk and a premium assessment based on the seriousness of the conditions.

Having the ability to underwrite many kinds of risk for long-term care coverage gives the agent some latitude in writing a greater number of prospects. The better long-term care producers will provide significant detail with their applications upon which an underwriter can place the risk in the proper rate class. Impaired risk underwriting is an important and necessary service for the better long-term care agents. There is a lot of energy spent by the agent in finding and interviewing the prospect and identifying the need. Tighter underwriting means fewer approvals and a higher ratio of prospecting to closes must be accomplished to be successful in the market.

Having several substandard classes is no guarantee of policy placement. The extra premium assessment must be fair and reasonable for the risk being accepted. The individual still might not accept too high a premium on the policy if he or she feels the cost isn't worth the coverage. Since long-term care underwriting and policy pricing is in its infancy, some guesswork is involved in developing the rates for these substandard risks. This is another of the delicate balances long-term care insurers must negotiate in writing the long-term care risk.

Underwriters may also have the flexibility today to adjust daily benefit amounts, elimination periods and/or benefit periods in order to feel comfortable with issuing a risk. Coverage that may be ratable due to medical history with a 30-day elimination period and a lifetime benefit period, may be issuable standard at 60 days – 5 year coverage. This process will also take time to fine-tune based on actual claims results.

Would access to genetic information help the underwriting process? Most underwriters would tell you this data would be extremely valuable, but the chances of accessing this information are meager at the moment. In the case of Alzheimer's disease, which has seen a number of genetic breakthroughs lately, this knowledge would undoubtedly be helpful.

Depression has always been problematic for underwriters of disability-based products. There's such a fine line here to walk, and predictability of outcomes are not necessarily measurable based on the size and scope of the depression history. Small problems can still lead to claims, while apparently larger difficulties may never present a formal insurance problem. The particulars of a case and the quality of information provided can have a lot to do with the underwriting outcome. An applicant whose condition is controlled by ongoing treatment may be rated standard, if other factors are favorable. Someone in otherwise good health may be rated preferred if they have recovered from a situational depression several years back.[3]

The residence of the insured could also play a part in an underwriting decision. For example, someone in good health in an independent living facility will likely see normal underwriting practices. Applicants from Continuing Care Retirement Communities (CCRCs) are different. What these individuals can qualify for depends on the type of contract signed and thus it is a good policy to include a copy of it with the application. The underwriter will, in all likelihood order a face-to-face assessment in addition to reviewing the contract terms as to what the potential insured has bought into with the CCRC living situation, now and into the future.[4]

Claims Results

While it may be too soon for reliable claims results, there is data coming in about experience to date in this market. Industry analysts warn about the important link between underwriting and claims. The more accurate the underwriting job done up front, the better the chance that the policy is priced properly. Make some mistakes and the entire block of business suffers, with across-the-board rate increases seemingly the only way out. While those increases may help future control of the policy block's loss ratio, the financial damage may already have been done. This is why any discussion of claims is preceded by a review of underwriting considerations, as noted above.

Some insurers today are feeling the pinch of some dementia and Alzheimer's claims that claims analysts say could have been alleviated somewhat by the more frequent use of either telephone or face-to-face assessments. Therefore, expect to see more of these.

Product development in long-term care has passed through several generations. With nearly 40 years of marketing some kind of long-term care plan, claims are now starting to be more of a factor. The same energy that companies put into designing their plans to best fit customers' needs must now be directed towards the creation of sound claims management strategies. As these procedures are constructed, finding the right care equation for the client has to be weighed against the quality, timeliness and cost of the services the patient needs.

Claims experience monitoring guidelines are also helpful for insurers as a baseline for managing their block of business. For example, for a carrier to be 100 percent certain that its actual experienced claims are not off by more than 10 percent due to random fluctuation, the company must insure 128,000 lives each year for a 3-year period. Alternately, insuring 32,000 lives each year for a 5-year period would come fairly close to producing cumulative credible experience.[5] This may explain why some insurers bailed out of the market, without the necessity of seeing actual claims results, if they felt they did not have a sufficient number of lives on the books for claims predictability purposes.

A recent LTC industry meeting saw the distribution of industry claims survey that revealed the following:[6]

- Most people were happy with their policy and the way claims were being paid. 25 percent found it difficult to understand what was covered.

- 20 percent felt the insurer could have provided better customer support.

- 25 percent reported they wished they had bought a higher daily benefit.

- Most indicated they couldn't afford care on their own in the absence of insurance.

- Half of the people indicated they would be in an institution if it weren't for the benefits the policy provided.

- Of the people who had private LTC insurance, those with the " disability" model were the most satisfied.

- Insureds reported more favorably on weekly or monthly home health care benefits.

- 79 percent of claimants had 2 or more ADL limitations.

- For more than 70 percent of claimants, insurance paid all the costs of care.

- Average age of claimant was 80.

- 15 percent of claimants did not meet either the 2 ADL or cognitive triggers. These people were older, more likely to live alone, less likely to be married, less likely to have informal support. The majority had 1 ADL limitation, and most had multiple ADL limitations. (Would non-TQ policies have paid this under medical necessity?)

At claims time, the primary assessment of the insured must include evaluation of health, functionality, behavior, emotion, environment, Medicare eligibility and finances in addition to the assessor's own personal observation of the claimant. The hands-on approach to long-term care claims is even more necessary as there may be several levels of care to coordinate. The evaluator must determine the best interests of the patient and balance those concerns against the limits of the policy.

The role of a policy's care coordinator can be a difficult one. These individuals are often seen as protecting only the insurer's interests. But they can be instrumental in helping the insured and family negotiate their way through today's health care maze. Seniors, the people most likely to need long-term care, are already dealing with early hospital discharge courtesy of Medicare's Diagnostic-Related Grouping (DRG) system. So, once discharged, where do they turn next for assistance? Depending on the severity of the problem, the insured may be least able to make these decisions. Family members are often caught off-guard and forced to make some quick – and often incorrect – choices about the next care steps. Here is where the care coordinator for a long-term care insurer can be of the most assistance.

Meeting with the doctor and discovering the care required is the first step. Who administers and where the care is received are two questions that the care coordinator can help to answer. A carefully constructed plan can be of both high quality and reasonable cost. The coordinator can then contact potential caregivers, some of whom may be contracted with the insurer to provide the care at a discount price. Arrangements are made and the insured is hopefully on the way to recovery.

The coordinator puts a face to the insurer that can create a positive atmosphere for an insured and family at claim time. So often, claims are a faceless enterprise, laden with paperwork, where the decline or modification of what the insured would like is handled via phone, fax or letter. The care coordinator is there to answer all questions and help put the family's mind at ease, if possible. This hands-on approach to claims is a lifesaver for the family and claimant.

HIPAA Effects

Claims handling has also been affected by the Health Insurance Portability and Accountability Act of 1996. In Chapter 13 on "Tax-Qualified Plans," the presence of a 90-day certification of the loss of two or more ADLs was required for benefit eligibility using this trigger. Claim forms have now been modified accordingly. Typically, a statement is present on one of the claims pages that says:

> "I certify that the above named insured's (1) functional capacity is expected to require or has required substantial assistance with at least 2 of the ADLs listed for a period of 90 days, or (2) cognitive impairment requires substantial supervision to protect such insured from threats to health and safety."

A licensed health care practitioner – including a properly licensed social worker – must sign this statement. As you can see, the 90 day certification added in HIPAA language to the first benefit eligibility trigger is front and center in this statement.

As noted earlier, states have been adding statutory language warning LTC claims departments not to challenge that certification. In the early post-HIPAA stages, there were reports of a couple of insurers getting a second opinion, but claims handlers run a risk in doing so now in some states.

The claim form will also indicate the primary diagnosis for which long-term care services are being prescribed. In addition, the type of residence recommended by the health professional will also be indicated. There will also be a listing of ADLs and the type of assistance needed with each. An example of a claim form can be found in Figure 18.1.

FIGURE 18.1

Individual Long-Term Care Claim Form

You must complete this form in full.
Please print or type all information except where signature is required.
Please return the completed form to the insured or authorized representative.

Name of Insured   Policy Number   Social Security Number

Name of Licensed Health Care Practitioner:

Address:

Telephone Number: Fax Number:

1. Primary Diagnosis:

2. Concurrent Diagnosis:

3. What type of long-term are you recommending?

Nursing Facility ☐	Rehabilitation Facility ☐	Home Health ☐
Assisted Living Facility ☐	Hospice ☐	Adult Day Care ☐

    Certification Dates: to
    Plan of Treatment:

4. Please indicate the level of assistance your patient needs with the activities of daily living (ADLs).

	Independent	Supervision/ Cueing	Physical Assistance	Totally Dependent
Eating	☐	☐	☐	☐
Bathing	☐	☐	☐	☐
Dressing	☐	☐	☐	☐
Toileting	☐	☐	☐	☐
Transferring	☐	☐	☐	☐
Continence	☐	☐	☐	☐
Ambulating	☐	☐	☐	☐
Manage	☐	☐	☐	☐
Medications	☐	☐	☐	☐
Housekeeping	☐	☐	☐	☐
Meal Preparation	☐	☐	☐	☐

FIGURE 18.1 (continued)

5. Has any form of cognitive impairment been diagnosed?   Yes ☐   No ☐
   If yes, what specific diagnostic tests were administrated?

---

6. Are you the proprietor or employee of the recommended
   Long-Term Care provider?   Yes ☐   No ☐

"I certify that the above named insured's (1) functional incapacity is expected to require or
had required substantial assistance with at least 2 of the first 6 ADLs named above for a
period of 90 days, or (2) cognitive impairment requires substantial supervision to protect
such insured from threats to health and safety."

Signature of Licensed Health Care Practitioner   Title   Date

---

If two or more ADLs are listed in the columns other than "Independent" and there is a certification that a continued need for assistance will last 90 days, a claim under that ADL benefit trigger may be valid.

The claimant may not always have to sign the form. The insured's authorized representative may sign if the insured cannot. Many of these claims may necessitate invoking the durable power of attorney, whereby someone else has taken over the affairs of the insured. Understanding this, insurers allow this individual to sign the form.

The underwriting and claims process involved with long-term care is in a constantly developing state. More in-depth experience will further help to shape these activities in time. For now, there is much learning on the job and patience is required on all sides of the insurance agreement while more accurate knowledge is obtained.

Chapter Notes

1. Source: Administration on Aging, 2001 Profile of Older Americans.
2. Marilee Driscoll, "Underwriting Has Role In Choosing Products For LTC Planning," *National Underwriter*, November 12, 2001, pg. 25.
3. Linda Koco, "Picture Brightening For Clients With History of Depression," *National Underwriter*, November 12, 2001, pg. 4.
4. Source: General Cologne RE, April 2001 LTC Underwriting Bulletin.
5. Peggy L. Hauser, FSA, and Dawn E. Helwig, FSA, "LTC Experience Monitoring: How God Were Your Estimates," *The Disability Newsletter*, Milliman USA, November 2001, pg. 1+.
6. Highlights of "A Descriptive Analysis of Patterns of Informal and Formal Caregiving among Privately Insured and Non-privately Insured Disabled Elders Living in the Community".

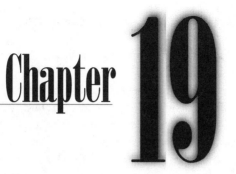

Chapter 19

Employer-Based Long-Term Care Insurance

"Executive ability is deciding quickly and getting someone else to do the work."

– John G. Pollard

The Human Resources Department of a medium to large business usually is considered the "pulse" for knowing what is going on with the average American. Each day, employees encounter situations that are often referred to the Human Resources Department. If there is a emerging pattern or trend, this department is bound to spot it.

The recent "boomer-echo" phenomenon, where workers in their 30's and 40's are having children, has resulted in the need for many large firms to arrange some type of day care for their employees. In so doing, life for the employees is much more convenient and the employer receives a fair amount of productivity in return.

But another pattern has started to surface. It's appeared in situations like that of a Massachusetts man whose mother moved in with him and his wife in 2000 after her dementia worsened. He wakes up his mother each morning, fixes meals, takes her to the doctor and gets her ready for adult day care, so he can go to work.[1]

Employees as Caregivers

The latest trend that employers are noticing is the employee as caregiver for an aging parent or relative. According to the National Alliance for Caregiving, more than 22 million American households (nearly one in four) are currently providing assistance to elderly individuals, spending around 18 hours per week furnishing this care, with an expected caregiving period of 4.5 years. Odds are the caregiver is female, and going it alone in her caregiving responsibilities. By 2007, that total households figure may grow to 39 million. According to a MetLife study, it's already costing businesses between as much as $29 billion in lost productivity. That figure doesn't even include the lost wages, Social Security and pension contributions, and career opportunities of the caregiver.[2]

Since this affects the employer's bottom line, this type of trend generally calls for a plan of action. On-site day care centers or child care allowances helped employees with children. But would the same type of arrangement assist the caregiver of an aging parent or relative? Could employers afford a similar program for employees that are caregivers?

Compounding the problem is the unpredictable nature of adult caregiving. For example, the adult requiring assistance may not necessarily be close by. It's a tough psychological burden, too. While child-rearing often brings more pleasure to the employee, adult caregiving can be depressing as one watches a parent or family member deteriorate in front of his or her eyes.

Those balancing caregiving and work are likely to arrive late, leave early, take extra-long lunch breaks, or miss work altogether. Efficiency falls. Stress rises. All this contributes to what a business consultant calls "presentee-ism," where employees are physically present, but they're also making sure the home health aide has shown up.[3]

Employers and Health Costs

The market downturn and the generally difficult economic times has employers in cut-back mode. In this oppressive environment, anything is fair game to be let loose. It may be an employee benefit, or employees in general, or a company division, or a poorly performing company within the corporate structure.

While employees worry about their falling retirement balances, employers are directing their attention to rising health insurance costs, and especially retiree health care costs. In a 2003 survey, 86 percent of employers chose controlling health care spending as one of their top five priorities.[4]

Included in this desire to reign in health care costs is the growing shift in responsibility from employer to employee in selecting and paying for health care benefits. Medium to larger size companies – the most likely to be affected by the demands on an employee's time for adult caregiving – have largely instituted a variety of managed care health plans from which to choose. These managed care health plans range in benefit flexibility, out-of-pocket expenses and cost. Flexible benefit cafeteria plans have further shifted the responsibility of benefit choice to the employee while employers have frozen their contribution level for benefits. Moreover, in the future, retired employees will see less and less benefits from their employers. Benefits will have to be accumulated during the employee's working years.

Employees have very little idea of the overwhelming potential of out-of-pocket health care spending in retirement. In 2003, the Employee Benefit Research Institute in Washington, D.C. ran the numbers. A 65-year-old retiree without employer-based health benefits who lives to age 100 with medical inflation averaging 14 percent annually, will need about $1.5 million to prefund lifetime out-of-pocket medical expenses. If the person had employer-based health benefits past age 65, that number decreases to $500,000, but currently only about 27 percent of those over age 65 have employer-based health care. If inflation and longevity are not as high as the previous example illustrated, a 65-year-old retiree who lived until 80 in a medical inflation world of 7 percent annually, would only need about $47,000 if employer-based health insurance was still present, $116,000 without it. It seems likely that the 27 percent statistic for those who have employer-based health care over age 65 will continue to drop.[5]

Another reason that health care costs have captured employer's attentions is that some workers who may have otherwise chosen to retire early or work part-time, have instead stayed in the workforce full-time. And, according to a 2001 study by the University of Michigan, a large number of these individuals, typically in the age 50-61 age bracket continue to work despite suffering from serious medical conditions like hypertension, heart disease, diabetes, and arthritis. These individuals are more likely to access health care. Boomers, playing financial catch-up ball late in the second half of work life, will probably affect those numbers adversely.[6]

So now it's not just the health of the employee on the mind of the budget-razing employer. Eighty percent of 1,200 organizations surveyed by Eckerd

College's Human Resource Institute in 2000 said they either "did not know or had to guess at the percentage of caregivers in their workforce."[7] One thing is for certain: employers know it's a growing problem.

Work/Life Programs

Currently, about 30 percent of U.S. firms offer elder care aid, with benefits ranging from toll-free referral lines that provide tips to long-term care insurance for workers, their spouses, their parents, and in-laws.[8] The eldercare referral service is a growing employee benefit trend. About 15 percent of employers offered such a feature in 2000, 19% did so in 2001 and that is up to 21 percent in 2002.[9]

Another interesting trend that has surfaced has been the growing number of working men who have had to take on caregiving roles. Changing family dynamics, along with more women in the work force, have brought more males into this elder care responsibility. Men's growing involvement should increase corporate awareness. Already, males in decision-making positions with personal experiences of elder care are making changes. For example, after his mother had a stroke, a senior vice-president of Human Resources led the company to hire an on-site geriatric care manager in 1999, and nearly 750 employees have utilized this service since its inception.[10]

Another solution for employees has been flex-time. This allows employees to work on a schedule that keeps them productive but also allows them the time needed to care for an aging adult. Many employees have a difficult time admitting they're caregivers, believing that this entails giving someone injections, changing bandages, or bathing someone. But shopping for an adult, cleaning and helping them with everyday chores, including doctor's visits, *is* caregiving. It demands time, and there's precious little of it in an average workday.

Flex time is critical. Time demands almost require it. Working caregivers miss time at work. They may be on the phone handling some of these tasks during work hours. They turn down promotions. This caregiving need has to affect productivity.

According to benefit consultants Hewitt and Associates, 74 percent of Fortune 500 companies offered flex-time – up from 54 percent in 1990 when flex-time was related more to child-care. The most common arrangements are flex-time (59 percent of firms), part-time employment (48 percent), work at home (30 percent), job sharing (28 percent), compressed workweeks (21 percent), and summer hours (12 percent).[11]

The Family and Medical Leave Act, passed in 1993, requires employers of a certain size of company to allow as many as 12 weeks of unpaid leave for the care of a seriously ill family member. With some employers offering little flexibility for an employee-caregiver, this Act may be the only way to take a leave and have a job (and preserved seniority) when ready to come back. However, the key word here is unpaid. Many individual employees can't afford to go without a paycheck for any length of time – not even one week, let alone twelve. Some companies are more understanding and in a better financial position to help finance some time off for an employee in a caregiving situation. But the majority of firms are not.

Based on 2001 data from the U.S. Census Bureau, there are nearly three million three-generation households in the United States.[12] This means a substantial number of working age adults who must juggle a work and caregiving schedule that can be extraordinarily demanding.

Employers realize that flex-time and other work/life programs alone won't solve the problem. As such, employers have begun seeking out and offering long term care insurance for their employees – many on a group basis. While most of the discussion in this book to date has centered on individually purchased policies, the emergence of employer-based long term care is directly related to the decreasing productivity caused by employees' growing need to take care of adult family members.

Take Care of Your Own Finances

There is a "catch" to the long term care insurance coverage offered on a group basis through employment. The majority of it is voluntary group – employees can choose whether they want the coverage or not. The employer makes it available (usually on a lower cost basis than if the employee purchased an individual plan) and may even contribute to a portion of its cost if the employee elects the coverage. The employee, however, has to pay a substantial part of the premium.

Employers are simply saying to employees – take care of your own finances. We'll help, with salary and a generous amount offered for employee benefits to be spent as the employee sees fit. But employees must choose wisely and begin to invest in their own future, too, and not rely on their employer for financial matters.

Employers seem to like the voluntary nature of the product. This is in line with the flexible benefits approach to employee benefits: let the employee decide. It may mean some extra paperwork and accounting for the employer, but most believe its worth it. Employers have been going this route with 401(k)s and cash balance pension plans with financial/retirement counseling services for these programs. Clearly, this is a different approach to employee benefits.

Female Business Owners

Despite the increasing number of working male caregivers, the female is still the most likely to carry this mantle. The number of women-owned businesses has been on a meteoric rise, currently at 6 million plus, employing 9.2 million people and generating $1.15 trillion each year.[13] Women have generally been the most empathetic to the long-term care need. Not only are they more likely to face (or be already involved in) caregiving tasks, they understand their own longevity and what the financial price tag to longer life will be. They are personally vulnerable to either side of the long-term care problem, and are good candidates to approach about solving this need.

They may also, as business owners, feel strongly about making long-term care insurance available as a financing solution to their employees. Caregiving chores will not just affect an employee, but the entire firm. The loss of an employee to death means you can replace that employee. Disability is a different story, especially with some of the protections afforded by the Americans with Disabilities Act. So is caregiving, as the time loss may be sporadic or specific (Family Medical Leave Act), but it's usually disruptive and will affect the bottom line.

Do not forget about this growing employer market segment, especially when long-term care might be the center of employee benefit discussions.

Group Long-Term Care

Historically, group coverage predated individual policies in the insurance marketplace. Both group life and group disability were forerunners of individual policies. This is not the case with group long term care.

The individual product for long term care surfaced first. After the introduction of Medicare, a few companies led by CNA introduced nursing home coverage for skilled care on a short-term basis. The year was 1965. The first group long term care plan would not be developed until 1987.

The reason it took so long to develop a group long term care product was the claims experience needed to price a product. Group plans carry a lower premium cost than individual policies do, yet if actuaries felt uncomfortable with the pricing of an individual policy, how easy could it be to lower the premium for a group plan? What benefits do you streamline out of individual LTC to help with this pricing dilemma?

Moreover, long term care was not a primary concern in the 1960's and 70's. It is only a recent trend as the population starts to age more rapidly and has forced employees to become caregivers for the aging adult. Thus, there was no employer motivation to offer this type of coverage – there was no market demand for group long term care.

It was employers that first realized the issue of group long term care was becoming a reality. A number of large corporations, including IBM and AT&T went to insurers offering this coverage and requested the design of a group long term care policy. The problem for insurers hadn't altered much since 1965. How do you price this type of policy when the data remains scarce?

Reluctant to pursue group long term care on a mass-market basis, the earlier group policies were developed specifically for larger firms. For example, John Hancock worked with IBM's benefits team to assemble a voluntary group product. A 16-page brochure announcing the program was mailed to all employees, including an offer to receive a free videotape about the new product. In addition, premiums were published for ages 20 to 95 and were divided into three program options: $50 a day, $100 a day, and $150 a day.

A further departure from the traditional group insurance product, this voluntary program gave access to coverage not only to employees but to employee's parents and relatives. Employees that were around 25 years old felt they had little need for this product but had parents in their 50's and even grandparents in their 70's and 80's that might have an interest in this type of program. Retirees of the company also had an opportunity to buy this coverage and many seized the opportunity to purchase long term care benefits.

In February of 1991, a *New York Times* article indicated that AT&T started mailing out long term care product announcements to 119,000 managers. By this time, companies like Ford Motors, American Express, Monsanto, Proctor & Gamble, and the states of Maryland and Nevada had already ventured into the group long term care product market.

Growth in this new group market was steady in the beginning. In 1988, group long term care represented 1.8 percent of all long term care policies sold. According to the Health Insurance Association of America, by mid-1990, there were 153 employer-sponsored plans. By that time, some 700,000 employees were offered the opportunity to purchase coverage as a voluntary employee benefit. At that time, 79,500 people were covered, 60 percent of them active employees, and the balance was retirees or family members. Thus, by 1991, group long term care was up to 8.7 percent of all long term care policies sold.[14]

However, in 1991, group long term care sales peaked. Since then, a steady decline in results has limited further progress of this type of insurance model. Outside analysts like the Life Insurance Marketing Research Association (LIMRA) have determined the reason for the decrease in the sale of group long term care based on a couple of factors. First was the lengthy Congressional debate surrounding the Clinton national health care program. Employers were not only concerned how long term care would be affected by a national health care program, but the uncertainty of the impact on an employer's overall health care costs brought employee benefit expansion to a grinding halt. Second, the status of the tax ramifications of long term care coverage was not at all clear – let alone the tax effect of the employer providing this benefit for employees. This not only made employers reluctant to consider this coverage, it relegated group long term care to a voluntary status, with premiums paid solely by the employee.

The result was a four percent sales decrease in 1993 followed by a 79 percent drop in 1994.[15] Obviously, the uncertainty documented above had much to do with this reversal in the growth of group long term care.

The passage of the Health Insurance Portability and Accountability Act of 1996 (HIPAA) clarified the rules for employers. C-Corporations were allowed to deduct 100 percent of premiums as a corporate expense (self-employed, partners, and S-Corp. owners were allowed a 45 percent deduction in 1998 – it's now 100 percent up to a scheduled amount that's indexed each year). These premiums paid would not be considered compensation to the employee. In addition, benefits when received were free of income taxation. For employers sitting on the fence wondering what the tax consequences would be, it was time to act.

It took a little time, but employers responded. Group plan sales jumped 56 percent in 1999, with participants increasing 126 percent that same year.[16] In 2000, plan sales dropped by 6 percent, but more people were taking advantage of the programs, increasing 19 percent despite the overall sales drop. 1.2 million U.S. residents now accessed long-term care through employer-based plans.[17] In

2001, new employer-sponsored LTC group plans grew by 10 percent, but number of participants was down by 1 percent and premiums by 6 percent. By this time the top 5 insurers offering employer-sponsored long-term care insurance accounted for 81 percent of the total in-force premium, making it a highly specialized sale.[18]

In Chapter 14, I outlined the results from the new Federal LTC Plan offered by the country's largest group employer – the Federal government. Over 250,000 applications received, twenty percent of the *total* number of employer-based LTC participants as of 2001, and that was in just a six-month open enrollment period.

The U.S. Chamber of Commerce is offering an association long-term care program that they expect could reach as many as 100 million member employers, employees of member companies, and dependents.[19]

The state of Michigan offered a group LTC program to its 62,000 eligible employees in 2001. While average participation rates in group plans nationally range between 5 and 8 percent, Michigan had a 16 percent employee participation rate in their employee LTC program. With funding from a state grant, Michigan spent about $2.7 million to create public awareness of long-term care, making sure that everyone eligible not only knew about the benefits being offered but also understood the consequences of not having long-term care insurance.[20]

One agent believes the target business prospects are those whose work force averages about 40 years old and earns at least $40,000 annually. White collar companies dominated by professionals – such as financial services firms are likely to have interest in this type of coverage. Other businesses to consider are pharmaceuticals, computer, communication services, education, chemical, manufacturing, publishing, utilities, and transportation. For true group coverage, prospective companies should have at least 500 lives.[21]

One shouldn't pre-judge a group. Recently, I assisted with an enrollment at a construction firm. The majority of the workers were under age 40 and male, on the surface not a likely group of candidates to be interested in long-term care. It was an unusual firm of its type though in terms of longevity, both as a company (over 75 years in business) and employees (majority had been with the firm at least 5 years). There was also far more interest when enrollment started with several personal stories arising about caregiving situations. The results were far better than predicted.

As a worksite product, long-term care could be characterized as "improving." In 2001, long-term care insurance had the greatest single product growth rate with a 77 percent increase over 2000. Of course, it's not hard to see this kind of high double digit growth when LTC remains only a 2 percent total of the entire worksite sales results.[22]

Contrary to initial expectations, it is employees and spouses who make up about 90 percent of the employer group business, and not retirees, parents and grandparents.[23] Long term care coverage may be of more importance to the single employee rather than the employee with family since the caregiving role is less likely to be shared with another.

More education needs to be done here, because this is only solving one part of the problem: an employee or spouse disability. But caregiving is likely to be for parents, grandparents, or in-laws, and this word just isn't getting out of the workplace. Of course, if these relatives live elsewhere, it presents logistical problems for enrollment, but agents must help employees (and employers) work through these issues.

This brings us to one of the keys to success in the employer-based market: a strong buy-in on the part of senior management. Unless the decision-makers and influence-peddlers are behind the launch of this employee benefit initiative, there is a strong possibility the enrollment will fall flat. In a small firm, this is especialy helpful, but in a large firm it is critical. Large-sized businesses compartmentalize the work and the management of its employees. If one manager thinks the LTC program is a lousy deal, his or her entire department could agree with that thinking. If all of the managers are enrolling, there is a good chance this could carry some positive weight with the rest of the workforce.

One way to secure this buy-in is through the implementation of a key employee LTC plan.

Key Employee Benefit

Employers may be offering long term care coverage to improve recruiting and retention. The top employees carefully review their benefits before choosing a firm. Disability income insurance producers have an advantage here in discussing this concept with an employer.

Back in the 1970s, singer-songwriter Harry Chapin wrote a song with the lyrics "All My Life's A Circle." This is never truer than it is in the insurance industry. What you learn at one time often comes back to help you in surprising ways in the future.

So it is with disability income and long-term care in the corporate market. There has always been a good living to be made helping employers establish and fund a sick pay plan for their employees. To not do this is to risk adverse tax consequences should an enterprising IRS auditor wonder why the boss was paying an employee who was listed as absent.

The employer certainly appreciates this help. More important, we have shown many employers how to carve out key employees from this mix, extend them lengthy sick pay time and fund it with an individual DI policy. Key employees can be selected without discrimination concerns utilizing such plan criteria as years of service, job title or income or any combination thereof. The plan can be written down on a simple one-page document, this program communicated to the key employees affected, and all without any filing requirements for the beloved IRS.

Flash forward a few years in the post-HIPAA long-term care environment. Tax clarification for the corporate owner saved this market from extinction. And, let's face it, employers are always looking for ways to retain *key* people. They see long-term care as a potential nightmare for their employees, especially during retirement, and they want nothing to do with any funding responsibility for that after the employee retires from the firm.

As one successful LTC agent puts it, "We're living longer, and everyone knows it. Just ask the CEO and CFO about their families. They understand that when they retire, their assets will need to last 30 or 40 years. These executives are retiring with lump sum retirement accounts that are vulnerable to investment risk, tax risk, and, yes, unfunded health care risk – including that of their spouses. The risk of one of them needing care can be as high as 65 percent, and the unfunded financial risk today is often $100,000, that could grow to $250,000 - $500,000 per person in 20 or 30 years."[24]

Enter key employee LTC. Once again, the same carve-out procedures can be used. If you've already set up a plan with this business, you can add LTC to it. If not, use the same criteria to establish a program for just the key employees the employer wants to cover with a tax-qualified long-term care insurance program.

However, there are two significant differences between the LTC and the DI plans here. Even if the employer pays for the LTC policy for the key employee

(C-Corporations get the full deduction; in 2003, S-Corp owners, partners and sole proprietors can deduct 100% of the premium up to the individual deductibility limits – see Chapter 13), the benefits of a tax-qualified LTC plan (the only policies that allow deductibility) are received *income-tax free*. That's a substantial difference from the disability income policy where a deductible premium translates into taxable benefits at claim time.

Second, if the employer (C-Corporation most likely due to the unlimited deductibility) buys a policy from an LTC insurer offering the ability to pay up the premiums in a short period of time (10 years, or paid up at age 65), this is a great story to tell a key employee. Imagine the attraction for a key employee who has an employer paying for his or her long-term care and receiving a paid-up policy (no future rate increases to worry about) that is a critical wealth protection vehicle with which to go into retirement. It may well soften the blow for retirees as employers are finding it nearly impossible to fund retiree health insurance. And it may likely help employers retain key people for a number of years.

It is likely that limited pay policies may be more popular with both consumers and insurers in the future. Rate stability laws (See Chapter 14) are forcing more accurate pricing work up front, thus minimizing future rate increases. On a 10-pay or paid-up-at-age 65 LTC plan, there is no opportunity to raise premiums once the limited pay period is over. This shouldn't scare insurers the same way any more, since they are pricing for the long haul now, and thus more of these types of limited pay options may arise in the future.[25]

It's a great opportunity to explore a market that has been underserved. Key employees are often older, experienced people and they may well be aware of some long-term care events that have happened to someone they know. Paid-up LTC provides the best of all taxable worlds for employer and employee, along with having vital protection for the future.

Group Premiums

Employer-sponsored plans are usually paid for by the employer. This is not the case with the majority of group long term care programs to date. The employee selects the plan and premium amount that best fits his situation. If the employer contributes at all, it is generally in the form of a subsidy, covering only a portion of the employee's costs. There are usually more generous contributions made on behalf of key employees.

Still, employee benefit dollars remain lean.. Additionally, the cost of group long term care, while less expensive than individual long term care, is still higher in relation to the premiums for individual plans than group life and disability is to their individual counterparts.

The plan, as noted, can be implemented on a voluntary basis (employee-pay-all) or as a simple base plan with buy-up options. The cost of a base plan is a real bargain, usually $10 per month, per employee. In general, group is becoming a much better premium deal. An average annual cost of an individual policy is $2,500, while an average group annual cost is $600.[26]

Annual group insurance rates, on average, for a three-year-policy are $259 for a 40-year-old; $482 for a 50-year-old, and $1,136 for a 60-year-old. Assuming premiums are paid until age 75, a 40-year-old will pay $259 a year over 35 years for a total of $9,065(assuming no rate increases). A 60-year-old will pay $1,136 a year over 15 years, totaling $17,040 (assuming no rate increases). With investment portfolios shrinking, employees may be thinking about buying LTC insurance when they are younger, at the peak of their earnings, and while rates are relatively low.[27]

Since many of the plans are voluntary, a step-by-step chart allows the employee to select the plan specifics and premium. Figure 19.1 is an example of one insurer's step-by-step guide:[28]

FIGURE 19.1

A GUIDE IN SELECTING A VOLUNTARY PLAN

Steps	Example	Your Premium
Step 1: Find your current age in the following chart.	This person is age 30.	Your age: _____
Step 2: Determine the coverage you want and find the "Monthly Premium per $10 Daily Benefit".	This person wants a daily benefit of $100, a 60 day elimination period, $75 home health care option, inflation and return of premium benefits. The monthly premium per $10/day benefit is $1.98.	Your coverage: $____ daily benefit ____ elimination period ____ home health care ____ inflation ____ ret of prem.

Steps	Example	Your Premium
FIGURE 19.1 (continued)		
Step 3. Figure your monthly premium by multiplying the amt. from Step 2 by the number of $10/day benefits you want. For example, someone who wants $40 in daily benefits would have 4 units of $10 daily benefit.	This person multiplies: $1.98 from Step 2 times 10 (for $100 in daily benefits) = $19.80 total monthly premium	$_____ (amount from Step 2) times ____ (for $_____ in daily benefits) = $____ total monthly premium

As you can see, there is no mention of a benefit period. In this case, there was a fixed benefit period with no options to select a different period of time, shorter or longer. Group benefits are generally meant to be streamlined to a certain extent while individual products let you tailor your own program. Given the voluntary nature of group long term care it has remained more flexible than traditional group insurance – choosing an elimination period and a benefit level is not the norm in group coverage. Since group health insurance products are allowing the employee to choose what type of coverage (HMO, PPO, POS, etc.) and how much to spend (varying co-payment and coinsurance choices) the employee benefit decision making responsibility has shifted from employers to employees.

The average age of the buyers for group long term care will continue to be in the age 40 to age 60 range. The policy is still an excellent buy at these ages and the sense of urgency is greater than for the younger individual early in a working career.

Rates will continue to be adjusted as insurers evaluate their group claims experience. Until more policies are sold, however, the validity of their results is still suspect.

Insurers, however, are clear in their message: long term care can be important irrespective of age. Protecting your income and assets is essentially what insurance is all about. Long term care is another cog in the protection wheel.

Since HIPAA, product development has increased in the group area. Obviously, tax clarification has helped. It is vital for agents to remember that tax-qualified (TQ) long-term care insurance plans are the only policies specified in the tax code. For employers and employees to benefit from the favorable tax law regarding employer-based LTC products, you must use TQ plans.

Group Policy Provisions

Traditionally, group coverage has maintained a streamlined approach to benefits. Interviews to enroll employees into a group program have typically been much shorter in length than the time one would spend with an individual for individual coverage. The employee enrollment is usually done on company time, while the individual appointment may be over a meal or the kitchen table.

As such, benefits must be easy to explain in a short period of time. Rather than give the employees a wide variety of choices that must be carefully explained, group plan parameters are often pre-set. In group life insurance, the amount is fixed at, for example, $15,000. In group disability income, the product may call for 60 percent coverage of salary, beginning on the 91st day and continuing to age 65.

Group insurance plans are not usually voluntary. Payment of premium can be made by either the employer paying the full premium, or a requirement of a certain level of participation.

Group long term care may also be streamlined, but generally the benefits are not unlike the typical individual program. Since the passage of HIPAA, tax-qualified plans have ensured that benefit triggers will be identical especially since the employee knows the favorable tax consequences of this program. Only one of the plan design choices may be pre-set. For example, the elimination period may be fixed at 90 days, but the employee can choose the daily benefit and the length of time benefits are payable, and may even have the option to buy a lower elimination period. Or the fixed design element is the benefit period that is set at four years, and the employee then chooses the daily benefit amount and the elimination period, with the possibility of buying a longer benefit period, too.

Chapter 12, "Provider-Aided Design," and Chapter 13, "Tax-Qualified Plans," reviewed the basic policy features found in individual policies. Many of these features also appear in group versions of the coverage, further explanation of the closer similarity in pricing between individual and group. But there are a few provisions that may be different.

Coordination of benefits – One would be more apt to find a coordination of benefits provision in a group plan than in an individual plan. HIPAA did determine that expense-incurred individual policies must include a Medicare coordination provision. Group policies have typically had this provision, even more so now that TQ plans are used in employer-based situations. Benefits in the policy are offset by dollars received from Medicare, and possibly other group long term care plans. This primary coverage versus secondary coverage is typical of group plans.

As an example, an employee could be covered at work and also on a spouse's group long term care plan. At claim time, if the employee needed long term care, the policy at his or her place of employment would be the primary coverage and the spouse's coverage secondary, paying for costs not covered by the primary plan.

Portability – Group plans often offer a conversion privilege for employees to have the option of exercising if they should leave their place of employment. The conversion would be made to a different policy that normally would not be as generous in benefits as the original plan. So far, however, group long term care plans are more likely to offer a portability rather than a conversion feature. This means the employee can elect to take the identical coverage when departing the firm and continue to pay for it on some basis other than payroll deduction.

This made sense up until now, especially since most of the premium has been paid for by the employee. Thus, the employee in a sense already *owns* the coverage. Portability simply lets the employee keep the coverage.

COBRA requires employers to offer the continuation of health insurance coverage for terminated employees. This does not apply to long term care policies. The portability provision of many group long term care programs eliminates the need for any type of COBRA consideration.

Nonforfeiture – Since many of the larger group long term care plans were not off-the-shelf products, they contained features that a company may have specifically desired. One of these benefits was non-forfeiture. For example, a nonforfeiture feature might allow an employee who has paid premiums for ten consecutive years and then ceases payment to retain 30 percent of the original daily benefit amount.

With the passing of HIPAA, non-forfeiture benefits are offered regularly in long term care policies, both individual and group.

Summary

A recent report published by the Health Insurance Association of America (HIAA) studied buying attitudes of those employees purchasing long-term care at the worksite. Some of the findings include:[29]

- Enrolled employees are slightly older, have higher incomes and more assets than non-enrolled employees and are more likely to be college educated. There is little difference between enrolled and non-enrolled employees in terms of marital status and gender.

- Enrolled employees are more likely to agree that it is important to plan now for future long-term care needs than non-enrollees. They are only half as likely to believe the government would finance the future cost of long-term care.

- Non-enrolled employees were more likely to believe they could rely on some other form of health insurance to pay for long-term care services if they needed them for more than six months.

- Enrolled employees were more likely than non-enrollees to have discussed the LTCI buying decision with others like a family member or co-worker.

- Non-enrollees overwhelmingly cited the cost of LTC coverage as the most important barrier to enrollment.

- Three out of five non-enrollees reported that confusion about which policy was right for them was an important factor in their decision not to enroll.

- Factors that would make non-enrollees more likely to take out coverage were (a) greater employer contribution to premium, and (b) option to deduct their costs from their income taxes.

Regarding the group policy designs, the report found:

- The vast majority of group LTC policies were comprehensive and reimbursable (expense-incurred) plans.

- The average daily benefit sold was $124/day.

- The average home care daily benefit was 60 percent of the nursing home daily benefit amount.

- About 88 percent of the policies included some type of inflation protection.

- The average premium in the group LTC market was $722, compared to $1,677 on an individual sale.

There are some important lessons in these results. Agents need to spend some time with potential enrollees reviewing the coverage. Home health care needs to be a higher percentage of daily benefit amount. More encouragement to the employer to contribute some dollars to the cost of the plan would further help enrollment.

Employers want employees and retirees to take control of their own finances. Combining a 401(k) plan with a group long term care plan is a significant step in shifting responsibility for financial security retirement to the employee. The 401(k) plan, a popular retirement program, allows the employees to build up substantial amounts of retirement income. Long term care is the protection of the retirement income from the high cost of health care services, most often needed during the retirement years.

Chapter Notes

1. Maggie Jackson, "Family issues blur gender roles, affect workplace," *Boston Globe*, January 5, 2003.
2. Jill Elswick, "Benefit programs reach out to employee caregivers," *Employee Benefit News*, July 2002, pg. 39+.
3. David Brauer, "When Your Parents Need You," *My Generation*, March-April 2002, pg. 14.
4. Gary S. Mogel, "Employers: Top Priority Is Controlling Health Insurance Costs," *National Underwriter*, February 17, 2003, pg. 27.
5. "EBRI Reports On Retiree Medical Costs," *National Underwriter*, March 3, 2003, pg. 18.
6. "The Baby Boomer Challenge," *Employee Benefit Plan Review*, June 2001, pg. 6+.
7. Jill Elswick, "Benefit programs reach out to employee caregivers," *Employee Benefit News*, July 2002, pg. 39+.
8. David Brauer, "When Your Parents Need You," *My Generation*, March-April 2002, pg. 14.
9. Jill Elswick, "Benefit programs reach out to employee caregivers," *Employee Benefit News*, July 2002, pg. 39+.
10. Maggie Jackson, "Family issues blur gender roles, affect workplace," *Boston Globe*, January 5, 2003.
11. Source: Hewitt and Associates, "Hewitt Study Shows Work/Life Benefits Hold Steady Despite Recession," May 13, 2002.
12. Source: U.S. Census Bureau, American Housing Survey for the United States: 2001.
13. Maggie Leyes, "Women Business Owners," *Advisor Today*, November 2002, pg. 38+.
14. Data from the Health Insurance Association of America's annual review of long-term care insurance.
15. LIMRA International, "Group Long-Term Care Sales and In-Force Change in Number of Participants, 1991-1994," *National Underwriter*, June 5, 1995, p. 7.
16. Timothy J. Murphy, "Increasing Group LTC Sales, *Life Insurance Selling*, February 2002, pg. 24+.
17. Allison Bell, "Group LTC Plans Cover 1.2 million," *National Underwriter*, May 21, 2001, pg. 5.
18. Source: LIMRA International, as reprinted in National Underwriter's LTC E-Wire, July 2002.

19. Allison Bell, "Group LTC Insurance Poised To Take Off," *National Underwriter*, May 21, 2001, pg. 4+.

20. Robert E. O'Toole, "Employer and Association Sponsored LTCI Plans," *HIU Magazine*, September 2002, pg. 13+.

21. Timothy J. Murphy, "Increasing Group LTC Sales," *Life Insurance Selling*, February 2002, pg. 24+.

22. Bonnie Brazell, "2001 Worksite Report Card," *Benefits Business Magazine*, 4th Quarter 2002, pg. 20+.

23. Ron Panko, "Hope for a Healthy Marketplace," *Best's Review*, April 2002, pg. 83.

24. Debra C. Newman, CLU, ChFC, "Capture the Exec LTC Market," *Advisor Today*, June 2002, pg. 60.

25. Claude Thau, "Making the Case For Limited Pay Long Term Care Insurance," *National Underwriter*, January 20, 2003, pg. 32.

26. John Smeykal, "Long-Term Care: The Next Employee Benefit," *HIU Magazine*, November 2001, pg. 44+.

27. Timothy J. Murphy, "Increasing Group LTC Sales," *Life Insurance Selling*, February 2002, pg. 24+.

28. This guide is from the Principal Financial Group's long-term care offering to its employees..

29. Source: HIAA, "Who Buys Long-Term Care Insurance in the Workplace 2000-01?" Executive Summary, November 2001.

Chapter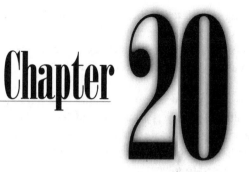

Taxation and Legislation Issues

"The mystery of government is not how Washington works, but how to make it stop."

– P.J. O'Rourke

Aside from health insurance, long-term care insurance, with its short history, has been the most heavily regulated product in the insurance industry. Life insurance, annuities, disability income insurance – none of these have been scrutinized the way long-term care insurance has been.

Much of the attention is due to the fallout from the industry's Medicare supplement fiasco. This disaster taught state insurance departments to be over-protective when it comes to any products that affect seniors. There is no sense in provoking a Congressional push to take over regulation of the insurance industry. The McCarran-Ferguson Act (i.e., state regulation) can easily be repealed by a Congress unified in its efforts.

Long-term care insurance regulation has been driven primarily by the National Association of Insurance Commissioners (NAIC) and initially was largely product oriented in nature. As outlined earlier in this book, attention focused on eliminating "gatekeepers" – caveats that can cut down on filed claims considerably. At the time this regulation was helpful in making products both useful and competitive. More recent attention has focused on rates, specifically substantial rate increases that have been filed in growing numbers. Having a comprehensive long-term care product is fine, but unless it is accompanied with common sense pricing up front, regulators will be staring down the barrel of rate increase requests that will force many consumers (especially older ones) to drop their policies just as they are close to utilizing them.

Tax clarification for long-term care insurance finally emerged with the passage of the Health Insurance Portability and Accountability Act of 1996 (HIPAA). While it cleared up some of the tax questions policyholders, employers, and insureds had, this federal legislation has also created nearly as many problems as it attempted to solve.

The NAIC

State regulation of long-term care insurance (or any insurance product) has its own set of problems. The NAIC does its best to encourage some uniformity in regulation, but with 50 states, that is virtually impossible to ensure. Still, as a unit, the NAIC has been very proactive when it comes to long-term care insurance regulation over the past 15-20 years. Highlights of NAIC Regulation include:[1]

1987	First NAIC Model Act
1989	Prohibition of post-claims underwriting
1990	Regulation of replacement policies
1990	Requirement to assess suitability
1995	Specification of minimum benefit triggers
1996	HIPAA clarifies tax deductibility of premiums and exclusion of benefits as taxable income
2000	NAIC amendments revise rules for state approval of initial rate filings and rate increases

The primary focus today continues to be on suitability and rates. Suitability includes a requirement that a consumer have the option to complete a worksheet regarding financial and other information to be sure that the individual applicant has an appropriate need for long-term care insurance. Questions relating to income on the worksheet are, as follows:[2]

> **FIGURE 20.1**
>
> # WORKSHEET
>
> **How will you pay each year's premium?**
>
> _____ From my income   _____ From my savings/investments   _____ My family will pay
>
> Note: Have you considered whether you could afford to keep this policy if the premiums went up, for example, by 20 percent?
>
> **What is your annual income?**
>
> _____ under $10,000   _____ $10-30,000   _____ $30-40,000   _____ $40-50,000
>
> _____ $50-60,000   _____ $60-70,000   _____ over $70,000 _____   actual _____
>
> How do you expect your income to change over the next 10 years?
> _____ no change   _____ Increase   _____ Decrease   Percentage of change _____
>
> Note: If you will be paying premiums with money received only from your own income, a rule of thumb is that you may not be able to afford this policy if the premiums will be more than 7 percent of your income.
>
> **Questions relating to assets:**
>
> Not counting your home, about how much are all of your assets (your savings and investments) worth?
>
> _____ under $20,000   _____ $20-30,000   _____ $30-50,000   _____ over $50,000
>
> How do you expect your assets to change over the next 10 years?
>
> _____ Stay about the same   _____ Increase   _____ Decrease
>
> Percentage of Change _____
>
> Note: If you are buying this policy to protect your assets and your assets are less than $30,000, you may wish to consider other options for financing your long-term care.

While 30 states had suitability standards as of January 2001, monitoring and enforcement are not easy. The insurer is the vital entity here, as underwriters will be reviewing the worksheets. If they are aggressive about returning long-term care insurance applications when the person's answers indicate their finances are below the accepted guidelines, this will help keep coverage geared towards those with adequate income and assets to protect. Consumers have the option of completing the form, and can opt out if they choose to do so. About all regulators can hope to accomplish here is to give consumers some financial standards to self-determine whether long-term care insurance is the right financing source.

Fifteen states, as noted in Chapter 14, have approved the new Rate Stability amendments to the Model Act. At least that many more are considering adoption. This does not guarantee that the policyholder will never see a substantial rate increase, but it should discourage deliberate under-pricing to achieve market share. It will certainly affect new business premiums, and it may further dissuade people who are borderline under the financial standards from opting for insurance.

Several insurers are battling lawsuits charging they concealed from customers the likelihood of premium increases in their long-term care policies. One lawsuit also alleges that a carrier knew some of its long-term care policies were under-priced at the time of their sale and that it would repeatedly need seek rate increases to pay out claims and stave off big losses.[3]

Right or wrong, this is not the kind of publicity the industry needs. The NAIC knows that, and is trying to protect the consumer's rights and the insurer's ability to meet future obligations to this customer.

A recent survey by the AARP Public Policy Institute in Washington, D.C. assessed how the current system was regulating long-term care insurance. Thirty-five (70 percent) state insurance departments scored a top rating (5 out of 5) in terms of extensiveness of long-term care insurance regulation.[4]

The state of Oklahoma has a formal program called the Senior Health Insurance Counseling Program (SHICP), designed to aid consumers with, among other products and topics, long-term care insurance. Volunteer counselors have been recruited across the state to answer consumer questions on a timely basis. Not surprisingly, Oklahoma's present insurance commissioner, Carroll Fisher, is a former insurance agent. So is Bill Smith, the Director of the SHICP program. They understand the types of questions consumers ask, having previous experience working with them in an insurance-related capacity.

The NAIC will continue to be the focal point for future long-term care insurance regulation.

Post-HIPAA

HIPAA was supposed to clear up all of the tax confusion that had been a part of the long-term care insurance market for years. In addition, clarification of its tax status was supposed to send long-term care insurance sales skyrocketing. The message from HIPAA was to be: take personal responsibility for your potential long-term care costs. (See Chapter 13, on tax-qualified plans for a complete discussion of HIPAA.)

By early 1997, several months after HIPAA was signed into law by President Clinton, insurers were reporting increases in sales. In a way, this was inadvertently misleading. The last quarter of 1996 brought substantial sales increases in part because people could buy policies with a triple-trigger method of qualifying for benefits rather than the new law's two-trigger eligibility process and still receive the tax-favored status HIPAA bestowed.

State regulators wrestled with the problems of folding HIPAA federal legislation into their own statutes, especially as some of the new law contradicted their state's laws. The NAIC worked diligently to help solve some of the difficulties HIPAA created. About the only thing that was clear was that the future of non-qualified long-term care taxation must still be unraveled by the Treasury Department.

Many are pleased about the inclusion of tax-favorability for both accelerated death benefits and viatical settlements in the HIPAA law. (For a complete description of these programs, see Chapter 17.) Prior to the law, for example, a terminally ill patient with less than two years to live could incur significant taxation upon selling his policy for a lower face amount. If that person had a $100,000 life insurance policy and was able to sell it to a viatical company and receive $75,000 immediately, the $75,000 would be includable in income to the extent it exceeded the person's basis in the contract, thus reducing the amount available for expenses. With HIPAA, the $75,000 payable to the terminally ill individual is not taxed, so the full amount can go for medical and living expenses.

Accelerated death benefits may be an even better way to receive proceeds from a policy and still have a portion of the face amount of the policy left for heirs. Its tax favored status has insurers highlighting an accelerated death benefit clause in their life insurance plans as a key policy feature.

HIPAA's latest long arm affect on long-term care insurance is in its privacy regulations, many of which are now finally coming into focus. For a law that was directed primarily at health insurance, it sure has stirred up a lot of muddy water on long-term care.

Long-term care insurance comes under the banner of policies that must subscribe to a practice to protect consumer information. That means, for the most part, keeping it out of the hands of insurance agents and brokerage managers. Agents are going to have access to medical information – they do take the application after all. But once these details are sent to the home office, the correspondence is now between applicant and insurer.

The list of protected information relates to individual customer information collected for the purposes of evaluating the insurance risk, primarily name and address, information provided on an application, health and medical information, financial information, and information collected from a third party for an insurance company (like an attending physician statement).

There has been a time-honored tradition of giving an agent an overview of the reasons for a rating or declination of a risk. This is intended to help the agent either place a substandard case or communicate the decision to not accept the case. That is less likely to happen today. Agents will not receive specific customer information normally used to shop cases that were previously declined or not placed, even if the consumer authorizes this work. The agent must obtain another application from another insurer to start the practice all over again.

Recently, insurers have been mailing out new privacy letters to existing policyholders, advising they need permission to make the insured other offers about various products the company has, or communicate about other products and services from other business connections. While many individuals probably threw this letter away without reading it, others may have celebrated the elimination of promotional material from the insurance company. It will be interesting to see how many policyholders actually write back.

There is probably more to HIPAA that we have not seen yet that could affect future marketing of long-term care insurance.

Legislation

Congress receives a multitude of lobbying attention each year. There are many issues that compete for the legislator's eye every day, whether Congress is in session or not. While one should not conclude that lobbying efforts dictate the federal legislative agenda, it would be naive to believe they do not have an influence. In the most recent report on lobbyist spending, finance, insurance, and real estate remained the broad economic sector's most willing donors.[5] Exactly what that buys is pure speculation, especially in regards to long-term care.

So what are the chances that lingering long-term care questions will be answered by the current Congress? Arguably, long-term care had its day in the Washington sun in 1996 when HIPAA was passed. The chances of further wide-sweeping legislation like that is minimal at best. Long-term care's primary issues come down to:

- expanded individual premium deductions for long-term care insurance;

- inclusion of long-term care in a Section 125 plan;

- lifting the moratorium on partnership programs; and

- clarifying the non-tax qualified policy tax status.

Time has changed priorities somewhat. Since HIPAA, focus on health issues on Capital Hill (with the exception of Medicare) has been on two subjects: children, and patients' rights under managed care. Neither of these issues helped to bring Congress back to clarifying unresolved long-term care questions. Efforts have been made every year since HIPAA passed, but the only fast track any of these issues (primarily above-the-line long-term care insurance premium deductibility) had was in 2001, and it was derailed by September 11, when everyone's priorities changed overnight.

President Bush's various budget proposals have included a phased-in above-the-line deduction for long-term care insurance premium along with a caregiver tax credit (up to $3,000).

The problem for Congress in considering these issues is how to pay for them. Bills that included some of the above wish-list items could not even get through in those brief years of budget surpluses. How are they going to survive when competing against dollars for Homeland Security and war with Iraq?

Partnership programs would seem to be the most likely issue to see some headlines in 2003. States are bursting their Medicaid budgets with a vengeance, and long-term care costs are a significant culprit. A number of states are at the ready when it comes to these programs, and aside from some promotional costs, it is not a budget-killer. Just the opposite, ultimately, if it can postpone or eliminate Medicaid spending because someone had private long-term care insurance instead.

The rest of the list is not promising. The above-the-line deduction has been packaged with a caregiver credit in the past and will likely be so in the future. In August 2002, the House of Representatives actually passed a bill that had an above-the-line deduction for long-term care insurance premiums in it. The deduction was to be phased in over 10 years, starting with 25 percent of the premium in 2003-2005, and working its way up to 50 percent by year 2012. But the consumers that could take the deduction were limited to individuals with adjusted gross incomes up to $20,000, and couples up to $40,000.[6]

These were exactly the people the NAIC was trying to warn *not* to buy long-term care insurance, when they completed their personal worksheets. These folks did not have sufficient assets and income to make the purchase of long-term care insurance a worthwhile protective action. Yet, here Congress was giving them the opportunity, providing they didn't take the NAIC's advice, to deduct some of the premium they could not afford to pay in the first place.

No matter. The Senate didn't bother with the bill, and it drifted off, like a Tibetan prayer flag, to Congressional heaven.

When Congress realizes that its own Federal government is encouraging taxpayers to take their own steps to addressing future long-term care expenses (the long-term care plan for federal employees), they may have a newfound ability to make the requested clarifications of long-term care insurance under HIPAA. This would be a significant step forward in helping to cover the needs of the chronically ill, and head off a future problem of a magnitude that will then necessitate more difficult actions that may be nearly impossible to make.

States

Individual states, as we have seen with suitability and rate stability, are more likely to take action on their own. Much as they did with health insurance and managed care, states are looking at issues that take time to come to federal resolution. Medicaid costs, rising primarily due to long-term care expenditures, have caused many state legislative bodies to encourage private long-term care insurance as an alternative financing solution.

A number of states have enacted tax deductibility or credits for long-term care insurance premiums to enable their residents to save money in state taxes. The following states all have either a credit or deduction for individuals and, in some states, employers, in an effort by states to encourage long-term care insurance purchases: Alabama, California, Colorado, Hawaii, Idaho, Indiana, Iowa, Kentucky, Maine, Maryland, Minnesota, Missouri, Montana, New York, North Carolina, North Dakota, Ohio, Oregon, Utah, Virginia, West Virginia, and Wisconsin.[7]

In addition to balancing Medicaid budgets, states' legislative priorities in 2003 involve pharmaceuticals, long-term care, access to health insurance, and health provider issues as their top five health policy issues to be debated.[8] The LTC focus could range from licensing assisted living facilities to adoption of rate stability amendments.

The value of long-term care savings accounts has been debated in states like California and Michigan. These would be companions to Medical Savings Accounts, constructed on a similar basis.[9] MSAs, of course, have not done that well, in their early years, and it's debatable if long-term care would enjoy any greater popularity under this concept.

In Colorado, a 2002 Resolution encouraged people to privately finance long-term care to help ensure the long-term viability of the state's safety net for the truly needy.[10] An excerpt from the Resolution said:

WHEREAS, The government provides a safety net for the impoverished; but it cannot afford to pay for long-term care for everyone who will need it; and

WHEREAS, Failing to protect household assets by planning for long-term care with private insurance can have dire consequences that result in the loss of those assets; and

WHEREAS, It is imperative that people begin now to plan for their long-term care needs; and

WHEREAS, Private long-term care insurance can help pay for most of the cost of long-term care, as well as provide protection against inflation; and

WHEREAS, increasing the number of private options for long-term care is not only important, but essential for the well-being of Coloradans; now, therefore

"Be it Resolved by the Colorado House of Representatives, the Senate concurring herein:

"That the General Assembly strongly encourages all Coloradans to investigate the costs of long-term care and the benefits of having private long-term care insurance; and

"That the General Assembly strongly encourages all Coloradans to actively pursue the purchase of appropriate long-term care insurance since the government can provide assistance for long-term care only to the most destitute, and not to all those who will need it; and

"That the General Assembly urges the private sector to increase the number of options for privately funded long-term care in Colorado."

If that's not a call to action, then we are all asleep at the wheel. States are desperate to stop the Medicaid bleeding, and resolutions like these and ones trying to enact Partnership programs are a recognition that the private insurance industry is being asked to be as active as possible in getting the word out about long-term care insurance, and the states will help promote it.

As Resolutions like this are publicized, other state cutbacks are drawing the wrath of its residents. In Ohio, the intention to freeze Medicaid payments for nursing home residents in 2003 was met with protest.[11] In Minnesota, more than 1,300 AARP members and volunteers rallied at the State Capitol to bring attention to budget cuts they said would result in a reduction of one million home-delivered and congregate meals per year to seniors and the closure of approximately 100 dining sites, and reduced access to services that allow for block nursing care in nursing homes.[12] Easy answers are not forthcoming.

States may enact a number of provisions in the future encouraging the sale of long-term care insurance. But the key questions can only be addressed by Congress and the Treasury Department. When this will occur is anyone's guess.

The Courts

Courts have played an increasingly larger role in the long-term care industry. With a law as large as HIPAA, that was to be expected. Since the IRS has chosen not to tax non-qualified long-term care benefits yet, court cases have dealt with a variety of other issues.

In 2001, the U.S. District Court for the Western District of Pennsylvania ruled that providing unequal health care coverage to Medicare-eligible retirees and to retirees younger than age 65 violated the Age Discrimination in Employment Act (ADEA). Essentially, the County of Erie, PA began offering over-age-65 retirees a Medicare coordinated health insurance plan, while retirees under age 65 (and not yet eligible for Medicare) had a PPO plan with arguably better coverage since it did not coordinate with Medicare. Unfair, argued a class action lawsuit filed by the Erie County Retirees Association. Agreed, said the Court in its ruling.[13] This may have a ripple effect on offering retirees any health care benefits in the future, giving people something else to fund in the way of out-of-pocket health costs during retirement.

In 2002, the U.S. Court of Appeals for the Second Circuit upheld a ruling regarding the limitation of home health care benefits for an individual who had multiple sclerosis and whose employer changed insurers during the claim. The new insurer agreed to pay for home health care beyond the new policy's limitations for a temporary period of time, and when it stopped paying (way past the point of their contractual obligation), the person sued. The claimant lost, as the Court would not (this time) force the plan to go farther than it already did. The plan would have paid for some nursing home care, but not home care.[14] One agent's comment about the matter was that it would have been easier and less expensive if long-term care insurance had been in place prior to the multiple sclerosis diagnosis. The option of home care would have been there.

Finally, lawsuits against nursing homes are growing in astronomical numbers. The costs of nursing home litigation are substantial, and these legal battles divert resources from resident care, further fueling quality issues. This is a 1990s phenomenon, and is one of the fastest-growing areas of health care litigation. Florida is a flash point for this type of lawsuit. The state, citing concerns about the financial viability of long-term care facilities, recently enacted sweeping reforms designed to stem the volume and cost of nursing home lawsuits. The average recovery amount among paid claims – resolved both in and out of court – was around $406,000 per claim, nearly twice the level of a typical medical malpractice claim. Texas was singled out as the second most prolific in these claims.[15]

Costs, costs, costs. That's where the legislative focus is and where it will remain when it comes to long-term care. Nursing home care is expected to increase from $98.9 billion in 2001 to $178.8 billion in 2012 when Boomers will be hitting Social Security retirement age. Home health care spending is projected at $68.9 billion, up from $33.2 billion in 2001. Medicaid spending is expected to go from $118.4 billion in 2001 to $338.7 billion in 2012.[16]

It's hard to believe that journey will be made without legislative incident.

Chapter Notes

1. Source: Henry J. Kaiser Family Foundation: "Regulation of Long-Term Care," published 2003.

2. Information taken from CNA's Personal Worksheet used in the state of Maryland, 2002.

3. Vicki Lankarge, "NAIC hopes to end surprise long-term care price hikes," *Insure.com*, February 2003.

4. Jim Connolly, "Regulators Push Ahead On LTC Manual," *National Underwriter*, May 13, 2002, p. 41.

5. Source: Influence, Inc. "Top Spenders," a report on Lobbyists spending in Washington, 2000 edition.

6. Steven Brostoff, "Insurers Lukewarm On LTC Bill Passed By The House," *National Underwriter*, August 5, 2002, p. 3.

7. Source: National Association of Health Underwriters, 2002.

8. "Medicaid, Pharmaceuticals, LTC Are Top Health Priorities, States Say," *HIU Magazine*, February 2003, p. 46.

9. Allison Bell, "California Insurance Industry Cool To Long-Term Care Savings Accounts," *National Underwriter*, September 3, 2001, p. 45.

10. "Colorado Confronts LTC Crisis," *LTC Bullet*, Center for Long-Term Care Financing, April 25, 2002.

11. "Ohio Health Care Association Says Governor's Plan Harms Frail Elderly and Disabled," *PR Newswire*, January 18, 2003.

12. 1,300 Rally To Keep Older Minnesotans Healthy and Independent," *PR Newswire*, April 2, 2002.

13. Source: *Employee Benefit Plan Review*, 2001: Erie County Retirees Association, et al. v. the County of Erie, Pennsylvania, et al (No. Civ. A. 98-272 Erie).

14. Source: Employee Benefits Institute of America, e-letter, April 4, 2002, Fay v. Oxford Health Plan, 2002 U.S. App. LEXIS 5133 (2d Cir. 2002).

15. David G. Stevenson and David M. Stuttert, "The Rise of Nursing Home Litigaqtion," *Health Affairs*, March/April 2003, p. 219.

16. Stephen Heffler, et al, "Health Spending Projections For 2002-2012," *Health Affairs* (web exclusive), February 7, 2003.

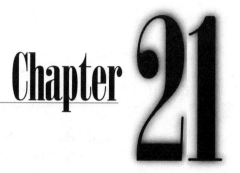

Chapter 21

The Agent's Checklist

"Trust everybody, but cut the cards."

– Finley Peter Dunne

"Idealism increases in direct proportion to one's distance from the problem."

– John Galsworthy

T oday's long-term care product is burdened with risk for the insurance agent. Despite rigid NAIC regulation and recent federal legislation, there can be significant differences within a policy's definitions, benefits, and features. Tax-qualified plans are marketed alongside non-qualified plans and the differences in benefits and possibly taxation is significant. It is imperative for the agent and financial planner to carefully review the complete policy specifications before making any recommendations.

The ultimate goal of a consumer-oriented sale of long-term care insurance is to make sure "insureds get the benefits they expect when the insurable event occurs."[1] This requires education – for both the agent and consumer.

Consumer education is what potentially separates the insurance agent from other individuals offering financial planning services to someone. There is a tremendous amount of consumer confusion in the marketplace as evidenced by the earlier noted results from HIAA's Consumer Buying Characteristics, discussed in Chapter 19.

The following is a checklist, provided by Long-Term Care Partners, LLC, who is administering the Federal long-term care plan, that consumers should follow (and agents should be aware of) in their consideration of long-term care insurance:[2]

- Don't assume you have coverage. Other types of health insurance coverage at best only provide short-term help for these expenses.

- Educate yourself. There is a lot of information on the web and in print on the subject of long-term care.

- Discuss your plans with your family. Could you depend on your family? Are they aware of their potential caregiving responsibilities if you need long-term care?

- Consider a range of options. Comprehensive coverage gives you a lot of treatment choices.

- Don't be penny-wise and pound-foolish. Sometimes the least expensive plan is not the wisest choice because coverage may be limited, provide few options, and may require a substantial rate increase later on.

- Buy only what you need. Understand what the risks are and the length of most long-term care situations. A four or five year benefit may be adequate in 90 percent of the possible claim scenarios.

- Buy when you are young. Those who can buy in their 40s and 50s can select better plans for a much lower price than they would pay if they waited to purchase.

- Keep pace with inflation. Be sure plan benefits are protected from inflation so they will be adequate to meet future needs.

- Don't overlook your employer or an affinity organization. This is the fastest growing segment of the long-term care insurance market and it may entitle you to a discount if you are part of these plans.

- Purchase from a stable company. Check the ratings and rate increase history on long-term care products of the insurers you are considering.

Obviously, the first thing we must do is uncover and then sell the need for the product. Long-term care insurance, despite its publicity, is a product that must still be sold to a prospect. It is unlikely it will develop into a policy that consumers simply call in for on a regular basis. Yet when the need is shown – if it exists – the sale is often made. Many people are experiencing what long-term care expenses and emotions are first-hand. This does not mean they know enough to pick up a phone and call to secure coverage for themselves. Yet when approached by an agent discussing the possible need for it, there is an openness not found with some other insurance programs. The above checklist is typical of the considerations consumers are being advised to make when considering this coverage, and should be a guide for agents reviewing the concepts and coverage specifics of LTC with a prospect.

The Public Is Interested

While consumers scramble to keep their retirement funds from sinking into oblivion, there will not be many secure retirements if long-term care health care costs are factored into the equation. There are so many people slouching towards retirement at a time when apparently fewer dollars will need to be stretched for a much greater length of time.

Certainly baby boomer attitudes about retirement change as they begin crossing the age 50 threshold. Analysts say boomers are setting aside only a small portion of what they will need to keep up their current lifestyles in retirement. Only five percent of people over age 50 have purchased a long-term care policy, according to LIMRA International.[3] Long-term care insurance should be a part of any retirement planning, especially if every retiree dollar is counted on to hold on to a standard of living.

The impending age wave poses huge challenges for America. Our retirement and health care security programs are highly vulnerable. But compared to other developing countries, the United States is relatively better positioned to face the challenges of an aging society. The U.S. ranked in the lowest age vulnerability index group, according to a 2003 report. The report says, "Of all the developed countries, the U.S. faces the most favorable demographic future. With the highest fertility rate and one of the highest immigration rates, it will be far and away one of the youngest countries in the world by 2040. Given this demographic advantage, together with a modest Social Security benefit formula, a relatively high rate of elder employment, and a well-developed private pension system, the United States could easily have ranked number one in the index. But it did not, mostly due to the high projected growth in government health care benefits.[4]

But we can beat this rap. Long-term care insurance has the potential to divert a fiscal crisis away from Medicare and Medicaid. If consumers understand the importance of their own personal responsibility on this issue, and the tremendous burden they will be placing on family members (not just the U.S. health system), they will have an opportunity to act.

But not without education. This is the agent's strong suit, understanding and being able to explain the need based on the analysis of the individual's specific situation. Having evaluated the various policies that are available, an agent must be prepared to make comparisons on behalf of the prospect once the specifics of his given situation are known.

Agents should not underestimate the value of product research. Knowing who has been in the long-term care market for some time and what their experience is can be as important as knowing how to analyze a client's needs. Prospects will be looking to you for guidance; many of them may never have heard of the company you are recommending. If you have done the proper research, however, this dependency will not be misplaced.

Long-term care needs are costly and for that reason agents and consumers need to be careful of the low-priced plans that might be available for sale. The disability income insurance industry had to rebound from the negative results of selling liberal benefits for an overly competitive premium. Loss ratios are eating some of the largest DI companies' bottom lines away and the push is on to save claims dollars, creating some difficult public relations situations for agents and their insureds.

The long-term care market can ill afford a public relations disaster with senior citizens. The new NAIC Rate Stability laws are an effort to avoid just that future.

Don't get caught in the "premium trap." Selling low premiums can create several difficulties:

1. Benefits may not be as strong as claimed, which the client won't discover until filing for benefits.

2. Benefits may well be as strong as claimed and the pricing may be inadequate to handle the claims.

3. The insurer may be forced to raise premiums significantly later on, turning the policy from one that is a bargain to one that is unafford-

able – perhaps at the very time the client may need the policy benefits. This has already happened in the industry – be careful! To assist in the evaluation of specific policy features, Figure 21.1, a policy checklist, focuses on key policy issues.

FIGURE 21.1

POLICY CHECKLIST

Feature

Policy:_____
Insurer:_____
Premium:_____

1. Elimination Period
2. Benefit Period
    Years: _____
    Pool of Money: _____
3. Specified Daily Benefit: $_____
    Indemnity - per diem ____
    Expense-incurred ____
4. Stand-alone indemnity/expense incurred plan
    Life insurance-based long-term care
    Annuity-based long-term care
5. Tax-qualified plan
    Non-qualified plan
6. Covered services: Amount of each:
    Nursing home $_____
    Home health care $_____
    Adult day care_____ $_____
    Assisted living facility care $_____
    Respite care $_____
    Hospice care $_____
    Bed Reservation benefit   Days_____
    Medical Help benefit $_____
    Caregiver training $_____
7. Definitions
    HIPAA definition of chronically ill - double trigger
    Triple trigger - non-qualified plans
    ADLs - HIPAA defined six activities, 90-day certification
    ADLs - non-qualified plans
    Cognitive impairment defined
    Renewability provision
    Pre-existing conditions
    Exclusions
    Contingent non-forfeiture
    Waiver of Premium
    Restoration of benefits

FIGURE 21.1 (continued)

8. Optional Benefits
    Inflation protection
        Simple or compound?
        Interest percentage?
        Any limit on increases?
    Guarantee of insurability benefit
    Spousal benefits
        Survivor benefit
        Shared benefits
        Joint waiver of premium
    Return of premium
        When?
        Does policy continue?
    Non-forfeiture benefit
9. Other
    Spousal discount?
    Group or affinity discount?

As noted, in addition to evaluating the policy, it is important to evaluate the insurance company standing behind the product. How long has the insurer been selling long-term care insurance? Does the company sell other health insurance products? What is its current experience with long-term care claims? What are the company's financial ratings? Has it ever raised long-term care premiums? (Note: This disclosure is part of the NAIC Suitability rules and can be found on the Personal Worksheet a consumer must complete.)

Financial ratings are available from several sources – A.M. Best, Standard & Poor's, Moody's, and Duff & Phelps. One of the problems in using all of these analysts' ratings is that they differ in identification. Figure 21.2 will assist in categorizing these ratings:

FIGURE 21.2

QUALITY FINANCIAL RATINGS

Description of Rating	A.M. Best	Standard & Poor's	Moody's	Fitch
Superior	A++, A+	AAA	Aaa	AAA
Excellent	A, A- AA-	AA+, AA, Aa3	Aa1, Aa2, AA-	AA+, AA,

FIGURE 21.2 (continued)

Description of Rating	A.M. Best	Standard & Poor's	Moody's	Fitch
Very Good	B++, B+	A+, A, A-	A1, A2, A3	A+, A, A-
Good		BBB+, BBB BBB-	Baa1, Baa2, Baa3	BBB+, BBB BBB-
Fair	B, B- BB-	BB+, BB, Ba3	Ba1, Ba2, BB-	BB+, BB,
Marginal	C++, C+	B+, B, B-	B1, B2, B3	B+, B, B-
Weak, Highly Vulnerable	C, C-	CCC, CC,	Caa1, Caa2, Caa3, Ca, C	CCC+, CCC, CCC-, CC, C
Below Minimum Standards	D			
Under Regulatory Supervision	E	R		DDD, DD, D
In Liquidation	F			
Rating Suspended	S			Rating Watch

If a company has been assigned some type of "A" rating, there is a certain comfort level about its future ability to meet policyholder obligations. The "A" ratings should be consistent, however, among the rating services. The "B" ratings with A.M. Best for example, should be evaluated carefully and companies carrying the rating B++ or B+ should only be used, in my opinion, when there is an accompanying "A" rating from other services, or the insurer is demonstrating a continued upward rating trend over the past several years.

Long-term care insurance is a form of health insurance and, as such, this will make it difficult for carriers specializing primarily in this market to reach the "superior" rating category. Agents should also check the company's risk-based capital ratio for further evaluation of the carrier. Long-term care insurance and disability income insurance carry higher risk factors than most other product lines for the purposes of calculating risk-based capital, so acceptable ratios must be present.

Study the company's annual report. Look at the assets and especially the capital and surplus numbers. See if the carrier is diversified into other lines, or is primarily a long-term care insurer. Ask yourself as you read, "would you buy or sell this insurer's stock if you were an investor?[5] An agent I know was presenting a long-term care insurance quote to a wealthy physician in South Florida. The doctor wanted long-term care insurance as he did not want his assets spent for long-term care costs. At the interview, the physician showed the agent a competing quote from a small insurer that was lower in price than the one he was proposing. The agent happened to carry a Financial Ratings Guide with him, so he looked up the company as the doctor waited patiently. After perusing the financial numbers quickly, the agent observed that the physician's net worth was higher than this small insurer he was considering. The doctor tossed the other quote. Rule of thumb: When the insurer's financial picture is worse than the prospect's, consider another company.

Agents as a Resource

In addition to a policy evaluation, the consumer could request information from the insurance agent or financial planner regarding community resources and additional details on long-term care providers and facilities. In addition to doing your own research in your local area, Figure 21.3 is a checklist of outside services and potential support systems within a community or state:

FIGURE 21.3

SERVICES CHECKLIST

Service Needed	Resources
Elder social programs and volunteering	Senior centers, day care, nutrition sites, senior companions, YMCA/YWCA, AARP talent bank
Chore Services	Local aging social services, area churches or synagogues, fraternal orders, youth groups, neighborhood organizations
Elder Law	Elder law attorneys, local bar association, Legal Aid, banks
Bereavement support	Church and synagogue groups, AARP Widowed Persons Service, National Assoc. of Military Widows
Transportation	City elderly transportation services, handicapped transportation services, Red Cross, churches or synagogues

FIGURE 21.3 (continued)

Service Needed	Resources
Housing	Retirement communities, public housing, foster homes, intermediate and skilled care facilities, nursing homes, house sharing, group homes, American Association of Homes for the Aged
Homemaker Services	Visiting Nurse Association, Social service agencies, private homemakers, Red Cross, Home health care agencies
Home Health/Personal Care	Home health care agencies, Visiting Nurses Association, Red Cross, private duty nurses, public health nurses
Nutrition	Meals on Wheels, Nutrition sites at senior centers, Home-delivered meals, Weekend meals programs
Adult-sitting	Adult day care centers, Live-in attendants, social service agencies, foster homes
Handicapped services	Disease-specific organizations (American Cancer Society, for example), local office administering Americans with Disabilities Act
Mental Health	City Mental Health Department, geriatric social workers, Alzheimer's association, crisis intervention units, psychiatric hospitals
Hospice	Hospice Association, Visiting Nurses Assoc., Cancer Society, local church or synagogue, local hospital social services department

Adult caregivers may ask you for information relating to any of these subjects. Keeping a file of resource material will give you a value-added service that many agents and financial planners may not offer.

Figure 21.4 lists national information hotlines that can assist you in building a resource library:

FIGURE 21.4

INFORMATION HOTLINES

AARP Information Services	1-800-424-3410
Elder Care Locator	1-800-677-1116
National Family Caregivers Association	1-800-896-3650
Medicare	1-800-633-4227
National Health Information Center	1-800-336-4797
National Meals on Wheels Foundation.	319-358-9362
National Institute on Aging	1-800-222-2225
Hospice Helpline	1-800-658-8898
Alzheimer's Association	1-800-272-3900
Alzheimer's Disease Education & Referral Ctr.	1-800-438-4380
Arthritis Foundation	1-800-283-7800
American Heart Association	1-800-242-8721
Women's Health Information	1-888-694-3278
National Cancer Institute	1-800-422-6237
Department of Veteran's Affairs	1-800-827-1000
American Diabetes Association	1-800-342-2383
American Society on Aging	1-800-537-9728
SeniorNet	1-800-474-8836
Visiting Nurses Association of America	617-737-3200

There are numbers available for Area Agencies on Aging that are listed in Appendix B at the back of this book. But states vary in who handles various long-term care services. Know the information well for the state in which you are selling. This is the type of resource information that can truly assist your clients and make your services even more worthwhile.

In addition to telephone resources and pamphlets that can be obtained from these organizations, there are a number of books available which address caregiving and elder care. Titles which may be of interest:

1. Barg, Gary, *The Fearless Caregiver: How to Get the Best Care for Your Loved One and Still Have a Life of Your Own* (Capitol Cares, 2003)

2. Carr, Sasha, and Choron, Sandra, *The Caregiver's Essential Handbook* (McGraw Hill, 2003)

3. Cooney, Eleanor, *Death in Slow Motion: My Mother's Descent into Alzheimer's* (Harper Collins, 2003)

4. Frolik, Lawrence, and Kaplan, Richard L., *Elder Law in a Nutshell* (3rd Edition, West Law School, 2002)

5. Lieberman, Trudy, et al, *Consumer Reports Complete Guide To Health Services For Seniors* (Three Rivers Press, 2000)

6. Miller, Sue, *The Story of My Father: A Memoir* (Knopf, 2003)

Working in the long-term care market can be a very productive and rewarding experience. You may be encountering some of the issues discussed in this book within your own family. Remember that the key to success in this market is to recognize both the emotional and technical aspects of the sale. Many situations are delicate at best and it will take a few sales interviews to understand the variety of potential circumstances that can surround the long-term care issue. Continue to read and keep up with the latest information, both social and product.

Stay abreast of legislative changes and clarifications. There may yet be word on non-qualified plans and it is conceivable further legislation modifying some of the changes made in HIPAA could be passed. Stay active on the state level to monitor any long-term care legislation activity. Remember, consumer education is critical today. People want to know more, especially about retirement planning. Be their resource and you will find this to be a rewarding market.

Your prospect's understanding of the need will develop through your work. The conversation you have today could result in another dream protected, another future saved. How many people can make that claim about their jobs?[6]

Developing clients in this market will keep you in good stead for some time to come. Unquestionably, long-term care is an insurance market with a future.

Chapter Notes

1. Stephen Piontek, "Making Consumer-Oriented LTC Sales," *National Underwriter*, February 18, 2002, p. 24.
2. "LTCI Checklist," *Advisor Today*, January 2003, p. 29.
3. Jennifer Douglas and Anita Potter, "Producers and Insurers Eye LTC Future," *National Underwriter*, January 20, 2003, p. 24.
4. Source: Center for Strategic and International Studies and Watson Wyatt Worldwide, "The 2003 Aging Vulnerability Index: An Assessment of the Capacity of Twelve Developed Countries To Meet The Aging Challenge," by Richard Jackson and Neil Howe, as noted in the *LTC Bullet*, April 9, 2003, by the Center for Long-Term Care Financing.
5. Linda Koco, "How Producers Choose LTC Carriers," *National Underwriter*, January 20, 2003, p. 4.
6. Kirk Okumura, "Breaking into Long-Term Care," *Advisor Today*, November 2001, p. 18.

Appendix A

Companies Selling Long-Term Care Insurance in 2000 and 2001

Reprinted with permission of the
Health Insurance Association of America

Company names that are italicized are affiliates or subsidiaries of the company above them.

Aetna Life & Casualty[1]
Aid Association for Lutherans
AIG Life Insurance Company
American General Life Insurance Company
Allianz Life Insurance Company of North America
Life USA, Incorporated
Allstate Life Insurance Company
Lincoln Benefit Life Insurance Company
American Family Life Insurance Company of Columbus (AFLAC)
American Family Mutual Insurance Company
American Fidelity and Liberty Insurance Company
American Fidelity Assurance Company
American General Life and Accident[3]
American Heritage Life Insurance Company
American Republic Insurance Company
Bankers Life & Casualty Company
California Public Employees' Retirement System (CalPERS)[1]
Catholic Order of Foresters
Central States Health and Life Company of Omaha

Cincinnati Financial Corporation
Combined Insurance Company of America
Conseco Health Insurance Company
Conseco Senior Health Insurance Company
Continental Casualty Company (CNA)[2]
Continental General Insurance Company
COPIC Insurance Company
Country Life Insurance Company
CUNA Mutual Group
Equitable Life Insurance Company of Iowa[3]
Farmland Life Insurance Company[3]
First Penn Pacific Life Insurance Company[3]
GE Capital Assurance Company
GE Capital Assurance Company of New York
Golden Rule Life Insurance Company[3]
Grange Life Insurance Company[3]
Great American Life Insurance Company
Great Republic Life Insurance Company
Guarantee Trust Life Insurance Company
Guaranty Income Life Insurance Company[3]
Guardian Life of America
Hartford Life Insurance Company[4]
IDS Life Insurance Company
IDS Life Insurance Company of New York
John Hancock Mutual Life Insurance Company[2]
Kanawha Insurance Company
Kansas City Life Insurance Company[3]
Life and Health Insurance Company of America
Life Investors Insurance Company of America
AUSA Life Insurance Company
Bankers United Life Assurance Company
Monumental Life Insurance Company[4]
PFL Life Insurance Company
Transamerica Life Insurance Company[4]
Lincoln National Life Insurance Company[4]
Lutheran Brotherhood
Massachusetts Mutual Life Insurance Company[2]
MedAmerica Insurance Company[2]
Medico Life Insurance Company
Mutual Protective Insurance Company
Metropolitan Life Insurance Company[2]
Mutual of New York

Mutual of Omaha[2]
National States Life Insurance Company
New York Life Insurance Company
Northwestern Mutual Life Insurance Company
Pan-American Life Insurance Company[3]
Penn Treaty Insurance Company
Network American Life Insurance Company
Physicians Mutual Insurance Company
Prudential Insurance Company of America[2]
Pyramid Life Insurance Company
Security Mutual Life Insurance Company[3]
Southern Farm Bureau Life Insurance Company
Southwestern Life Insurance Company
Standard Life & Accident Insurance Company
State Farm Mutual Insurance
State Life Insurance Company
Sunset Life Insurance Company[3]
Teachers Insurance and Annuity Association (TIAA)[2]
Teachers Protective Mutual Life Insurance Company
Trustmark Insurance Company
Union Labor Life Insurance Company
United American Insurance Company
United Farm Bureau Family Insurance Company[3]
United Security Assurance Company of Pennsylvania
United Teachers Associates Insurance Company
Universal American Financial Corporation
American Pioneer Life Insurance Company
American Progressive Life and Health Insurance Company of New York
UNUM Provident[2]
US Life Corporation[3]
All American Life Insurance Company[3]
WEA Insurance Group[2]
WellPoint Health Networks, Inc.
Woodmen Life and Accident Insurance Company

Blue Cross and Blue Shield Plans, By State

C.S.A. (subsidiary of Blue Cross and Blue Shield of Arizona)
Anthem Blue Cross and Blue Shield of Conecticut[2]
Blue Cross and Blue Shield of Delaware
All Nation Life Insurance Company
    (subsidiary of Blue Cross and Blue Shield of Delaware)

Blue Cross and Blue Shield of Florida
Hawaii Medical Service Associaiton[2]
Regence Blue Shield of Idaho
Anthem Blue Cross and Blue Shield of Indiana
Wellmark, Incorporated
       (affiliated with Blue Cross and Blue Shield of Iowa)
Blue Cross and Blue Shield of Kansas
Anthem Blue Cross and Blue Shield of Kentucky
Blue Cross and Blue Shield of Maryland, Inc.
BCBCM, Inc. (subsidiary of Blue Cross and Blue Shield of Minnesota)[2]
Blue Cross and Blue Shield of Montana
Blue Cross and Blue Shield of the National Capital Area
Corporate Diversified Services, Inc.
       (subsidiary of Blue Cross and Blue Shield of Nebraska)
Combined Services Inc.
       (subsidiary of Blue Cross and Blue Shield of New Hampshire)
Horizon Blue Cross and Blue Shield of New Jersey
Blue Cross and Blue Shield of North Carolina
Blue Cross and Blue Shield of North Dakota
Anthem Blue Cross and Blue Shield of Ohio
Regence Blue Cross and Blue Shield of Oregon
Blue Cross and Northeastern Pennsylvania[2]
Independence Blue Cross (Philadelphia, Pennsylvania)
Blue Cross and Blue Shield of South Carolina
Wellmark, Incorporated
       (affiliated with Blue Cross and Blue Shield of South Dakota)
Regence Blue Cross and Blue Shield of Utah
Trigon Insurance Company
       (subsidiary of Blue Cross and Blue Shield of Virginia)[2]
Premera Blue Cross (formerly Blue Cross of Washington and Alaska)
Regence Blue Shield (Tacoma, Washington)
United Wisconsin Services Inc.
       (subsidiary of Blue Cross and Blue Shield United of Wisconsin)
Blue Cross and Blue Shield of Wyoming

---

1.   Provides an employer-sponsored plan only.
2.   Provides an individual and an employer-sponsored plan.
3.   Provides long-term care coverage as part of a life insurance policy only.
4.   Provides an individual plan and a plan offered as part of a life insurance policy.

Appendix B

State Agencies on Aging

Alabama
Department of Senior Services
RSA Plaza
770 Washington Avenue, Suite 470
Montgomery, AL 36130-1851
(800) 243-5463
(334) 242-5743

Alaska
Commission of Aging
Division of Senior Services
P.O. Box 110209
Juneau, AK 99811-0290
(907) 465-3250

Arizona
Department of Economic
Security
Aging and Adult Administration
1789 West Jefferson Street, #950A
Phoenix, AZ 85007
(602) 542-4446

Arkansas
Division of Aging & Adult
Services
Donaghey Plaza South, Suite 1417
P.O. Box 1417, Slot S-530
Little Rock, AR 72203-1437
(501) 682-2441

California
Department of Aging
1600 K Street
Sacramento, CA 95814
(916) 322-5290

Colorado
Division of Aging and Adult
Services
Department of Human Services
1575 Sherman Street,
Ground Floor
Denver, CO 80203-1714
(303) 866-2636

Connecticut
Division of Elderly Services
25 Sigourney Street, 10th Floor
Hartford, CT 06106-5033
(860) 424-5298

Delaware
Services for Aging & Adults with
Physical Disabilities
Dept. of Health & Social Services
1901 North DuPont Highway
New Castle, DE 19720
(800) 223-9074
(302) 577-4791

District of Columbia
Office on Aging
441Fourth Street, NW, 9th Floor
Washington, DC 20001
(202) 724-5622

Florida
Department of Elder Affairs
4040 Esplande Way, Suite 152,
Bldg. B
Tallahassee, FL 32399-7000
(800) 96ELDER
(850) 414-2000

Georgia
Division of Aging Services
Department of Human Resources
2 Peachtree Street N.E., 9th Floor
Atlanta, GA 30303-3142
(404) 657-5258

Hawaii
Executive Office on Aging
250 S. Hotel Street, Suite 109
Honolulu, HI 96813-2831
(808) 586-0100

Idaho
Commission on Aging
P.O. Box 83720
Boise, ID 83720-0007
(208) 334-3833
(312) 814-2916

Illinois
Department on Aging
421 E. Capitol Avenue, #100
Springfield, IL 62701-1789
(800) 252-8966

Indiana
Bureau of Aging and
In-Home Services
402 W. Washington Street, #W454
P.O. Box 7083
Indianapolis, IN 46207-7083
(800) 545-7763
(317) 232-7020

Iowa
Department of Elder Affairs
200—10th Street
3rd Floor
Des Moines, IA 50309-3709
(515) 281-3333

Kansas
Department on Aging
New England Bldg.
5035 Kansas Avenue
Topeka, KS 66603-3404
(785) 296-4986

Louisiana
Governor's Office of Elderly Affairs
P.O. Box 80374
Baton Rouge, LA 70806-0374
(225) 342-7100

Maryland
Department of Aging
301 W. Preston Street
Baltimore, MD 21201-2374
(410) 767-1100

Michigan
Office of Services to the Aging
611 W. Ottawa Street
N. Ottawa Tower, 3rd Floor
P.O. Box 30026
Lansing, MI 48909
(517) 373-8230

Mississippi
Div. of Aging & Adult Services
750 N. State Street
Jackson, MS 39202
(800) 948-3090
(601) 359-4925

Kentucky
Office of Aging Services
Cabinet for Family and Children
275 East Main Street
Frankfort, KY 40621
(502) 564-6930

Maine
Bureau of Elder & Adult Services
35 Anthony Avenue
State House, Station 11
Augusta, ME 04333
(207) 624-5335

Massachusetts
Executive Office of Elder Affairs
1 Ashburton Place, 5th Floor
Boston, MA 02108
(800) 882-2003
(617) 727-7750

Minnesota
Board on Aging
444 Lafayette Road
St. Paul, MN 55155-3843
(651) 296-2770

Missouri
Division of Senior Services
Dept. of Health & Senior Sciences
615 Howerton Court
P.O. Box 1337
Jefferson, MO 65109-1337
(800) 235-5503
(573) 751-3082

Montana
Division of Senior and Long-Term
Care/DPHHS
111 Sanders, Room 211
P.O. Box 4210
Helena, MT 59620
(800) 332-2272
(406) 444-4077

Nevada
Department of Human Resources
Division for Aging Services
State Mail Room Complex
3416 Goni Road, Bldg. D-132
Carson City, NV 89706
(775) 687-4210

New Jersey
Division of Senior Affairs
P.O. Box 807
Trenton, NJ 08625-0807
(800) 792-8820
(609) 984-3436

New York
State Office for the Aging
2 Empire State Plaza
Albany, NY 12223-1251
(800) 342-9871
(518) 474-5731

North Dakota
Department of Human Services
Aging Services Division
600 South 2nd Street, Suite 1C
Bismarck, ND 58504
(800) 755-8521
(701) 328-8910

Nebraska
Division on Aging
P.O. Box 95044
1343 Main Street
Lincoln, NE 68509-5044
(800) 942-7830
(402) 471-2307

New Hampshire
Division of Elderly & Adult
Services
State Office Park South
129 Pleasant Street,
Brown Bldg. #1
Concord, NH 03301
(603) 271-4680

New Mexico
State Agency on Aging
La Villa Rivera Bldg.
228 East Palace Avenue,
Ground Floor
Santa Fe, NM 87501
(800) 432-2080
(505) 827-7640

North Carolina
Division of Aging
2101 Mail Service Center
Raleigh, NC 27699-2101
(919) 733-3983

Ohio
Department of Aging
50 W. Broad Street, 9th Floor
Columbus, OH 43215-5928
(800) 282-1206
(614) 466-5500

Oklahoma
Department of Human Services
Aging Services Division
312 N.E. 28th Street
Oklahoma City, OK 73125
(405) 521-2327

Pennsylvania
Department of Aging
Forum Place
555 Walnut Street, 5th Floor
Harrisburg, PA 17101-1919
(717) 783-1550

Rhode Island
Department of Elderly Affairs
160 Pine Street
Providence, RI 02903-3708
(401) 222-2858

South Dakota
Office of Adult Services & Aging
700 Governor's Drive
Pierre, SD 57501-2291
(605) 773-3656

Texas
Department on Aging
4900 North Lamar, 4th Floor
Austin, TX 78751
(800) 252-9240
(512) 424-6890

Vermont
Dept. of Aging and Disabilities
103 S. Main Street
Waterbury, VT 05671-2301
(802) 241-2400

Oregon
Seniors & People with Disabilities
500 Summer Street, N.E., 2nd Floor
Salem, OR 97310-1015
(800) 232-3020
(503) 945-5811

Puerto Rico
Governor's Office of Elderly
Affairs
Call Box 50063
Old San Juan Station, PR 00902
(787) 721-5710

South Carolina
Office of Senior & LTC Services
P.O. Box 8206
Columbia, SC 29202-8206
(803) 898-2501

Tennessee
Commission on Aging & Disability
Andrew Jackson Bldg., 9th Floor
500 Deaderick Street
Nashville, TN 37243-0860
(615) 741-2056

Utah
Division of Aging & Adult
Services
120 North 200 West
Salt Lake City, UT 84145-0500
(801) 538-3910

Virginia
Department for the Aging
1600 Forest Avenue, Suite 102
Richmond, VA 23229
(800) 552-3402
(804) 662-9354

Washington
Aging & Adult Services
Administration
Dept. of Social & Health Services
P.O. Box 45050
Olympia, WA 98504-5600
(360) 725-2310

Wisconsin
Bureau of Aging & Long Term
Care Resources
1 West Wilson Street, Room 450
Madison, WI 53707
(800) 242-1060
(608) 267-2536

West Virginia
Bureau of Senior Services
Holly Grove, Bldg. 10
1900 Kanawha Blvd. East
Charleston, WV 25305
(304) 558-3317

Wyoming
Division on Aging
6101 Yellowstone Road,
Suite 259B
Cheyenne, WY 82002-0710
(800) 442-2766
(307) 777-7986

Appendix C

Sample Outline

Long-Term Care Coverages

NOTE: This is a sample outline of the coverages offered under a typical long-term care policy. It does not represent the coverage offered by any single company or policy and is intended for instructional purposes only.

1. POLICY – This policy is an individual policy of insurance. [This language is also often used in group contracts.]

2. PURPOSE OF OUTLINE OF COVERAGE – This outline provides a brief description of the important features of the policy. You should compare this outline to other outlines of coverage for other policies which are available. This is not a contract of insurance, but only a summary of coverage. Only the actual policy contains governing contractual provisions. It is the actual policy which sets forth in detail the rights and obligations of both you and the insurance company. Therefore, if you purchase this coverage or any other coverage you should read your policy carefully.

3. TERMS UNDER WHICH THE POLICY MAY BE RETURNED AND THE PREMIUM REFUNDED – If, for any reason, you are not satisfied with your policy it can be returned within 30 days to either our Home Office or to the agent from whom it was purchased. You will receive a refund of any premium that you have paid. Except for a refund of any premium paid beyond your date of death, the policy does not provide for a refund of any unearned premium upon *surrender* of the policy.

4.   THIS IS NOT A MEDICARE SUPPLEMENT POLICY – If you are eligible for Medicare, review the Medicare Supplement Buyer's Guide available from the insurance company. Be advised that neither the insurance company nor its agents represent Medicare, the federal government, or any state government.

5.   LONG-TERM CARE COVERAGE – Policies of this type are designed to provide coverage for one or more necessary diagnostic, preventative, therapeutic, rehabilitative, maintenance, or personal care services provided in a setting other than an acute care unit of a hospital, such as in a nursing home, in the community, or in the home.

Coverage for actual expenses are subject to policy limitations, elimination periods, and other requirements.

6.   BENEFITS PROVIDED BY THIS POLICY –

A.   IMPORTANT TERMS DEFINITION –

1.   *Activities of Daily Living (ADLs)* – The activities of daily living (ADLs) used to qualify for benefits under this policy are: (1) Bathing; (2) Continence; (3) Dressing; (4) Eating; (5) Toileting; and (6) Transferring. Bathing is washing in a tub or shower and getting into and out of the tub or shower without assistance. Continence is controlling bowel and bladder functions voluntarily or maintaining a reasonable level of personal hygiene when not able to control bowel or bladder functions. Dressing is putting on and taking off all necessary items of clothing and prosthetic devices including getting these items out of and returning them to their usual storage places. Eating is moving prepared food from a container into the body. Toileting includes getting to and from the bathroom, transferring to and from the toilet, cleansing oneself and adjusting one's clothing. Transferring is defined as changing positions such as from the bed to a chair, from a chair to an upright position, and from an upright position to a chair or a bed. To qualify for benefits, one must be certified by a licensed health care practitioner as being unable to perform, without substantial assistance from another person, at least 2 of the 6 ADLs listed above for a period of at least 90 days.

2.   *Severe Cognitive Impairment (Alzheimer's and Other Organic Brain Disorders)* – This is a deterioration in intellectual capacity to the extent that one requires substantial supervision for

3. *Spousal Benefit Transfer Rider* – With the purchase of this rider for each spouse, you are increasing the Lifetime Benefit Amount. Benefits will be charged against your Lifetime Benefit amount until it is exhausted and then they will be charged against your spouse's Lifetime Benefit amount. If a spouse dies, the surviving spouse will inherit the total remaining combined pool of Lifetime Benefit amount. If a spouse cancels the rider, the rider for the second spouse is automatically cancelled.

7. **EXCEPTIONS, LIMITATIONS AND REDUCTIONS –**

This policy does not cover losses due to (1) war or an act of war; (2) intentionally self-inflicted injury, whether inflicted while sane or insane; (3) to the extent covered under Medicare or any other government program except Medicaid; (4) to the extent provided by a family member or person who ordinarily lives in the family home; (5) a mental illness or nervous disorder without evidence of organic disease. (Loss due to Parkinson's disease, Alzheimer's disease and senile dementia are covered.); (6) a stay in a hospital, a hospice, or a care facility that treats primarily the mentally ill, drug addicts, or alcoholics, only in some contracts.

This policy will not pay benefits for a loss due to a pre-existing condition which is not disclosed in the application unless the loss begins more than six months after the policy is in force. Losses due to a pre-existing condition shown on the application are covered immediately.

NOTE: THIS POLICY MAY NOT COVER ALL OF THE EXPENSES ASSOCIATED WITH YOUR LONG-TERM CARE NEEDS.

8. **RELATIONSHIP OF COST OF CARE AND BENEFITS –**

Because the cost of long-term care services is likely to increase over time, you should consider whether and how the benefits of this policy may be adjusted. Unless you elect one of the options listed below, the benefits under your policy will not increase over time.

Your benefits may increase over time if you select one of the following optional riders: (1) the Inflation Protection Rider – Automatic Equal Increases Option; or (2) the Inflation Protection Rider – Automatic Compound Increases Option.

If you select the Inflation Protection Rider – Automatic Equal Increases Option, the maximum daily facility benefit and the maximum home and

one's own health and safety and the safety of others. To qualify for benefits, the severe cognitive impairment must be certified by a licensed health care practitioner.

3. *Elimination Period* – This is the number of days in which you received covered long-term care services before benefits are payable. Such days do not need to be continuous but must be accumulated within a continuous 730-day period. The elimination period must be satisfied only one time. The more common elimination periods available are 0, 20, 30, 90, 100, 180, or 365 days.

4. *Inability to Perform Activities of Daily Living (ADLs)* – Dependence upon another because of the need, which is due to injury or sickness or frailty, for regular human assistance or supervision in performing normal activities of daily living.

5. *Long-term Care Facility* – A long-term care facility is one which is licensed by the state as either a skilled nursing facility, an intermediate nursing facility or a custodial care facility. It must have 24-hour nursing services which are provided under the supervision of an R.N., L.V.N. or L.P.N. and it must keep a daily record on each patient.

6. *Home and Community-Based Care* – Home health care, adult day care, and assisted living facilities are also available for skilled, intermediate, custodial, hospice, and respite care.

7. *Pre-Existing Condition* – Any condition for which you received medical advice or treatment in the six months before the effective date of the policy.

B. **BENEFIT LIMITS –**

1. The maximum daily facility benefit is equal to $_____.

2. The maximum daily home and community-based care or alternate care benefit is equal to ____% of the maximum daily facility benefit amount.

3. The maximum lifetime benefit, or total amount the policy will pay during your lifetime for all benefits, is equal to $_____.

4. The elimination period is _____ days.

C.   HOME AND COMMUNITY-BASED CARE BENEFITS –

To receive home and community-based care benefits, you must require covered services while the policy is in force due to certification by a licensed health care practitioner (1) as being unable to perform, without substantial assistance from another person, at least 2 of the 6 ADLs listed above for a period of at least 90 days or (2) as requiring substantial supervision to protect yourself from threats to health and safety due to severe cognitive impairment.

1.   *Caregiving Training Benefit* – The policy will pay the expenses incurred for caregiving training if you require a long-term care facility stay or home or community-based care. The expenses cannot exceed five times the maximum daily home and adult day care benefit. This benefit is not subject to the elimination period.

2.   *Home, Adult Day Care and Assisted Living Facility Benefit* – For every day that you receive home and community-based care in your home, adult day care center, hospice facility, or assisted living facility, the policy will pay the lesser of: (1) the maximum daily home and community-based care benefit or (2) the total of (a) expenses incurred for adult day care; (b) expenses incurred for services provided by a medical social worker, home health aide, or homemaker; and (c) expenses incurred for occupational, physical, respiratory or speech therapy or nursing care services provided by a registered nurse, licensed practical nurse or a vocational nurse.

3.   *Respite Care Benefit* – The policy will pay the lesser of the maximum daily home and adult day care benefit or the expenses incurred each day for respite care for up to 21 days each calender year.

4.   *Hospice Care Benefit* – The policy will pay actual charges up to 50% of the maximum daily facility benefit and is limited to the maximum benefit period of 180 days.

D.   LONG-TERM CARE FACILITY BENEFITS –

To be eligible for long-term care facility benefits you must require a stay in a long-term care facility that begins while the policy is in force due to certification by a licensed health care practitioner (1) as being

unable to perform, without substantial assistance from another person, at least 2 of the 6 ADLs listed above for a period of at least 90 days or (2) as requiring substantial supervision to protect yourself from threats to health and safety due to severe cognitive impairment.

The long-term care benefit is equal to the lesser of the maximum daily facility benefit or the charges made by the facility for the care, including room and board. The long-term care benefit will be paid when you are charged for your room in the long-term care facility while you are temporarily hospitalized. This benefit is limited to 21 days in each calendar year.

E.   ALTERNATE PLAN OF CARE BENEFIT –

If you require a stay in a long-term care facility the policy will pay for alternate services, devices, or types of care under a written alternate care plan. This plan must be developed by health care professionals and must be agreed to by you, your doctor, and the insurance company. The plan must be medically acceptable. Benefits paid under the alternate care plan count against the policy's lifetime maximum benefit.

F.   AMBULANCE BENEFIT –

The policy will pay up to $250 per trip by ambulance to or from a long-term care facility for up to four trips in each calendar year.

G.   OPTIONAL BENEFITS –

1.   *Inflation Protection Rider – Simple Automatic Increase Option* – The maximum daily facility benefit and the maximum home and community-based care benefit will be increased by 5 percent of the amounts shown on the schedule of benefits. The increase will take place on the policy anniversary. The maximum lifetime benefit will be increased proportionately.

2.   *Inflation Protection Rider – Automatic Compound Increase Option* – The maximum daily facility benefit and the maximum home and community-based care benefit and the remaining maximum lifetime benefit will be increased by 5 percent of the benefit in effect on the previous anniversary of your policy.

adult day care benefit will be increased by 5 percent of the amounts shown on the schedule of benefits. The maximum lifetime benefit will be increased proportionately. If you select the Inflation Protection Rider – Automatic Compound Increases Option, the maximum daily facility benefit and the maximum home and adult day care benefit and the remaining maximum lifetime benefit will be increased by 5 percent of the benefit in effect on the previous anniversary of your policy.

If you do not select one of these optional benefits, you may request increases to your daily benefits on any policy anniversary date subject to health underwriting and the payment of an additional premium.

9. **TERMS UNDER WHICH THE POLICY MAY BE CONTINUED IN FORCE OR DISCONTINUED –**

1. *Renewal* – This policy is guaranteed renewable. This means that your coverage will continue for life as long as you pay the policy premium in a timely fashion. We cannot change the coverage or benefits without your consent. We can change the premium rate but only if we give you 31 days prior written notice and we change the premium rate for everyone who has this policy form in your policy rating group in your state.

2. *Waiver of Premium* – After you receive at least 60 consecutive days of covered care or services including any days that you are hospitalized or the days used to satisfy the elimination period, we will waive the premium on this policy on a monthly basis. We will apply any unearned premiums to your policy following the end of the Waiver of Premium period. You will be responsible for premium payments starting with the first premium due date on or after the date that payment of benefits ceases.

10. **ALZHEIMER'S DISEASE AND OTHER ORGANIC BRAIN DISORDERS –**

This policy covers loss due to Alzheimer's disease, Parkinson's disease, senile dementia or other organic brain disorders.

11. **PREMIUM –**

The total premium for this policy is $_____.

The portion of the premium for the Inflation Protection Rider – Automatic Equal Increases Option, if selected, is $_____.

The portion of the premium for the Inflation Protection Rider – Automatic Compound Increases Option, if selected, is $_____.

12. **ADDITIONAL FEATURES –**

    1.   **Medical Underwriting** – Medical underwriting is used for this policy. Your eligibility for coverage is based on the answers to the medical questions in the policy application and any additional information that may be needed to complete our evaluation of your application.

    2.   **Unintentional Lapse Protection** – Under this policy, you have the right to name an individual to receive notification when your policy will lapse due to non-payment of premium. The notice will be sent no earlier than 30 days after the premium due date. The policy will not be terminated until 30 days after this notice is sent.

    3.   **Nonforfeiture Benefit/Shortened Benefit Period** – Under this policy, coverage will continue on a limited basis during your lifetime if you stop paying premiums after the policy has been in force at least 3 years. The benefits payable for any long-term care facility stay or home and community-based care which begins after the date that coverage under the policy would otherwise terminate in the absence of this nonforfeiture provision will be subject to the following limits:

        a)   The daily benefit amounts will be same amounts available at the time the policy would have lapsed.

        b)   The maximum amount paid under this provision will be the greater of: (1) an amount equal to all of the premiums paid, excluding waived premiums; or (2) an amount equal to 30 times the maximum daily facility benefit in effect at the time of termination.

Glossary of Terms

Accelerated Death Benefit. An option in a life insurance policy that will pay all or part of the policy face amount prior to death. This benefit can pay the cost associated with catastrophic medical conditions which can include the need for nursing home confinement.

Activities of Daily Living. Functional routines that relate to one's ability to live independently. These activities consist of bathing, dressing, feeding, toileting, continence, and mobility.

Adult Congregate Living Facility. Residential or apartment housing, which can include a minimum amount of assistance with the activities of daily living.

Adult Day Care. Services provided to individuals who cannot remain alone, including health and custodial care and other related support. This care is rendered in specified centers on a less than 24 hour basis.

Adult Day Care Facility. An institution designated to provide custodial and/or minimum health care assistance to individuals unable to remain alone, usually during working hours when the caregiver is employed.

Alternate Plan of Care. A long-term care insurance policy feature that allows for substantial flexibility in designing a recovery and/or maintenance program for a claimant, using as many types of long-term care assistance as needed on a reasonable cost basis delivered in an agreed-upon setting.

Asset Spend-down. Procedure where an individual's income and assets are diminished in order to attain the minimum required levels of the various states' eligibility requirements for Medicaid assistance.

Assisted Living Facility. Residence for long-term care patients that is generally less expensive than a nursing home. Residents can also receive some long-term care services in this type of facility.

Benefit Period. The length of time for which benefits under a long-term care insurance contract will be paid (i.e.; four years or lifetime).

Bereavement Counseling. A support service designed to assist family members of terminally ill patients to cope with their grief. This service is often available under a hospice care program and a benefit may be payable under a long-term care insurance policy.

Care Coordinator. A person designated by an insurer to organize a plan of care at claim time between the insured, medical providers, and family members.

Caregiver. A person providing assistance to a dependent person due to medical reasons or the inability to conduct routine activities of daily living.

Centers for Medicare and Medicaid Services. The federal agency that administers Medicare, Medicaid, and other federal programs.

Chronically Ill. This is the definition under which an individual qualifies for favorable tax treatment for long-term care expenses, whether self-insured or reimbursed by an insurance company. To be chronically ill, the person must be either unable to perform two of six activities of daily living for at least 90 days or suffer a severe cognitive impairment.

Cognitive Impairment. One of the measurements used to determine eligibility for long-term care benefits in a policy, it is the deterioration or loss of one's intellectual capacity, confirmed by clinical evidence and standardized tests, in the areas of: (1) short and long term memory; (2) orientation as to person, place and time; and (3) deductive or abstract reasoning.

Cohorts. A grouping of individuals based on their values and characteristics formed by the period of time they came of age. Understanding this orientation is important in relationship selling.

Comprehensive Benefits. A long-term care insurance plan that offers a wide variety of coverage for long-term care insurance services. These plans are modeled after the NAIC model policy of 1988. These policies could be both tax-qualified and non-qualified plans.

Contingent Nonforfeiture. This policy feature is included in policies conforming to the NAIC's Rate Stability amendments. It provides a choice of paid-up and other policy scenarios that the insured can choose from if the insurer exceeds the limits of cumulative future rate increases.

Continuing Care Retirement Communities. This campus-type environment offers houses, apartments, communal dining facilities, a nursing facility, recreation, a library, and other services. An entry fee and a stipulated monthly payment are required.

Custodial Care. The most common type of long-term care service rendered, it provides assistance with activities of daily living and is generally performed by a trained aide in a variety of settings, most often in the home.

Custodial Care Facility. A facility that is licensed by the state to provide custodial care, including assistance with activities of daily living and a nursing staff to oversee the administering of medication.

Daily Benefit Amount. The specified amount of benefit payable for long-term care services. The dollar amount may vary by service such as $100 a day payable for a nursing home confinement and $75 a day payable for home health care, or $130 a day for nursing home and $195/day for home health care.

Diagnostic Related Grouping. Medicare uses this grouping as a guide for the treatment of Medicare recipients and payment to providers. This guide governs the length of a hospital stay for each illness or injury. Hospital discharges often force individuals not well enough to go home to be admitted into a skilled nursing facility.

Elimination Period. In a long-term care insurance policy, this is a period of time during which no benefits are payable and is sometimes referred to as a deductible. Examples of elimination periods are 15 and 100 days.

Employer-Sponsored plans. This is group long-term care insurance first introduced in 1987. The earlier plans were voluntary, portable products with benefits and premiums similar to individual long-term care coverage. Development of true group long-term care insurance plans is underway.

Expense incurred. A method under which daily benefit amounts are paid based on the actual expenses incurred for the necessary long-term care service.

Gatekeepers. Also called "safety nets", these specific qualifications must be met before becoming eligible for any specific benefit payment under a long-term care insurance policy. These qualifications set by insurance company have largely been eliminated through the NAIC's model policy and state regulation.

Geriatric Case Manager. An individual assigned to handle the various needs of a person unable to do for themselves. This qualified individual can coordinate every aspect of an aging adult's care from interviewing and hiring household help to paying bills, and often serves as the eyes and ears of other family members not located in the immediate area.

Guaranteed Renewable. The renewal provision of a long-term care insurance policy, ensuring that the policy cannot be canceled by the insurer nor can policy provisions be changed without the insured's consent. Policy premiums, however, may be adjusted upward based on the company's experience for an entire class of business.

Health Care Surrogate. An individual designated in a medical durable power of attorney to make medical decisions on behalf of another person.

Health Insurance Portability and Accountability Act (HIPAA). This federal legislation, passed in 1996, clarified the tax treatment of long-term care insurance, defining the parameters under which benefits and expenses are received tax-free.

Home Care. This is a type of long-term care service, provided in the home, generally consists of activities of daily living assistance, and is rendered by a trained aide.

Home Health Care. A program of professional, paraprofessional, and skilled care usually provided through a home health care agency to a person at home. This care is often prescribed by a physician as medically necessary and can include nursing services, physical, speech, respiratory, and occupational therapy.

Home Health Care Agency. An organization providing home health care or home care, state licensed or accredited as required, keeps clinical records of all patients, and is supervised by a qualified physician or registered nurse.

Hospice Care. A coordinated program for control of pain and symptoms for the terminally ill, which may also provide support services to family members.

Inflation Protection Benefit. This optional benefit is designed to help preserve the value of the daily benefit amount. It automatically increases the daily benefit annually on a simple or compounded basis either by a stipulated percentage amount or an index measurement.

Instrumental Activities of Daily Living (IADLs). These are primarily homemaker services such as preparing meals, shopping, managing money, using the telephone, doing housework, and taking medication.

Intermediate Care. Occasional nursing services, preventive or rehabilitative, performed under the supervision of skilled medical personnel.

Intermediate Care Facility. An institution licensed by the state to provide patient care for those requiring constant availability and support, but very little in the way of skilled care. This facility may also provide custodial care services.

Life Insurance-Based Long-term Care Insurance. This is a form of long-term care coverage where benefits are wrapped inside a life insurance policy. Benefits can be provided for both long-term care insurance and death, with cash values also available for withdrawal.

Life Settlements: The sale of a life insurance policy for a portion of its face amount value. A terminal illness is not required here, but instead a life expectancy of 10-15 years or less.

Long distance caregiving. A difficult position in caring for a family member while located in another area and not available for day to day assistance.

Long-term Care Insurance. A specific type of insurance policy designed to offer financial support in paying for necessary long-term care services rendered in a variety of settings.

Long-term Care Rider. This is an optional benefit that can be added to a life insurance, annuity, or disability income policy to provide benefits for long-term care.

Managed Care. A type of claims management system for long-term care insurance policies using pre-selected providers who have agreed to treat insurance company claimants on a reduced cost basis.

Medicaid. The joint federal and state welfare program administered by the states to provide payment for health care services, including long-term care, for those meeting minimum asset and income requirements.

Medicare. Federal program organized under the Health Insurance for the Aged Act, Title XVIII of the Social Security Amendments of 1965, it provides hospital and medical expense benefits, including long-term care services, for those individuals over age 65 or those meeting specific disability standards.

Medicare Catastrophic Act. Federal legislation enacted January 1, 1989, it expanded long-term care benefit payments provided under Medicaid and also changed some Medicaid requirements. The Medicare changes in the Act were repealed that same year effective January 1, 1990. The Medicaid changes stayed intact.

NAIC Model Policy. Recommended minimum policy standards as designated by the insurance industry watchdog, the National Association of Insurance Commissioners (NAIC), originally established in 1988 and amended thereafter. States have the choice to adopt part, all, or none of the standards for their own regulation. HIPAA legislation, passed by Congress in 1996, re-defined some of the provisions of the model policy.

NAIC Rate Stability. This amendment to the NAIC Model Policy requires insurers to maintain higher loss ratios, certify their filed rates as intended for lifetime at that level, and institutes a contingent nonforfeiture benefit that must be offered an insured if cumulative rate increases exceed a scheduled table limit.

NAIC Suitability. This amendment to the NAIC Model Policy requires insurers and agents to seek the most appropriate buyers for long-term care insurance by requiring applicants to complete a Personal Worksheet on finances and, among other requirements, to disclose the company's rate increase history.

90-day ADL Certification. A new requirement under HIPAA which requires certification by a licensed health professional that the loss of at least two of six activities of daily living will last a minimum of 90 days. The certification must be made to facilitate insurer claim payments.

Nonforfeiture Benefits. This long-term care insurance policy feature enables the insured to continue long-term care coverage in some form after the insured has ceased making premium payments. A cash return, a paid-up policy, or an extended term feature are typical nonforfeiture benefits.

Non-Qualified Plans. This term refers to all long-term care insurance policies that do not meet the required definitions under HIPAA federal legislation. There could be adverse tax consequences for these plans sold from January 1, 1997 forward.

Partnerships. A joint public and private sector program that allows residents of a state to buy an approved long-term care insurance policy that will pay benefits during a long-term care claim and enable these residents to conserve some assets that would otherwise have to be spent down to access Medicaid. States introducing partnerships so far are Connecticut, New York, Indiana, and California, but several other states are expected to introduce their versions in the near future, should the Federal Government remove its impediment placed in the OBRA'93 law.

Per Diem. A method for paying the daily benefit amount that is based on an elected amount and not on the actual expenses incurred. Long-term care insurance policies that are tax-qualified have capped the tax-free per diem amount that may be elected for 2003 at $220 per day.

Pool of Money. Under a long-term care insurance program, this is a variation on the typical benefit period. Rather than designate a period of time over which benefits can be payable, this concept creates a lump sum of money to be used as needed during a long-term care claim. The claim ceases when services are no longer needed or the lump sum of money runs out.

Pre-existing condition. A diagnosed injury or sickness for which medical advice or treatment was sought prior to the effective date of the long-term care insurance contract.

Prospective Payment System. Introduced to Medicare in 1983, this is the program where payments are calculated and made to providers of medical services for Medicare eligible individuals based on the diagnostic related groupings.

Respite Care. Services provided for caregivers to permit temporary periods of relief or rest from caring for a person. These services can be provided by a home health care agency or other state licensed facility and may be reimbursable under a long-term care insurance policy.

Return of Premium. An optional benefit under a long-term care insurance policy that provides a return of all or a portion of premiums paid less claims paid, either on a specified policy anniversary, at policy surrender, or death of the insured.

Sandwich Generation. This term was coined when describing individuals caring for both dependent children and an aging parent or relative.

Skilled Care. A professional type of nursing assistance performed by trained medical personnel under the supervision of a physician or other qualified medical personnel. It is the only type of care eligible for reimbursement in a skilled nursing facility under Medicare.

Spousal Impoverishment Protection. Medicaid changes made as part of the Medicare Catastrophic Act of 1988, which provided an income and shelter allowance for the at home spouse whose partner is institutionally confined.

Standby Assistance. An individual is considered unable to perform an activity of daily living if someone must be in close proximity to him to help when he is attempting to perform the activity.

Subacute Care. Assistance provided by nursing homes for health services such as stroke rehabilitation and cardiac care for post-surgery that offers a lower cost alternative to hospital treatment of the same kind.

Swing beds. Hospital beds that may be designated as either acute care or skilled nursing, changing from one to the other to continue care to the individual without having to switch rooms or facilities.

Tax-qualified plans. These are long-term care insurance policies that meet the definition required by HIPAA and therefore are eligible for favorable tax treatment.

Transfers. In qualifying for Medicaid, transfers are moving assets to someone other than a spouse or to a trust for the purposes of qualifying for Medicaid. Transfers must be made 36 months before Medicaid application (or 60 months for certain transfers involving trusts).

Triple Trigger. This is the designation for the three ways to be eligible for benefits under a long-term care insurance policy including assistance with activities of daily living, cognitive impairment, or medical necessity. This definition is not available in tax-qualified plans.

Viatical Settlements. The purchase, on a reduced basis, of a life insurance policy owned by a terminally ill person.

Waiver of Premium. A policy provision of a long-term care insurance contract that suspends premium payment after a specified period of time during which the insured is receiving policy benefits for long-term care services. The suspension continues until recovery at which resumption of premium payment is expected.

Index

ORDER ADDITIONAL PREMIERE REFERENCES

Year after year, thousands of financial professionals rely on **The National Underwriter Company's** leading references for expert, accurate information. Use this handy order form to order additional copies of *The Long-Term Care Handbook* or to order complementary products.

These excellent resources will save time and enhance your reputation as a reliable expert.

To order, **call 1-800-543-0874** and ask for operator BB; **fax** your order to **1-800-874-1916**; or visit our **online store** at **www.NationalUnderwriterStore.com**.

PAYMENT INFORMATION AND GUARANTEE
Add shipping & handling charges to all orders as indicated. If your order exceeds total amount listed in chart, or for overseas rates, call 1-800-543-0874. Any order of 10 or more items or $250.00 and over will be billed for shipping by actual weight, plus a handling fee. Any discounts do not apply to shipping and handling. Unconditional 30-day guarantee. Product(s) damaged in shipping will be replaced at no cost to you. Claims must be made within 30 days from the invoice date. Price, information, and availability subject to change.

SHIPPING & HANDLING

ORDER TOTAL			S&H
$10.00	TO	$19.99	$5.00
$20.00	TO	$39.99	$6.00
$40.00	TO	$59.99	$7.00
$60.00	TO	$79.99	$9.00
$80.00	TO	$109.99	$10.00
$110.00	TO	$149.99	$12.00
$150.00	TO	$199.99	$13.00
$200.00	TO	$249.99	$15.50

SALES TAX (Additional)
Sales tax is required for residents of the following states:
CA, DC, FL, GA, IL, KY, NJ, NY, OH, PA, and WA.

The
NATIONAL
UNDERWRITER Company
PROFESSIONAL PUBLISHING GROUP

Please send me the following : (*please indicate quantity*)

_____ Copies of *The Long-Term Care Handbook* $29.95

_____ Copies of *The Long-Term Care Sales Power Kit* $69.95

_____ Copies of *The Annuity Handbook* $29.95

_____ Copies of *The Tools & Techniques of Employee Benefit and Retirement Planning* $52.95

_____ Copies of *Financial Planning for the Older Client* $39.95

☐ Check enclosed*   Charge My ☐VISA ☐MC ☐AmEx (check one)   ☐ Bill me

Make check payable to The National Underwriter Company. Please include the appropriate shipping & handling and any applicable sales tax.

Card # _____ CVV#** _____ Exp. Date _____

Signature _____

Name _____ Title _____

Company _____

Address _____

City _____ State _____ Zip+4 _____

Business Phone ( ) _____

E-mail _____

**For Visa/Mastercard, the three-digit CVV number is printed on the signature panel on the back of the card immediately after the card's account number. For American Express, the four-digit CVV number is usually printed on the front of the card above the card account number.

2-BB